LATE BIOLOGICAL EFFECTS OF IONIZING RADIATION
VOL. I

The following States are Members of the International Atomic Energy Agency:

AFGHANISTAN	HOLY SEE	PHILIPPINES
ALBANIA	HUNGARY	POLAND
ALGERIA	ICELAND	PORTUGAL
ARGENTINA	INDIA	QATAR
AUSTRALIA	INDONESIA	ROMANIA
AUSTRIA	IRAN	SAUDI ARABIA
BANGLADESH	IRAQ	SENEGAL
BELGIUM	IRELAND	SIERRA LEONE
BOLIVIA	ISRAEL	SINGAPORE
BRAZIL	ITALY	SOUTH AFRICA
BULGARIA	IVORY COAST	SPAIN
BURMA	JAMAICA	SRI LANKA
BYELORUSSIAN SOVIET	JAPAN	SUDAN
SOCIALIST REPUBLIC	JORDAN	SWEDEN
CANADA	KENYA	SWITZERLAND
CHILE	KOREA, REPUBLIC OF	SYRIAN ARAB REPUBLIC
COLOMBIA	KUWAIT	THAILAND
COSTA RICA	LEBANON	TUNISIA
CUBA	LIBERIA	TURKEY
CYPRUS	LIBYAN ARAB JAMAHIRIYA	UGANDA
CZECHOSLOVAKIA	LIECHTENSTEIN	UKRAINIAN SOVIET SOCIALIST
DEMOCRATIC KAMPUCHEA	LUXEMBOURG	REPUBLIC
DEMOCRATIC PEOPLE'S	MADAGASCAR	UNION OF SOVIET SOCIALIST
REPUBLIC OF KOREA	MALAYSIA	REPUBLICS
DENMARK	MALI	UNITED ARAB EMIRATES
DOMINICAN REPUBLIC	MAURITIUS	UNITED KINGDOM OF GREAT
ECUADOR	MEXICO	BRITAIN AND NORTHERN
EGYPT	MONACO	IRELAND
EL SALVADOR	MONGOLIA	UNITED REPUBLIC OF
ETHIOPIA	MOROCCO	CAMEROON
FINLAND	NETHERLANDS	UNITED REPUBLIC OF
FRANCE	NEW ZEALAND	TANZANIA
GABON	NICARAGUA	UNITED STATES OF AMERICA
GERMAN DEMOCRATIC REPUBLIC	NIGER	URUGUAY
GERMANY, FEDERAL REPUBLIC OF	NIGERIA	VENEZUELA
GHANA	NORWAY	VIET NAM
GREECE	PAKISTAN	YUGOSLAVIA
GUATEMALA	PANAMA	ZAIRE
HAITI	PARAGUAY	ZAMBIA
	PERU	

The Agency's Statute was approved on 23 October 1956 by the Conference on the Statute of the IAEA held at United Nations Headquarters, New York; it entered into force on 29 July 1957. The Headquarters of the Agency are situated in Vienna. Its principal objective is "to accelerate and enlarge the contribution of atomic energy to peace, health and prosperity throughout the world".

Printed by the IAEA in Austria
September 1978

PROCEEDINGS SERIES

LATE BIOLOGICAL EFFECTS OF IONIZING RADIATION

PROCEEDINGS OF THE SYMPOSIUM ON
THE LATE BIOLOGICAL EFFECTS OF
IONIZING RADIATION, Vienna, 1978
HELD BY THE
INTERNATIONAL ATOMIC ENERGY AGENCY
IN VIENNA, 13–17 MARCH 1978

In two volumes

VOL.I

QP82.2
I53
S93
v.I
1978

INTERNATIONAL ATOMIC ENERGY AGENCY
VIENNA, 1978

LATE BIOLOGICAL EFFECTS OF IONIZING RADIATION, VOL.I
IAEA, VIENNA, 1978
STI/PUB/489
ISBN 92—0—010678—1

FOREWORD

With the rapid rise in the peaceful uses of atomic energy in medicine, industry and power generation, concurrent efforts are being made to protect workers and the general population from exposure to external and internal radiation sources. The mechanisms of the biological effects of ionizing radiation are fairly well elucidated. From the health protection point of view certain hazardous somatic effects which can appear long after the time of exposure are of particular interest. These effects, termed late biological effects, may include possible induction of malignant neoplasms, various types of degenerative diseases, impairment of fertility and cytological abnormalities.

Research and surveys are continuing, under the various national, regional and international programmes, directed towards the gaining of further knowledge of the nature and extent of incidence of these hazardous effects; this work, an integral part of the radiation protection programme, aims to provide the relevant scientific bases for their prevention. Although much work has been done, there are still considerable ambiguities in the qualitative and quantitative aspects as well as in the mechanisms, not to mention the additional complications projected through the inevitable interactions of some chemical and physical agents co-existing in the environment. These factors associated with the late biological effects are of great significance in setting up guidelines for acceptable radiation exposure, and in evaluating the risk/benefit factor for the future promotion of peaceful nuclear applications.

The Symposium on the Late Biological Effects of Ionizing Radiation was convened in Vienna by the International Atomic Energy Agency from 13 to 17 March, 1978. The symposium was attended by about 250 participants from 33 countries and nine international organizations. The principal aim of the symposium was to review the current status of understanding of the late biological effects of ionizing radiation from external and internal sources. Furthermore, the international experts critically evaluated information obtained from epidemiological studies of relevant human population groups, such as atomic bomb survivors, patients receiving medical exposures as well as occupationally exposed radiation workers. Eighty-one papers were presented in 10 sessions which covered epidemiological studies on late effects in human populations exposed to internal and/or external ionizing radiation; quantitative and qualitative data from experimentation on animal models; methodological problems and modern approaches; factors influencing susceptibility or expression of late radiation injury; comparative evaluation of late effects induced by radiation and other environmental pollutants; and problems of risk assessment.

In addition, a discussion was held on the planning of further epidemiological studies of occupationally exposed populations in the light of the projected rapid growth of the nuclear power programme in Member States. The expert group recommended that a national registry system for the dosimetry and medical records of radiation workers be established and co-ordinated internationally in order to facilitate reliable epidemiological surveillance and risk-assessment of the population.

The dose-effect relationship, by which human risk estimates at low doses are derived by extrapolation, was also discussed. Several new models based on theoretical analysis and experimental data were proposed and compared with available human and animal data. The important matter of predicting the combined effects, where the picture is complicated by other environmental factors such as chemical pollutants, was discussed in several papers.

The full text of the papers, together with a record of the discussions, is published in these Proceedings. The symposium brought together international experts with a wide range of interests including the practicalities of radiological protection, health physics, epidemiology, oncology and other relevant medical practices, theoretical and experimental radiobiology, biophysics and dosimetry as well as the regulatory authorities of the national health services. The Proceedings are thus expected to serve as a major source of current information and reference material for the above specialities.

EDITORIAL NOTE

The papers and discussions have been edited by the editorial staff of the International Atomic Energy Agency to the extent considered necessary for the reader's assistance. The views expressed and the general style adopted remain, however, the responsibility of the named authors or participants. In addition, the views are not necessarily those of the governments of the nominating Member States or of the nominating organizations.

Where papers have been incorporated into these Proceedings without resetting by the Agency, this has been done with the knowledge of the authors and their government authorities, and their cooperation is gratefully acknowledged. The Proceedings have been printed by composition typing and photo-offset lithography. Within the limitations imposed by this method, every effort has been made to maintain a high editorial standard, in particular to achieve, wherever practicable, consistency of units and symbols and conformity to the standards recommended by competent international bodies.

The use in these Proceedings of particular designations of countries or territories does not imply any judgement by the publisher, the IAEA, as to the legal status of such countries or territories, of their authorities and institutions or of the delimitation of their boundaries.

The mention of specific companies or of their products or brand names does not imply any endorsement or recommendation on the part of the IAEA.

Authors are themselves responsible for obtaining the necessary permission to reproduce copyright material from other sources.

CONTENTS OF VOL. I

HUMAN STUDIES: EPIDEMIOLOGICAL STUDIES ON POPULATIONS
EXPOSED TO ATOMIC EXPLOSIONS (Session 1)

HUMAN STUDIES: LATE EFFECTS DUE TO MEDICAL EXPOSURE
(Session 3 and Session 5, Part 1)

HUMAN STUDIES: OCCUPATIONAL EXPOSURE
(Session 5, Part 2, and Session 7)

INDICATORS FOR LATE EFFECTS (Session 6)

HUMAN STUDIES:
EPIDEMIOLOGICAL STUDIES ON
POPULATIONS EXPOSED TO
ATOMIC EXPLOSIONS
Session 1

THE HYPOTHESIS OF RADIATION-ACCELERATED AGING AND THE MORTALITY OF JAPANESE A-BOMB VICTIMS

G.W. BEEBE
Radiation Effects Research Foundation,
Hiroshima,
Japan
and
National Academy of Sciences,
Washington, D.C.
and
Clinical Epidemiology Branch,
National Cancer Institute,
Bethesda, Maryland,
United States of America

C.E. LAND
Radiation Effects Research Foundation,
Hiroshima,
Japan
and
Environmental Epidemiology Branch,
National Cancer Institute,
Bethesda, Maryland,
United States of America

H. KATO
Radiation Effects Research Foundation,
Hiroshima,
Japan

Abstract

THE HYPOTHESIS OF RADIATION-ACCELERATED AGING AND THE MORTALITY OF JAPANESE A-BOMB VICTIMS.

The hypothesis that ionizing radiation accelerates aging is extremely difficult to investigate in man except at the level of mortality, where there are five significant series: (1) U.S. radiologists compared with other medical specialists; (2) British radiologists compared with the general population; (3) ankylosing spondylitics treated by X-ray versus those otherwise treated; (4) U.S. Army X-ray technicians compared with other medical technicians; and (5) the Japanese A-bomb survivors. Only the first of these provides any evidence in support of the hypothesis. Among the 82 000 Japanese A-bomb survivors being followed for mortality, there were 14 400

3

deaths from non-neoplastic diseases from October 1950 to September 1974, and this experience has been analysed for evidence of a non-specific mortality differential associated with radiation dose (kerma). Cause of death has been classified as follows: neoplastic diseases individually and in various groupings, tuberculosis, cerebrovascular diseases, cardiovascular diseases other than cerebrovascular, diseases of blood and blood-forming organs, diseases of the digestive system, all other non-neoplastic diseases, and all non-neoplastic diseases. Although there is clear evidence of a radiation effect for many forms of cancer, mortality from other diseases contains little suggestion of a relationship to radiation dose. A superficial association between mortality from diseases of blood and blood-forming organs and radiation rests entirely on the carcinogenic effect of radiation, especially the leukaemogenic effect. Some deaths from leukaemia were mistakenly certified to anaemia, and deaths attributable to solid tumours were sometimes misclassified when anaemia became a prominent feature of the terminal illness. Deaths from digestive diseases also seem related to radiation dose but only in the 1971—74 period and among the Hiroshima survivors; the excess is small but occurred in all age groups. Further investigation will be required to determine whether this is truly a late-radiation effect or the indirect result of the misclassification of deaths from cancer of the gastro-intestinal system. Thus far the mortality experience of the Japanese A-bomb survivors suggests that the life-shortening effect of whole-body human exposure to ionizing radiation derives from its carcinogenic effect, not from any acceleration of the aging process.

INTRODUCTION

The hypothesis that ionizing radiation accelerates the natural aging process grew out of experimental work on rodents in the late 1930s and 1940s [1, 2] in which life-shortening was found to be dose-dependent and irradiated animals appeared senescent. The hypothesis received considerable support from the 1956 report of the National Academy of Sciences on the Pathological Effects of Atomic Radiation [3], which contained Warren's data on the age at death of U.S. radiologists [4]. By 1957 radiation-induced premature aging had come to con-stitute an important line of experimental investigation [5—7]. In his 1957 review, however, Upton [7] noted that the non-neoplastic changes known to follow irradiation seemed insufficient to account for the life-shortening effect being observed, and that some of them bore little resemblance to spontaneous senile changes. Mole [5], citing the work of Henshaw, Evans, Lorenz, Neary, Thompson and others, raised important questions about the customary statistical index of mean survival-time, and remarked on the absence of really good data on cause of death. In 1958 Court-Brown and Doll [8] reported that they could find little excess mortality among British radiologists apart from that attributed to cancer. At the same time Warren's methodology was severely criticized by Seltser and Sartwell [9] who then proceeded to organize a study of their own contrasting cohorts of medical specialists as to age-specific mortality [10]. Meanwhile, experimental work on life-shortening proceeded with age-specific mortality rates being used in at least some studies, and with more attention being paid to cause of death [11–13]. Although Lindop and Rotblat [12] concluded that radiation caused non-specific life-shortening in their large mouse experiment, they remarked that the process was not identical with that of natural aging. Also, when Alexander and Connell [14] employed serial killing in their experiments they found that many diseases normally associated with senescence were not advanced in time and concluded that radiation-induced life-shortening could not be regarded as an acceleration of natural aging. Nevertheless, with Casarett's 1964 summary [15] of the field it appeared that the hypothesis was close to becoming theory. In their 1965 report, Seltser and Sartwell [10] reported that radiologists suffered higher mortality rates not only from cancer but also from cardiovascular-renal diseases, and from other non-neoplastic diseases, in comparison with other medical specialists. They interpreted their findings as supportive of the hypothesis of radiation-accelerated aging. More recently, the interpretation of much of the earlier experimental work was seriously questioned by Hoel and Walburg [16, 17]. Walburg's critical and systematic review of the literature [17], with re-analysis of some of the older data, led him to propose that radiation at moderate to low doses (under 300 rads of low LET radiation) shortens life principally, and perhaps exclusively, by induction or acceleration of neoplastic diseases. Meanwhile the follow-up of U.S. radiologists and other medical specialists has been continued, and in the 1975 reports the persistent excess mortality among radiologists from diseases other than neoplasia still seemed consistent with the hypothesis of radiation-accelerated aging [18, 19]. Most recently, Doll and his co-workers [20] have shown that ankylosing spondylitic patients not treated by X-ray have no significant excess cancer mortality, but do have higher mortality than normal expectation from the same non-neoplastic diseases for which excess mortality has been observed for the ankylosing spondylitic patients treated by X-ray. This suggests that the experience of the ankylosing spondylitic patients will provide little support for the hypothesis of radiation-accelerated aging. In its 1977 report, the United Nations Scientific Committee on the Effects of Atomic Radiation [21] takes the position that, except perhaps in the very high dose range, life-shortening rests almost entirely upon the induction of neoplasia.

The previous studies of A-bomb survivors relevant to the hypothesis of radiation-accelerated aging have been of several kinds:

(1) Cause-specific mortality based on death certificates;
(2) Postmortem studies of age-related changes; and
(3) Clinical tests and observations of a wide variety.

The on-going mortality study of A-bomb survivors, most recently reported on by Jablon and Kato [22] for the period 1950–70, has thus far provided no consistent evidence of radiation-induced excess mortality from diseases other than neoplasia. Postmortem observations have been at best suggestive, and clinical tests and observations have also been negative except for chromosomal aberrations (presumably a specific effect) and capillary abnormalities [23]. The representativeness of the experience of the A-bomb survivors as a basis for estimating risks of radiogenic disease has, however, been challenged by Stewart [24] and by Rotblat [25] on the grounds that the acute mortality may have served to select survivors who were more resistant to some of the late effects of radiation.

In this report we examine the mortality experience of the A-bomb survivors more closely than has been done before, using recently tabulated information on deaths through September 1974 [26], and explore the question of bias from the heavy acute mortality.

METHODS AND MATERIALS

The mortality of A-bomb survivors is being monitored by the Radiation Effects Research Foundation (formerly the Atomic Bomb Casualty Commission) on the basis of a cohort of 109 000 subjects, 82 000 survivors drawn from the Hiroshima and Nagasaki schedules from the nation-wide supplement to the 1950 Census, and 27 000 others, not in the city (NIC) when the bombs fell, drawn from rice ration lists and local censuses of 1950–53 [27–29]. Radiation dosimetry is based on the work of a group at the Oak Ridge National Laboratory [30] and shielding interviews of survivors [31], with confirmatory studies by a Japanese team at the National Institute of Radiological Sciences in Chiba [32]. Although tissue doses are becoming available from both dosimetry groups [30, 32], the analysis to be reported here is based on the T-65 dose in rads kerma, which is not a whole-body dose but represents the energy absorbed by a small volume of tissue located at the co-ordinates of the survivor, based on a shielding interview.

Mortality ascertainment rests on the Japanese family registration system, and is known to be virtually complete [27]. Deaths for the period 1 October 1950 − 30 September 1974 have been coded according to the eighth revision of the International Classification of Diseases of the World Health Organization. Expected deaths were calculated from corresponding age-, sex- and time-specific Japanese national death rates for age-groups under 10, 10–19, 20–34, 35–49, and 50+ in 1945, and for the not-in-city and T-65 dose groups 0, 1–9, 10–49, 50–99, 100–199, 200–299, 300–399, and 400+ rads. Statistical tests were based on contrasts of 0–9 rads versus the higher dose groups, including the contrast 0–9 versus 100+. In addition, a systematic analysis was made on the observed numbers of deaths with internally calculated expectations based on an extension of the Mantel-Haenszel procedure [33]. In this analysis tests of low dose versus high dose groups were also performed, but major reliance was

placed on tests of general homogeneity and of linear trend [26]. Although the
analysis of the 1950—74 mortality was primarily directed at the various forms
of cancer, the following groups of non-neoplastic diseases were tabulated
separately for the specific purpose of testing the hypothesis of radiation-
accelerated aging:

Disease Group	1965 ICD Code	No. of Deaths
Tuberculosis	010—019	1 440
Cerebrovascular diseases	430—438	5 679
Other circulatory diseases	390—429, 440—458	3 706
Diseases of blood and blood-forming organs	280—289	134
Diseases of the digestive system	520—577	2 031
Other non-neoplastic diseases	—	6 034
All non-neoplastic diseases	—	19 024
All non-neoplastic diseases except those of blood and blood-forming organs	—	18 890

The number of deaths from non-neoplastic diseases is thus quite large, 14 826
among the 82 000 A-bomb survivors, and 4198 among those not in the city
when the bombs fell.

The hypothesis of radiation-induced premature aging implies that exposure
to ionizing radiation will cause excess mortality not only from cancer but also
from many other diseases, i.e. that there will be life-shortening of a non-specific
nature. The reports of Seltser, Sartwell, and their colleagues [10, 18, 19] are
confirmatory in this sense; their 7th ICD groupings as to cause of death are:
diabetes; cardiovascular-renal diseases; stroke; hypertensive disease; and
pneumonia. We chose our list of diseases in an effort to test the hypothesis over
a broad range of specific diseases grouped so as to retain, for the most part,
numbers of deaths large enough to support fairly sensitive statistical tests. The
diseases that seem most relevant to a test of the hypothesis are the chronic
diseases of middle life and old age. Excess mortality from only a few chronic
diseases would not seem to confirm the hypothesis. Confirmation requires that
excess mortality be fairly general with respect to the chronic diseases of later
life, but not that it be uniform in magnitude or pertain to all such causes. Also,
ionizing radiation may have specific mortality effects other than carcinogenesis,
even if the hypothesis of radiation-accelerated aging is invalid.

Results are mainly presented for the two cities separately. There are two
reasons for this. First, the carcinogenic effects appear to be different for the
two cities, and this might also be expected for any non-specific life-shortening
effect. Second, we would like to exhibit dose-specific mortality in terms of

BEEBE et al.

TABLE I. DEATHS AND STANDARDIZED MORTALITY RATIOS FOR TUBERCULOSIS AMONG A-BOMB SURVIVORS AND NOT-IN-CITY SAMPLE, BY CITY, 1950—74

Exposure status and T-65 dose (rads)	Observed deaths Hiroshima	Observed deaths Nagasaki	SMR Hiroshima	SMR Nagasaki
NIC	184	107	0.90	1.49
0	333	80	0.94	1.50
1—9	186	118	1.11	1.71
10—49	159	74	1.22	1.88
50—99	34	16	0.99	1.06
100+	41	48	0.97	1.46
Total[a]	964	476	1.01	1.62
Test P				
0—9 versus 100+ rads (two-tailed)			>0.10	>0.10
General homogeneity, A-bomb survivors			0.06	>0.10
Linear trend, A-bomb survivors			>0.10	>0.10

[a] Includes those of unknown dose, 2.3% of survivors in Hiroshima, 5.2% in Nagasaki.

TABLE II. RELATIVE RISK (RR) OF DEATH FROM TUBERCULOSIS BY CALENDAR PERIOD, 1950—74, 100+ versus 0—9 rads

Calendar period	Hiroshima Deaths in 100+ rads group	Hiroshima RR	Hiroshima P^a	Nagasaki Deaths in 100+ rads group	Nagasaki RR	Nagasaki P^a
1950—54	16	1.15	>0.10	11	0.51	0.06
1955—58	9	0.87	>0.10	16	1.30	>0.10
1959—62	6	1.12	>0.10	5	0.57	>0.10
1963—66	3	0.54	>0.10	10	1.70	>0.10
1967—70	5	1.27	>0.10	2	0.83	>0.10
1971—74	2	0.72	>0.10	4	1.61	>0.10
Total	41	0.98	>0.10	48	0.90	>0.10

[a] Two-tailed test of 0—9 versus 100+ rads.

TABLE III. DEATHS AND STANDARDIZED MORTALITY RATIOS FOR
MORTALITY FROM CEREBROVASCULAR DISEASES AMONG A-BOMB
SURVIVORS AND NOT-IN-CITY SAMPLE, BY CITY, 1950–74

Exposure status and T-65 dose (rads)	Observed deaths		SMR	
	Hiroshima	Nagasaki	Hiroshima	Nagasaki
NIC	1016	266	0.75	0.86
0	1676	215	0.76	0.93
1–9	742	338	0.75	0.98
10–49	595	208	0.72	0.98
50–99	169	59	0.79	0.84
100+	173	105	0.80	0.90
Total[a]	4446	1233	0.76	0.93

Test P		
0–9 versus 100+ rads (two-tailed)	>0.10	>0.10
General homogeneity, A-bomb survivors	>0.10	>0.10
Linear trend, A-bomb survivors	>0.10	>0.10

[a] Includes those of unknown dose, 2.3% of survivors in Hiroshima, 5.2% in Nagasaki.

TABLE IV. RELATIVE RISK (RR) OF DEATH FROM CEREBROVASCULAR
DISEASE BY CALENDAR PERIOD AND BY CITY, 1950–74, 100+ rads
versus 0–9 rads

Calendar period	Hiroshima			Nagasaki		
	Deaths in 100+ group	RR	P[a]	Deaths in 100+ group	RR	P[a]
1950–54	19	0.96	>0.10	12	1.23	>0.10
1955–58	27	1.21	>0.10	13	0.78	>0.10
1959–62	29	1.06	>0.10	19	1.18	>0.10
1963–66	32	1.08	>0.10	28	1.17	>0.10
1967–70	36	1.10	>0.10	14	0.61	>0.10
1971–74	30	0.95	>0.10	19	0.85	>0.10
Total	173	1.06	>0.10	105	0.94	>0.10

[a] Two-tailed test of 0–9 versus 100+ rads.

TABLE V.   DEATHS AND STANDARDIZED MORTALITY RATIOS FOR
CIRCULATORY DISEASES OTHER THAN CEREBROVASCULAR AMONG
A-BOMB SURVIVORS AND NOT-IN-CITY SAMPLE, BY CITY, 1950–74

Exposure status and T-65 dose (rads)	Observed deaths		SMR	
	Hiroshima	Nagasaki	Hiroshima	Nagasaki
NIC	615	162	0.79	0.92
0	1127	137	0.89	1.05
1–9	502	202	0.89	1.02
10–49	394	140	0.84	1.15
50–99	127	52	1.05	1.30
100+	111	73	0.92	1.10
Total[a]	2906	800	0.86	1.05

Test P		
0–9 versus 100+ rads (two-tailed)	>0.10	>0.10
General homogeneity, A-bomb survivors	>0.10	>0.10
Linear trend, A-bomb survivors	>0.10	>0.10

[a]   Includes those of unknown dose, 2.3% of survivors in Hiroshima, 5.2% in Nagasaki.

TABLE VI.   RELATIVE RISK (RR) OF DEATH FROM CIRCULATORY
DISEASES OTHER THAN CEREBROVASCULAR, BY CALENDAR PERIOD,
AND BY CITY, 1950–74, 100+ rads versus 0–9 rads

Calendar period	Hiroshima			Nagasaki		
	Deaths in 100+ group	RR	P[a]	Deaths in 100+ group	RR	P[a]
1950–54	10	1.07	>0.10	13	1.82	>0.10
1955–58	14	0.97	>0.10	8	1.05	>0.10
1959–62	17	1.10	>0.10	7	0.76	>0.10
1963–66	16	0.80	>0.10	13	1.20	>0.10
1967–70	29	1.22	>0.10	15	0.98	>0.10
1971–74	25	1.02	>0.10	17	0.86	>0.10
Total	111	1.04	>0.10	73	1.06	>0.10

[a]   Two-tailed test of 0–9 versus 100+ rads.

standardized mortality ratios (SMRs), where the age-, sex- and time-specific
death rates for all Japan are taken as the standard, and since the two cities often
differ in their relationship to the national standard, and have very different
dose-distributions (Hiroshima being heavily weighted at the low-end of the dose
range), observed and expected deaths for the two cities cannot simply be added
together.

Results are generally shown by calendar period because we have no basis
for predicting what the latent period might be for any non-specific aging effect.
For those diseases for which the original tabulations were made in sufficient
detail, results are also shown by age in 1945, because an accelerated aging effect
might not apply with equal force to all age groups, and these necessarily differ
greatly in their contribution to mortality in the 1950–74 period.

RESULTS

Mortality from tuberculosis is summarized in Tables I and II. In Table I
the dose-specific SMRs for the two cities are at very different levels, as tuberculosis mortality in Nagasaki has been well above the national average. But in
neither city is the mortality from tuberculosis related to T-65 dose. The P of
0.06 in the test of general homogeneity of the Hiroshima exposure groups
reflects the RR of 1.22 for 10–49 rads. In Table II, which provides risk ratios
for mortality in the 100+ rads group relative to that of the 0–9 rads group in
each city, there is little evidence of a systematic relationship to radiation. There
was, however, a suggestive (P = 0.06) deficit of tuberculosis deaths in high-dose
Nagasaki survivors in the 1950–54 period.

Deaths from cerebrovascular diseases are given in Tables III and IV. The
SMRs in Table II are below unity for both cities, and especially so for Hiroshima.
There is, however, no evidence of a relationship with radiation dose in either
city. Relative risk ratios for the six four-year periods of the analysis appear in
Table IV, and these also lack any suggestion that cerebrovascular diseases have
been accelerated by higher dose of ionizing radiation.

Tables V and VI provide information about deaths from circulatory diseases
other than cerebrovascular diseases. Again the two cities deviate appreciably from
one another when their mortality is standardized by means of the death rates for
all Japan, Nagasaki having the higher rates. In Table V, covering 3706 deaths, the
SMRs show no evidence of variation associated with T-65 dose. In Table VI the
relative risk ratios for the individual four-year periods also reveal no systematic
relationship with radiation.

Deaths from diseases of the digestive system, numbering about 2000 in the
two cities combined, are shown in Tables VII and VIII. The SMR for Hiroshima
survivors (Table VII) exposed to 100+ rads is somewhat above the average for
those exposed to 0–9 rads, but not significantly so. Otherwise there is no

TABLE VII. DEATHS AND STANDARDIZED MORTALITY RATIOS FOR
DISEASES OF THE DIGESTIVE SYSTEM AMONG A-BOMB SURVIVORS
AND NOT-IN-CITY SAMPLE, BY CITY, 1950−74

| Exposure status | Observed deaths | | SMR | |
and T-65 dose (rads)	Hiroshima	Nagasaki	Hiroshima	Nagasaki
NIC	308	108	0.83	1.13
0	626	74	0.98	1.04
1−9	256	127	0.88	1.22
10−49	228	65	0.97	1.02
50−99	57	22	0.94	1.02
100+	71	40	1.13	1.08
Total[a]	1569	462	0.93	1.13
Test P				
0−9 versus 100+ rads (two-tailed)			>0.10	>0.10
General homogeneity, A-bomb survivors			>0.10	>0.10
Linear trend, A-bomb survivors			>0.10	>0.10

[a] Includes those of unknown dose, 2.3% of survivors in Hiroshima, 5.2% in Nagasaki.

TABLE VIII. RELATIVE RISK OF DEATH FROM DISEASES OF THE
DIGESTIVE SYSTEM BY CALENDAR PERIOD AND BY CITY, 1950−74,
100+ rads versus 0−9 rads

| Calendar period | Hiroshima | | | Nagasaki | | |
	Deaths in 100+ group	RR	P[a]	Deaths in 100+ group	RR	P[a]
1950−54	11	0.95	>0.10	8	0.83	>0.10
1955−58	8	0.72	>0.10	9	1.21	>0.10
1959−62	9	0.90	>0.10	7	1.07	>0.10
1963−66	14	1.56	>0.10	4	0.65	>0.10
1967−70	13	1.28	>0.10	4	0.54	>0.10
1971−74	16	2.01	0.04	8	1.52	>0.10
Total	71	1.19	>0.10	40	0.94	>0.10

[a] Two-tailed test of 0−9 versus 100+ rads.

TABLE IX.   DEATHS AND STANDARDIZED MORTALITY RATIOS FOR
DISEASES OF BLOOD AND BLOOD-FORMING ORGANS AMONG A-BOMB
SURVIVORS AND NOT-IN-CITY SAMPLE, BY CITY, 1950–74

| Exposure status | Observed deaths | | SMR | |
and T-65 dose (rads)	Hiroshima	Nagasaki	Hiroshima	Nagasaki
NIC	12	5	0.74	1.10
0	35	5	1.34	1.48
1–9	18	5	1.53	1.01
10–49	22	1	2.26	0.35
50–99	6	1	2.40	1.02
100+	13	11	4.6	5.5
Total[a]	106	28	1.51	1.45

Test P				
0–9 versus 100+ rads (two-tailed)			<0.001	<0.001
General homogeneity, A-bomb survivors			<0.001	0.002
Linear trend, A-bomb survivors			<0.001	<0.001

[a]   Includes those of unknown dose, 2.3% of survivors in Hiroshima, 5.2% in Nagasaki.

indication of variation with dose in either city. Table VIII contains the relative
risk ratios over time for the 100+ rads group, by city. The higher SMR for the
Hiroshima 100+ rads group is seen here to rest largely on the experience of
1963–66 and later years, with RR ratios of 1.56, 1.28 and 2.01 for the three
four-year intervals. Nothing of this nature is seen in Nagasaki, with its many
fewer deaths from these diseases.

For deaths from diseases of blood and blood-forming organs (Table IX),
the situation is quite different. In each city mortality from these causes is
markedly increased at the higher dose levels ($P < 0.001$). It will be recalled,
however, that these are death certificate diagnoses which, for these causes, are
confirmed by autopsy less than half the time [34]. When the 134 deaths among
A-bomb survivors coded to these causes were collated with the carefully studied
case-material of the Leukemia Registry [35], it was found that 66 had come to
the attention of Registry haematologists, nine of which were attributed to
leukaemia, six to other forms of cancer in which anaemia was an important
clinical feature of the terminal illness, and 19 to other diseases for which anaemia
was also a frequent complication. Table X gives the results of the review by
exposure status. The proportion reviewed by haematologists of the Leukemia

TABLE X. RESULTS OF HAEMATOLOGIC REVIEW OF DEATHS CERTIFIED TO DISEASES OF BLOOD AND BLOOD-FORMING ORGANS

| Exposure status and T-65 dose | Total person-years | Total deaths | Not in Registry | In Leukemia Registry, by Registry diagnosis | | | | |
				Total	Leukaemia	Other cancer	Diseases of blood Obs.-Exp.[a]		Other diseases
NIC	541.0	17	10	7	2	0	2	7.77	3
0–9	1166.0	63	33	30	0	1	18	16.7	11
10–99	392.7	30	15	15	0	3	9	5.65	3
100+	129.1	24	10	14	7	2	3	1.85	2
Total	2228.8	134	68	66	9	6	32	32.00	19

[a] Expectation based on distribution of person-years.

TABLE XI. DEATHS AND STANDARDIZED MORTALITY RATIOS FOR
DISEASES OTHER THAN NEOPLASMS, TUBERCULOSIS, AND THOSE OF
THE CIRCULATORY, DIGESTIVE AND HAEMATOPOIETIC SYSTEMS,
AMONG A-BOMB SURVIVORS AND NOT-IN-CITY SAMPLE, BY CITY,
1950–74

| Exposure status | Observed deaths | | SMR | |
and T-65 dose (rads)	Hiroshima	Nagasaki	Hiroshima	Nagasaki
NIC	1102	313	0.90	1.15
0	1814	245	0.88	1.23
1–9	806	352	0.87	1.12
10–49	593	205	0.78	1.03
50–99	149	55	0.79	0.85
100+	162	107	0.91	1.09
Total[a]	4715	1319	0.87	1.10
Test P				
0–9 versus 100+ rads (two-tailed)			>0.10	>0.10
General homogeneity, A-bomb survivors			0.05	>0.10
Linear trend, A-bomb survivors			>0.10	>0.10

[a] Includes those of unknown dose, 2.3% of survivors in Hiroshima, 5.2% in Nagasaki.

TABLE XII. RELATIVE RISK (RR) OF DEATH FROM ALL DISEASES
EXCEPT NEOPLASMS, TUBERCULOSIS, AND THOSE OF THE CIRCULATORY,
DIGESTIVE AND HAEMATOPOIETIC SYSTEMS, BY CALENDAR PERIOD
AND BY CITY, 1950–74, 100+ rads versus 0–9 rads

| Calendar period | Hiroshima | | | Nagasaki | | |
	Deaths in 100+ group	RR	P[a]	Deaths in 100+ group	RR	P[a]
1950–54	33	1.18	>0.10	20	0.91	>0.10
1955–58	27	0.99	>0.10	17	0.76	>0.10
1959–62	18	0.61	0.03	20	0.93	>0.10
1963–66	32	1.28	0.10	17	1.08	>0.10
1967–70	29	1.20	>0.10	14	0.85	>0.10
1971–74	23	1.03	>0.10	19	1.29	>0.10
Total	162	1.04	>0.10	107	0.94	>0.10

[a] Two-tailed test of 0–9 versus 100+ rads.

TABLE XIII. DEATHS AND STANDARDIZED MORTALITY RATIOS FOR
ALL DISEASES EXCEPT NEOPLASTIC AND HAEMATOPOIETIC AMONG
A-BOMB SURVIVORS AND NOT-IN-CITY SAMPLE, BY CITY, 1950–74

Exposure status and T-65 dose (rads)	Observed deaths		SMR	
	Hiroshima	Nagasaki	Hiroshima	Nagasaki
NIC	3 225	956	0.80	1.01
0	5 576	751	0.84	1.07
1–9	2 492	1137	0.83	1.08
10–49	1 969	692	0.80	1.07
50–99	536	204	0.85	0.95
100+	558	373	0.88	1.04
Total[a]	14 600	4290	0.83	1.06
Test P				
0–9 versus 100+ rads (two-tailed)			>0.10	>0.10
General homogeneity, A-bomb survivors			>0.10	0.03
Linear trend, A-bomb survivors			>0.10	>0.10

[a] Includes those of unknown dose, 2.3% of survivors in Hiroshima, 5.2% in Nagasaki.

TABLE XIV. EXCESS DEATHS FROM ALL DISEASES EXCEPT NEOPLASTIC
PER MILLION PERSON-YEARS PER RAD BY AGE IN 1945, BOTH CITIES
COMBINED, 1950–74

Age in 1945	Estimate	90 per cent confidence interval		P[a]
0–9	− 0.02	− 1.06,	1.02	>0.10
10–19	0.52	− 0.67,	1.72	>0.10
20–34	− 1.32	− 3.20,	0.56	>0.10
35–49	3.00	0.84,	6.86	0.10
50+	− 10.83	− 24.64,	2.97	0.10
All ages	− 0.24	− 1.68,	1.19	>0.10

[a] In test for linear trend.

Registry varies little by exposure status (P > 0.50). Changes in diagnosis, however, are quite strongly related to exposure status, especially changes to leukaemia
or other cancer. When the 32 deaths confirmed as due to diseases of blood and
blood-forming organs are compared with expectation based on the distribution
of person-years, X^2 on 3 d.f. = 7.09, for which P = 0.07. Even this suggestive
result, however, rests mainly on the difference between the NIC and the exposed,
not on the higher risk of these diseases among those exposed to higher T-65
doses. This is not to say that there is no relationship between dose and the
probability of dying from diseases of the blood and blood-forming organs, for
in a larger series there might be. In this material, however, the presumptive
evidence rests on the fact that these diseases, being easily confused with the
complications of other underlying diseases, are very poorly reported on the
death certificate.

   The residual group of deaths from natural causes is the subject of Tables XI
and XII. The SMRs of Table XI vary little by dose in either city. The test of
general homogeneity for Hiroshima, however, returns a P of 0.05, reflecting two
somewhat lower SMRs for the 10—49 and 50—99 dose groups. Similarly, the
relative risk ratios for the six four-year periods shown in Table XII provide no
support for the view that mortality from this group of miscellaneous diseases
(all except neoplasms, tuberculosis, circulatory diseases, digestive diseases and
diseases of the haematopoietic system) has varied with dose in a way suggestive
of accelerated aging by radiation.

   The SMRs for all diseases except neoplasms and diseases of the haematopoietic system are given in Table XIII. Consolidation of all the disease groups
of Tables I—XII produces no more evidence of a relationship with radiation dose than
was seen in the individual tables. The low P-value in the general test of homogeneity
for Nagasaki reflects a combination of both high and low SMRs, as follows:
50—90 rads, 0.95; 100—199 rads, 0.94; 200—299 rads, 1.19; 300—399 rads, 0.74;
and 400+ rads, 1.39. Table XIV provides age-specific regression estimates of
absolute risk in terms of excess deaths per million person-years per rad, but deaths
from blood and blood-forming organs are included here. These estimates are shown
together with their 90% confidence intervals and test results for both cities combined. They also contain no evidence that there may be an important acceleration
in disease among survivors at one or another location on the age range; none of
the estimates differs significantly from zero. In Table XV similar information
(including deaths from diseases of blood and blood-forming organs) is given for
the six four-year periods, by city. Here there is a suggestion that, in Hiroshima,
deaths from non-neoplastic diseases may now be greater among high-dose groups
than among low-dose groups, although over the entire period 1950—74 this is not
the case. In 1971—74 the excess achieved borderline statistical significance,
P = 0.05 in the test for linear trend. In the 100+ rads group there were 99 deaths
versus 90.6 expected, but of these 99 deaths three were certified as diseases of
blood and blood-forming organs.

BEEBE et al.

TABLE XV.   EXCESS DEATHS FROM ALL DISEASES EXCEPT NEOPLASTIC PER MILLION PERSON-YEARS PER RAD BY CALENDAR PERIOD AND BY CITY, 1950—74

Calendar period	Hiroshima			Nagasaki		
	Estimate	90 per cent confidence interval	p[a]	Estimate	90 per cent confidence interval	p[a]
1950—54	− 2.36	− 6.37, 1.65	>0.10	− 0.90	− 5.64, 3.84	>0.10
1955—58	− 2.30	− 6.83, 2.22	>0.10	0.16	− 5.01, 5.33	>0.10
1959—62	− 0.98	− 5.59, 3.61	>0.10	− 2.11	− 7.29, 3.05	>0.10
1963—66	1.88	− 3.07, 6.83	>0.10	1.63	− 3.91, 7.17	>0.10
1967—70	1.91	− 3.38, 7.21	>0.10	− 3.37	− 8.94, 2.19	>0.10
1971—74	5.66	− 0.13, 11.45	0.05	1.14	− 4.87, 7.16	>0.10
Total	0.14	− 1.82, 2.12	>0.10	− 0.57	− 2.76, 1.61	>0.10

[a]   In test for linear trend.

DISCUSSION

The lack of any strong evidence of radiation-induced premature aging among A-bomb survivors is in accord with the experience of British radiologists [8], but in marked contrast to the much larger experience of U.S. radiologists [10]. The three series differ in many ways, of which the most notable are:

(1)   The numbers of deaths from all causes:
       British Radiologists −   463
       U.S. Radiologists   −   1 519
       A-bomb Survivors   −   20 230
       100+ rads only   −   1 443
(2)   Average length of follow-up:
       British Radiologists (1 377): 18.7 years
       U.S. Radiologists (6 524):   16.0 years
       A-bomb Survivors (82 242):   21.2 years after 1950
(3)   Dose-fractionation, the radiologists having a low dose-rate, and the A-bomb survivors, a single exposure;

(4)   Age and sex composition, the radiologists being adult males and the
       A-bomb survivors including both sexes and all ages; and
(5)   Nature of contrast used to test for effect of radiation:
            British radiologists: mortality of general population, physicians,
                and men in social class I
            U.S. radiologists: members of the American College of Physicians
                and members of the American Academy of Ophthalmology
                and Otolaryngology
            A-bomb survivors: low dose versus high dose comparisons.

It should be noted that, although the sample of British radiologists is much smaller
than the U.S. sample, it includes an appreciable number who entered British
radiologic societies before 1920; 302 of the 463 deaths were of this earlier
cohort.   ·
        What reason, or combination of reasons, explains the differences in the
findings of the three studies is not clear. If there is any weakness in the study
of U.S. radiologists it lies in the choice of the comparison groups, but the same
might be said of the British study. The experience of the A-bomb survivors
permits the most powerful examination of the hypothesis in terms of size,
dosimetry and comparability of contrasting groups. The only question that has
been raised with respect to this experience is its representativeness. Stewart [24]
has argued that the number of recognized cancers in each age and sex group has
been affected by the high mortality rates which prevailed in the bombed cities
between the bombings and the dates marking the beginning of the observational
period. Her argument is applied to the findings in the in utero sample, in which
no excess cancer was found in the first 10 years of life [36], and to the children
in the Life Span Study sample whose observation for mortality began 1 October
1950. Quite recently, Rotblat [25] has suggested that the A-bomb survivors may
have experienced a favourable mortality rate from diseases other than malignant
neoplasms because 'only the fittest managed to get over the physical insults'.
He has also stated that the excess incidence of cancers of thyroid, breast and
lung among the A-bomb survivors is lower than would be expected from the
data on other human exposure, and that even the incidence of leukaemia among
the survivors may be too low because published Japanese data on the early entrants,
i.e. rescue workers and others who entered the cities after the bombings, suggest
that their incidence is higher than that of the A-bomb survivors exposed to
comparable doses [37].
        The A-bomb population is a highly selected one, of course, but that its
selection has made it unrepresentative with respect to the carcinogenic effect
in man has not been shown. In fact, so little precision attends quantitative
estimates of the carcinogenic effect of radiation upon specific tissues that few
direct comparisons may be made with estimates derived from different sources.

Each specific effect has at least a latent period and a maximum or a plateau, and may also have a period of subsidence if the leukaemia experience is any guide [38]. These parameters may all vary by age at exposure and by dose-rate. And, in the case of the A-bomb survivors, for many tissues there are as yet no adequate factors for converting the T-65 kerma dose to a specific tissue dose. Also, the differences between the two cities with respect to the radiation spectrum appear to have produced differences in specific cancer-induction rates [26]. Breast tissue is one for which information is available with which to convert the T-65 kerma dose to a tissue dose [39]. When this is done, for women aged 10+ in 1945, and from 1950 through 1969, the radiogenic increase in cancer incidence becomes 2.3 cases per million person-years per rad. This estimate, based on 231 cases, is well below the average values of 6.2 obtained by Boice and Monsen [40] in their report on breast cancer following fluoroscopic examinations of tuberculosis patients treated by pneumothorax, and 8.3 obtained by Shore and co-workers [41] in their recent report on women given X-ray therapy for mastitis. The latter estimates pertain to much younger women than the A-bomb survivors, and to a follow-up period starting 10 years after exposure. When comparisons are made in terms of both age at exposure to radiation and age at risk of cancer, the three series are rather similar:

Age at Exposure to Radiation	A-bomb Survivors	Tuberculosis Patients [42]	Mastitis Patients [43]
(Excess cancers per million person-years per rad after age 30)			
10–19	6.9	8.7	—
20–29	2.7	4.3	5.2
30–39	3.6	3.1	5.0

The situation is somewhat similar with respect to lung cancer, although the data are much less adequate because of the difficulty of accurately estimating the radiation dose received by uranium miners and because there may be a marked difference between Hiroshima and Nagasaki as to the lung cancer effect. The recent UNSCEAR report [21] gives estimates of 10–25 per million persons per rad for A-bomb survivors, 40–180 for uranium and other miners, and about 60 for ankylosing spondylitic patients, but contains an excellent discussion of the reasons why these estimates may not be directly comparable. Fairly comparable estimates may be deduced from the data of Doll and Smith given there. An excess of 31.5 deaths from lung cancer, in 6838 persons followed for 11.3 years starting six years after therapy with a bronchial dose in the range of 80–130 rads [44], yields an estimate of absolute risk of 3.1 to 5.1 excess cancers per million person-years per rad. If the comparison is made on the basis of

A-bomb survivors aged 35+ in 1945, those younger not yet having aged sufficiently to show the effect, and adjusted for under-reporting by death certificate
[34], and for the difference between T-65 kerma dose and tissue dose [32], one
obtains, for the two cities combined:

Age in 1945	Excess per million person-years per rad
35–49	1.9
50+	4.4

The significance of leukaemia incidence among so-called 'early entrants' is
doubtful. It is not a group that has been carefully enumerated, and there are two
features of the reports of Watanabe and his colleagues [37, 45, 46] that raise
serious questions about the validity of their estimates. One is the lack of any
published distribution of the cases over time, and Watanabe's characterization of
their occurrence as sporadic and lacking a peak, which is in sharp contrast to the
well-known peaking of incidence among the A-bomb survivors. The other, and
related, feature is that a comparison of the data given in the 1964 UNSCEAR
report [46] for the period 1950–62, in Hirose's report [45] for 1950–67, and
in Watanabe's report for 1946–72 [37], yields time-specific estimates as
follows, in terms of cases per 100 000 persons annually:

1950–62: 8.05 cases per 100 000 annually
1963–67: 14.0 cases per 100 000 annually
1968–72: 13.2 cases per 100 000 annually

With mortality in the immediate area of the hypocentre essentially 100%
except for the few who were very heavily shielded, and falling rapidly with
increasing distance from the hypocentre [47, 48], selection is an indubitable fact
and not an issue. Rather, the issue is: What was its effect on estimates of late
effects? There is a fairly extensive literature on the apparent influence of
medical selection but little information on the effect of catastrophic experiences.
The studies that have been made of medical selection, i.e. selection for fitness,
show that the effect varies in size and duration with the intensity of the selection
process, and that it wears off rather rapidly but differentially by cause of death.
Table XVI gives a summary of several large, well-studied experiences, one of
severe adversity.

BEEBE et al.

TABLE XVI. STANDARDIZED POST-WW II MORTALITY RATIOS (SMR) FOR U.S. ARMY VETERANS SELECTED IN DIFFERENT WAYS

Time period	SMR
A — Repatriated Pacific prisoners of war captured in the Philippine Islands: 312 deaths from all causes [48]	
1946—1949	1.52
1950—1953	1.27
1954—1957	1.06
1958—1961	0.89
1962—1965	1.07
B — U.S. Army Veterans separated from service in 1946: 3631 deaths from disease only [47]	
1947—1951	0.43
1952—1956	0.68
1957—1961	0.82
1962—1966	0.85
1967—1969	0.86
C — U.S. Army Veterans, controls for psycho-neurosis study: 960 deaths from all causes [49]	
1946—1950	0.62
1951—1955	0.71
1956—1960	0.87
1961—1965	0.90
1966—1969	0.96

(1)   The effect of medical selection for military service in the U.S. Army
      in WW II [49];
(2)   The effect of capture and long-term imprisonment upon the U.S. Army
      survivors of the fall of the Philippine Islands in 1942 [50]; and
(3)   The effect of pre-service screening on the post-war mortality of a
      control group of 10 000 men aged 28—32 on 1 January 1946,
      followed for 24 years [51].

In their study of U.S. WW II Army veterans Seltzer and Jablon [49] show that
the application of the physical standards for entry into the Army resulted in a
halving of the mortality rate for disease immediately after the war, followed by
a gradual increase in the direction of the United States average for men of their
age. Twenty years after entry into service the SMR was about 85% of that norm.
In contrast, for the repatriated prisoners of war, who suffered an almost 40%
mortality during the period from capture in 1942 to release in 1945, deaths
from all causes were 50% above the United States average for their age in
1946—49, and declined rapidly to reach normal in the period 1958—61 because
of trauma. The controls for a mortality follow-up study of men with psycho-
neurosis during WW II have a distinctly favourable mortality immediately after
the war, but in the third decade of follow-up their mortality was over 90% of
the United States average for their age. These examples exhibit the very different
nature of the effects of selection, but any selection for fitness wears off in time.
Only a direct examination of the experience of the A-bomb survivors can reveal
the effects of their selection for survival after 1 October 1950 when the census
was taken that provides the basis for the mortality sample of A-bomb survivors
[27]. For those exposed to greater amounts of radiation, mortality in the period
October 1945 through September 1950 continued to be well in excess of
expectation [52].

      If selection for survival to 1 October 1950 had an important effect on the
subsequent mortality of A-bomb survivors it should be possible to show:

(1)   That there was initially a large mortality deficit that was wearing off
      in the later years of the period 1950—74; and
(2)   That the effect depended upon dose or distance from the hypocentre.

      Table XV gives the experience over the time expressed in terms of absolute
risk estimates, and it does seem clear that some change was taking place over
time, at least in Hiroshima as the absolute risk estimates start at −2.36 in 1950—54
and increase steadily to 5.66 in 1971—74. Although only the latter is of suggestive
statistical significance by itself, the progression is impressive. This may be the
result of the selective influence of the early acute mortality, 1945—49, although
nothing like it is seen in Nagasaki. When the absolute risk estimates of Table XV

are scaled in terms of absolute numbers of deaths, however, any such effect is seen to be small. There follow the observed numbers of deaths from all except neoplastic diseases and the calculated deficit, or excess, corresponding to the absolute risk estimates of Table XV, by time-period, and for those exposed to 10 rads or more:

	50–54	55–58	59–62	63–66	67–70	71–74	Total
Observed deaths	438	538	472	578	553	525	3104
Calculated excess or deficit, deaths	–12.0	–10.6	–4.3	7.8	7.5	19.7	8.1

These differences seem too small to have influenced the response to radiation in any important way. Table XIII gives SMRs by T-65 dose and also shows no evidence of a differential by dose. Finally, Table XIV shows that within age groups there is little evidence of a systematic increase in SMRs of the kind that any important selective process would necessarily produce.

At most, then, there is some evidence that the selection of A-bomb survivors for fitness by 1 October 1950 favourably influenced subsequent mortality from non-neoplastic diseases in Hiroshima, but not in Nagasaki. Moreover, the indications are that the effect in Hiroshima, if real, was quite small in comparison with other experiences where the effects of selection are well documented. Although the analysis can hardly prove that the A-bomb survivors after 1 October 1950 are fully representative of all of humanity with respect to the effects of ionizing radiation, there can be no doubt as to their great usefulness as a guide to what may be expected in other exposures to other people. And, at least up to 1974, their experience very strongly suggests that the effects of ionizing radiation on mortality are specific and focal, and principally carcinogenic. It lends no support to the view that ionizing radiation causes premature aging in man or that the carcinogenic effect is merely part of a general acceleration of aging. Nevertheless, the experience of the A-bomb survivors should continue to be monitored for evidence of accelerated aging among the youngest members of the population as well as for carcinogenesis.

REFERENCES

[1]   RUSS, S., SCOTT, G.M., Br. J. Radiol. 12 (1939) 440.
[2]   HENSHAW, P.S., J. Natl. Cancer Inst. 4 (1944) 513.
[3]   NATIONAL ACADEMY OF SCIENCES, Report of Committee on Pathological Effects of Atomic Radiation, NAS, Washington, D.C. (1956).
[4]   WARREN, S., J. Am. Med. Assoc. 162 (1956) 464.

[5]   MOLE, R.H., Nature (London) **180** (1957) 456.

[6]   ALEXANDER, P., Gerontologia **1** (1957) 174.

[7]   UPTON, A.C., J. Gerontol. **12** (1957) 306.

[8]   COURT BROWN, W.M., DOLL, R., Br. Med. J. **2** (1958) 181.

[9]   SELTSER, R., SARTWELL, P.E., J. Am. Med. Assoc. **166** (1958) 585.

[10] SELTSER, R., SARTWELL, P.E., Am. J. Epidemiol. **81** (1965) 2.

[11] UPTON, A.C., et al., Cancer Res. **20** 8, Pt 2 (1960) 1.

[12] LINDOP, P.J., ROTBLAT, J., Long-term effects of a single whole-body exposure of
      mice to ionizing radiation: II. Causes of death, Proc. Royal Soc. (London), Ser. B
      (1961) 350.

[13] UPTON, A.C., et al., "Age-specific death rates of mice exposed to ionizing radiation
      and radiomimetic agents", Cellular Basis and Aetiology of Late Somatic Effects of
      Ionizing Radiation (HARRIS, R.J.C., Ed.), Academic Press, London (1963).

[14] ALEXANDER, P., CONNELL, D.I., "Differences between radiation-induced life-span
      shortening in mice and normal ageing as revealed by serial killing", Cellular Basis and
      Aetiology of Late Somatic Effects of Ionizing Radiation (HARRIS, R.J.C., Ed.),
      Academic Press, London (1963).

[15] CASARETT, G.W., Adv. Gerontol. Res. **1** (1964) 109.

[16] HOEL, D.G., WALBURG, H.E., Jr., J. Natl. Cancer Inst. **49** (1972) 361.

[17] WALBURG, H.E., Jr., "Radiation-induced life-shortening and premature aging",
      Advances in Radiation Biology **5** (LETT, J.T., ADLER, H., Eds), Academic Press,
      New York (1975).

[18] MATANOSKI, G.M., et al., Am. J. Epidemiol. **101** (1975) 188.

[19] MATANOSKI, G.M., et al., Am. J. Epidemiol. **101** (1975) 199.

[20] RADFORD, E.P., et al., New Engl. J. Med. **297** (1977) 572.

[21] UNITED NATIONS, Sources and Effects of Ionizing Radiation, United Nations
      Scientific Committee on Effects of Atomic Radiation, Report to the General Assembly,
      UN, New York (1977).

[22] JABLON, S., KATO, H., Radiat. Res. **50** (1972) 649.

[23] FINCH, S.C., BEEBE, G.W., J. Radiat. Res. Suppl. (1975) 108.

[24] STEWART, A., Health Phys. **24** (1973) 223.

[25] ROTBLAT, J., New Sci. (London) **75** (1977) 475.

[26] BEEBE, G.W., KATO, H., LAND, C.E., Life Span Study Report 8, Mortality Experience
      of Atomic Bomb Survivors, Radiation Effects Research Foundation Technical Report
      1−77, Hiroshima (1977).

[27] BEEBE, G.W., et al., Radiat. Res. **16** (1962) 253.

[28] JABLON, S., et al., Radiat. Res. **25** (1965) 25.

[29] BEEBE, G.W., et al., Radiat. Res. **48** (1971) 613.

[30] AUXIER, J.A., J. Radiat. Res. Suppl. (1975) 1.

[31] MILTON, R.C., SHOHOJI, T., Atomic Bomb Casualty Commission Technical Report
      1−68, Hiroshima (1968).

[32] HASHIZUME, T., MARUYAMA, T., J. Radiat. Res. Suppl. (1975) 12.

[33] MANTEL, N., HAENSZEL, W., J. Natl. Cancer Inst. **22** (1959) 719.

[34] STEER, A., et al., Atomic Bomb Casualty Commission Technical Report 16−73,
      Hiroshima (1973).

[35] ISHIMARU, T., et al., Radiat. Res. **45** (1971) 216.

[36] JABLON, S., KATO, H., Lancet ii (1970) 1000.

[37] WATANABE, S., "Cancer and leukemia developing among A-bomb survivors", Handbuch
      der allgemeinen Pathologie, Geschwülste. Tumors I, Morphologie, Epidemiologie,
      Immunologie (GRUNDMANN, E., Ed.), Springer-Verlag, Berlin (1974) 461.

[38] ICHIMARU, M., et al., Radiation Effects Research Foundation Technical Report 10–76, Hiroshima (1976).
[39] McGREGOR, D.H., et al., J. Natl. Cancer Inst. **59** (1977) 799.
[40] BOICE, J.D., Jr., MONSON, R.R., J. Natl. Cancer Inst. **59** (1977) 823.
[41] SHORE, R.E., et al., J. Natl. Cancer Inst. **59** (1977) 813.
[42] BOICE, J.D., Jr., Personal communication.
[43] SHORE, R.E., Personal communication.
[44] RADFORD, E.P., Personal communication.
[45] HIROSE, F., Acta Haem. Jaem. Jap. (1968) 765.
[46] UNITED NATIONS, Report of the Scientific Committee on the Effects of Atomic Radiation, General Assembly Official Record: Nineteenth Session, Suppl. No. 14 (A/5814), UN, New York (1964).
[47] SUZUKI, M. (Ed.), Medical Report on Atomic Bomb Effects, Part 1, National Research Council of Japan, Tokyo (1953).
[48] OUGHTERSON, A.W., WARREN, S. (Eds), Medical Effects of the Atomic Bomb in Japan, McGraw-Hill, New York (1956).
[49] SELTZER, C.C., JABLON, S., Am. J. Epidemiol. **100** (1974) 367.
[50] NEFZGER, M.D., Am. J. Epidemiol. **91** (1970) 123.
[51] KEEHN, R.J., et al., Psychosomatic Med. **36** (1974) 27.
[52] TACHIKAWA, K., KATO, H., Atomic Bomb Casualty Commission Technical Report 6–69, Hiroshima (1969).

DISCUSSION

Y. NISHIWAKI: In Japan, medical X-ray examination is compulsory in some schools, factories and companies. In certain diseases, such as tuberculosis and some diseases of the digestive system, extensive X-ray examinations may be conducted and repeated periodically. What is the magnitude of medical X-ray exposure of the populations you studied? Also what is the accuracy of diagnosis of the cases investigated and was diagnosis confirmed by pathological autopsy?

G.W. BEEBE: I can give no quantitative response to your question about initial X-ray, but there are two relevant observations I can offer. First, a very careful study has been made of the initial exposure of all patients in the Adult Health Study, with patients coming in for biennial examination being carefully interrogated about their interim history, including details of any X-ray exposure of course, in the RERF clinics. X-ray exposure is minimized, and a careful record is kept of all exposures and stored on tape. Second, the medical institutions of the community have co-operated in surveys of their equipment and procedures which have provided the basis for estimating typical dose values for specific procedures. With these two types of information it has been possible to compare the A-bomb survivors exposed to different A-bomb doses of radiation as to their medical X-ray exposure. These comparisons have at least shown that medical X-ray exposure is unrelated to A-bomb dose.

The quality of diagnosis varies greatly, as these are death certificate diagnoses. These are typically good for many but not all forms of cancer, good for tuberculosis and for cerebrovascular disease, not good for coronary heart disease, etc. The autopsy rate is low in Japan, but in this series a special effort has been made, for those dying in Hiroshima or Nagasaki, to procure autopsies. In consequence, the autopsy rate has varied from about 20% currently to 40-odd % in the mid-1940s when the programme was far more effective. But the autopsy report is made after the death certificate has been completed, and rarely has any corrective influence on the certification of cause of death. However, the autopsy programme has told us how accurate death certificates typically are, in terms of errors of both inclusion and exclusion.

H. KATO *(Chairman):* As the analysis of cause of death presented by Mr. Beebe is based on death certificates, one may wonder whether and how the accuracy of diagnosis of cause of death affects the results. In this regard, I should like to report the results of a recent analysis of the incidence of cardiovascular disease.

Besides the mortality data which Mr. Beebe presented, we have another set of data, namely data based on biennial physical examination of one fifth of the mortality cohort at RERF. The annual incidence rate for 1958−74 was determined using the standard criteria of the diagnosis.

The incidence rate for both cerebrovascular accident and coronary heart disease does not differ by radiation dose except for Hiroshima females, when the analysis was made by city and sex. For Hiroshima females, the incidence of both CVA and CHD increases with dose. As the risk factor of the disease, such as distribution of blood pressure and serum cholesterol, does not differ among dose comparison groups, it is still a mystery why the relationship to radiation was observed only in the case of Hiroshima females. However, these findings do in general support the results obtained from mortality statistics.

LATENT PERIODS OF RADIOGENIC CANCERS OCCURRING AMONG JAPANESE A-BOMB SURVIVORS

C.E. LAND
Radiation Effects Research Foundation,
Hiroshima,
Japan
and
Environmental Epidemiology Branch,
National Cancer Institute,
Bethesda,
Maryland,
United States of America

J.E. NORMAN
Radiation Effects Research Foundation,
Hiroshima,
Japan
and
Medical Follow-up Agency,
National Academy of Sciences —
    National Research Council,
Washington, D.C.,
United States of America

Abstract

LATENT PERIODS OF RADIOGENIC CANCERS OCCURRING AMONG JAPANESE A-BOMB SURVIVORS.

The latent period of a cancer caused by a given exposure to a carcinogen may be defined as the time between the exposure and the clinical appearance of the cancer. The concept of latent period is important both to risk estimation and to theories of carcinogenesis. It is rarely possible to observe latent period directly because of uncertainty about the cause of a given case, but it is sometimes possible to compare the distributions over time of cancers occurring in otherwise comparable populations affected by different levels of a carcinogen. This is particularly simple for radiation-related cancers in the Life-Span Study sample of Japanese A-bomb survivors and age-matched controls. Cancers of the lung and female breast, and acute and chronic granulocytic leukaemia have occurred at substantially higher rates among survivors exposed to high levels of radiation, and in sufficient numbers to permit conclusions to be drawn by comparing temporal distributions at diagnosis or at death. For these data latent period and dose response can be considered separately to an extent not possible with populations subjected to more than one exposure, or for which periods of follow-up vary. The investigation

shows that there have been at least two distributions of latent period for cancers caused by
a single exposure to ionizing radiation. In one, typified by leukaemia among A-bomb survivors
exposed during childhood, there was a marked wave of increased incidence following exposure.
Radiogenic leukaemias appear to have occurred earlier than so-called spontaneous leukaemias
among members of the same age cohorts. It is uncertain whether dose has had a differential
effect on latent period among radiogenic leukaemias. Another pattern of latent period, typified
by radiogenic cancers of the lung and female breast, shows no separation between the temporal
distribution of radiation-induced and spontaneous cancer, among members of the same birth
cohort. It is conjectured that fundamentally different mechanisms of carcinogenesis are
manifested in these two patterns.

INTRODUCTION

In analysing carcinogenesis data, it is often necessary to rely heavily upon
assumptions about the latent period, the time from the initiating exposure until
the clinical appearance of a resulting cancer. This is especially true when several
exposures have occurred, or when exposure has been continuous. Such assumptions
depend upon theories of carcinogenesis, which in turn may be influenced by new
data on latent periods. Unequivocal determination of the latent period of a given
instance of cancer requires that the causal relation be certain, and that the times
of the initiating exposure and the clinical appearance of cancer be known. Such
complete information is rarely available in epidemiological investigations, but
studies of certain cancers in Japanese A-bomb survivors come close enough for
many purposes. The relative risks of leukaemia and, for certain ages at exposure,
of lung cancer and female breast cancer are high among survivors exposed to high
doses of radiation, follow-up for these diseases has been nearly complete, and the
probable cause of most of the cases occurring in the high-dose group was a
single known exposure.

In a previous paper, the latency patterns of the above three cancers among
members of the extended Life-Span Study (LSS) sample of the Atomic Bomb
Casualty Commission (ABCC) and its successor organization, the Radiation
Effects Research Foundation (RERF), were explored by graphical methods [1].
In the present paper, a similar approach has been followed, using the most
recently available data on lung cancer and leukaemia mortality, and on leukaemia
and breast cancer incidence. More plentiful and more detailed data have permitted
the use of statistical tests sensitive to differences in average date of death,
diagnosis or clinical onset of disease, between cancers presumably caused by
radiation and cancers presumably unrelated to radiation.

It is shown below that there are at least two patterns of latent period for
cancers caused by a single exposure to ionizing radiation. In one, typified by
chronic granulocytic leukaemia among A-bomb survivors, there is a marked

difference in time to occurrence between radiation-caused and 'spontaneous' cancers among members of the same birth cohort. In another, typified by radiation-caused cancer of the lung and female breast, the age distribution of radiation-induced cancer is no different from that expected normally among similar persons free of cancer at the time of exposure. It is conjectured that these two patterns correspond to fundamentally different mechanisms of carcinogenesis.

METHODS AND MATERIALS

The data for this study were taken from published ABCC and RERF reports [2–5], and from intermediate tabulations used in the preparation of two of them [4, 5]. The ABCC-RERF research programme includes leukaemia registries of diagnoses among A-bomb survivors resident in the vicinities of Hiroshima and Nagasaki at the time of diagnosis, but depends mainly on the LSS sample, which includes 82 000 survivors resident in Hiroshima or Nagasaki on 1 October 1950, and 26 500 non-exposed residents taken from censuses of 1950–53 [6]. Personal histories of location and shielding at the time of the bombings (ATB) have been obtained for all but a very few LSS sample members, and reliable radiation dose estimates have been calculated for all but about 3500 [4, 7]. Dose estimates have also been assigned to leukaemia registry cases whenever sufficient information has been available, but only information on ground distance from the explosions was available to the authors of the present report for individual cases outside the LSS sample.

The Japanese family registry system provides death certificate information by place of family registry, as well as by place of death. This has facilitated nearly complete mortality follow-up for the LSS sample. Incidence studies based on this sample cannot attain such complete coverage, but bias analyses have revealed no tendency for reporting to be more complete in one exposure classification than in others [8]. The leukaemia registry, on the other hand, is not based on a fixed sample, and is subject to bias from the migration of survivors in and out of the reporting areas. The LSS clinical sub-sample data indicate that migration from the vicinities of Hiroshima and Nagasaki depends on age ATB but not on estimated dose [9]; however, they are uninformative about the migration of survivors who were not resident in either city in 1950 back into the leukaemia registry reporting areas since that time. By 1972, the leukaemia registry contained 126 definite and probable cases of leukaemia among A-bomb survivors estimated to have received kerma[1] doses of 100 rads or more, of

---

[1] kerma = kinetic energy released in matter; kerma doses refer to tissue kerma in air [10] at a location corresponding to the centre of the body.

whom only 58 were in the LSS sample, and 169 among survivors whose estimated kerma doses were less than 1 rad, including 23 in the LSS sample [3]. Besides migration, these figures reflect the greater geographic area covered by the leukaemia registry compared with the basis of the LSS sample, and the fact that tha LSS sample was constructed on a probability basis, with a much more thorough coverage of heavily exposed survivors than of the more numerous lightly exposed survivors.

The lack of a fixed population basis for the leukaemia registry is a sufficient reason for extreme caution in drawing conclusions from it about the relation between radiation dose and leukaemia incidence. The inclusion of leukaemia registry material in the present report is motivated by the need for more detail than can be provided by the less numerous LSS sample data. The fact that we are concerned only with the temporal patterns of leukaemia occurrence among different exposure groups of similar ages at the time of the bombings (ATB), and not primarily with leukaemia rates, removes some of the hazard from the use of leukaemia registry cases outside the LSS sample; another safety factor is that parallel analyses are presented based on LSS sample material. Nevertheless, it should be emphasized that comparisons involving the entire leukaemia registry depend on the assumption that the relative proportions of heavily exposed and lightly exposed A-bomb survivors in the reporting area have not changed markedly over time, within age-ATB groupings. For this reason, non-exposed leukaemia registry cases outside the LSS sample have not been included in these comparisons since a similar assumption with respect to the proportion of non-exposed residents, even within age cohorts, seems less supportable.

The definition of the LSS sample in terms of a population alive in 1950 necessarily restricts the number of leukaemias with onset before that date, a restriction that does not apply to the leukaemia registry.

The present report is concerned with comparisons of distributions of date of onset, diagnosis or death between groups of cancer cases that are either mostly radiation-caused or mostly unrelated to radiation for similar age cohorts ATB. In such comparisons, numbers of persons at risk are of interest because the likely proportion of radiation-induced cancers in a high-dose group can be deduced from a comparison of rates. Also, bias may be introduced into comparisons of temporal distributions by variation over time in the numbers of persons at risk, and given these numbers, it is possible to adjust for this bias. The age-specific comparisons presented here are not adjusted in this way, because such adjustment was found to make no difference with respect to comparisons based on LSS sample data, and because no such adjustment was possible for the non-LSS material.

The results presented here are in the form of curves giving the cumulative proportion of the cancers occurring in a given group as a function of time. For data from the LSS sample, each curve begins at zero in 1950, and reaches unity at the end of the period of observation for risk specified in the respective figure heading, whereas for leukaemia registry data the curves begin in 1946 and end in 1964. High-dose versus low-dose comparisons are made within age-ATB cohorts. For LSS data the 'high-dose' group consists of cases with an exposure of 100 or more rads (kerma or breast tissue dose) and the 'low-dose' group consists of cases among the non-exposed and among survivors exposed to under 10 rads. The leukaemia registry groups are defined in terms of distance: less than 1500 metres versus 1500–9999 metres. Survivors exposed at 1490–1499 metres received 25 rads on the average, including 3.2 rads from neutrons, in Hiroshima, and 108 rads, with negligible neutron component, in Nagasaki [7]. Those exposed under 1450 metres of course received higher doses. The number of relatively high-dose survivors in the 1500–9999 metre group is greatly outweighed by the very large number with small doses. Non-exposed cases are included in the LSS data but excluded from the leukaemia registry comparisons.

The graphical comparisons are supplemented by t-tests of the differences between means of the high-dose and low-dose distributions.

RESULTS

Leukaemia

Leukaemia is the cancer most strongly associated with radiation dose among the A-bomb survivors. At the death certificate level for the period 1950–74, the relative risk for the LSS sample component exposed to 100 rads kerma or more, compared with those not in either city ATB or exposed to 0–9 rads, and adjusted for age, city, and sex, was 12 [4]. By age ATB, the numbers of deaths and the relative risks were as follows:

Age ATB	0–9	10–19	20–34	35–49	50+
Low-dose (No.)	7	11	24	27	10
High-dose (No.)	15	11	17	12	8
Relative risk	41.3	9.8	16.3	6.0	12.8

The cumulative proportions of deaths occurring over time, as tabulated by 4-year intervals, are given in Fig.1 by exposure level and age ATB. For each cohort except the oldest, the high-dose curve is to the left of the low-dose curve, and markedly so for the 10–19 and 35–49 ATB cohorts.

The death certificate data of the LSS mortality series are complete and presumably free of bias, but the diagnoses have not been as thoroughly reviewed as those in the leukaemia registry series, nor are they as detailed as we should like in terms of type of leukaemia and date of onset. The experience with the

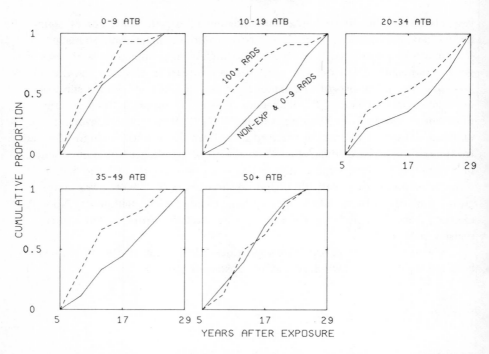

FIG.1.   Cumulative proportions over time (date of death), of leukaemia mortality in the LSS sample, 1950–74, by age ATB and radiation kerma.

LSS series has been that 89% of leukaemia deaths have been correctly detected on death certificates, and 83% of the tested death certificate diagnoses of leukaemia have been confirmed by autopsy [11]. The report by Ichimaru and co-workers of leukaemia incidence during 1950–71 is based on leukaemia registry cases in the LSS sample [3]. These authors report that the temporal patterns of onset of both acute types of leukaemia and of chronic granulocytic leukaemia (CGL) among the heavily exposed have followed characteristic wave-like patterns, the amplitudes being age-dependent for both types, but with displacement by age only for the acute types.

Table I gives numbers of cases and average dates of onset for cases in this series, by dose, age ATB and leukaemia type. For each type, the age-weighted average of onset times for high-dose leukaemia cases is significantly earlier than that for low-dose cases. However, only for ages 0–9 and 10–19 ATB are the age-specific differences statistically significant for acute leukaemia, and only for ages 20–34 ATB are there enough CGL cases to be tested. The cumulative curves for the acute leukaemia cases are given in Fig.2.

TABLE I. LEUKAEMIA INCIDENCE IN THE LSS SAMPLE, 1950–71,
by type, age ATB, and radiation exposure

	Age ATB					
	0–9	10–19	20–34	35–49	50+	Total
Acute leukaemia						
No. low-dose cases[a]	4	8	7	13	5	37
No. high-dose cases[b]	9	9	9	9	6	42
Relative risk	8.5**	8.7**	9.5**	19.6**	14.7**	11.7**[c]
Av. date of onset[d]						
Low-dose cases	15.4	17.9	17.6	15.9	14.9	16.4[c]
High-dose cases	9.3	9.8	14.5	14.0	17.4	12.1[c]
Difference (years)	6.1*	8.1*	3.1	1.9	− 2.5	4.3**
± SD	± 2.9	± 2.7	± 4.3	± 2.1	± 2.6	± 1.7
Chronic granulocytic leukaemia						
No. low-dose cases[a]	1	1	3	0	2	7
No. high-dose cases[b]	5	1	5	2	1	14
Relative risk	95.5**	9.8	20.3**	–	8.8	24.3**[c]
Av. date of onset[d]						
Low-dose cases	20.6	13.4	19.3	–	14.7	18.4[c]
High-dose cases	9.3	24.6	7.4	16.3	12.5	11.2[c]
Difference (years)	11.3	− 11.2	11.9**	–	2.2	7.2**
± SD	–	–	± 1.5	–	–	± 1.1

[a] Non-exposed and 0–9 rads kerma.

[b] 100+ rads kerma.

[c] Age-standardized.

[d] Years after the bombings.

*,** $p < 0.05$ or $p < 0.01$ in a two-tailed test.

    The leukaemia registry includes many cases among A-bomb survivors
outside the LSS sample. By using this material, we can increase the number of
leukaemia cases, including some with onset before 1950, but there are a number
of hazards, which are discussed in the methods section.

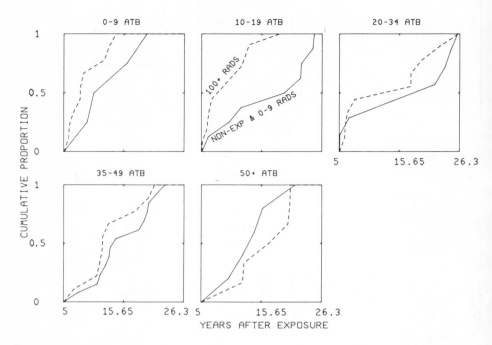

FIG.2. *Cumulative proportions (date of onset) of acute leukaemia incidence in the LSS sample,*
1950–71, by age ATB and radiation kerma.

Bizzozero and co-workers have listed leukaemia registry cases with onset
during 1946–64 by type and age ATB in three groups defined by exposure
distance (dose estimates were not given) [2]. By using only the two closer groups,
exposed at distances under 1500 metres or between 1500 and 10 000 metres,
we hoped to minimize the possibility of confounding between intensity of
exposures and variation over time of the numbers of survivors in the reporting
areas. Table II shows numbers of acute leukaemias and CGL in these two groups,
by age ATB, with mean dates of onset. The group closer to the explosions did
not have as high an average dose as the 100+ rad kerma group used in the
comparisons for the two LSS series, at least in Hiroshima, and therefore the
proportion of radiation-induced cases must be less. Nevertheless, the pattern of
earlier onset, overall, for high-dose than for low-dose cases continues to hold.
As in the LSS incidence series, the high-dose acute leukaemias appeared markedly
earlier than the low-dose acute leukaemias for survivors who were 0–9 and
10–19 years-old ATB, but not for older cohorts. In fact, the relationship is
reversed for the survivors who were 50 or older ATB. The pattern for CGL is

TABLE II. LEUKAEMIA INCIDENCE IN THE LEUKAEMIA REGISTRY, 1946—64,

by type, age ATB, and exposure distance

| | Age ATB | | | | | |
	0—9	10—19	20—34	35—49	50+	Total
	Acute leukaemia					
No. cases 1500—9999m	26	17	32	36	17	128
No. cases < 1500m	27	36	21	14	6	104
Av. onset date[a]						
1500—9999m	11.0	13.3	11.8	11.7	11.2	11.8[b]
< 1500m	8.7	9.2	10.6	11.8	.14.7	10.6[b]
Difference (years)	2.3	4.1**	1.2	− 0.1	− 3.5*	1.2*
± SD	± 1.3	± 1.4	± 1.3	± 1.3	± 1.6	± 0.6
	Chronic granulocytic leukaemia					
No. cases 1500—9999m	4	7	7	9	7	34
No. cases < 1500m	7	13	17	10	8	55
Av. onset date[a]						
1500—9999m	15.6	10.8	10.2	8.0	10.3	10.5[b]
< 1500m	9.4	8.9	6.2	6.8	6.9	7.4[b]
Difference (years)	6.2**	1.9	4.0**	1.2	3.4	3.1**
± SD	± 1.7	± 2.4	± 1.4	± 2.0	± 2.3	± 0.9

[a] Years after the bombings.

[b] Age-standardized.

*,** $p < 0.05$ or $p < 0.01$ in a two-tailed test.

much clearer than in the LSS series, because there are many more cases. It also seems more consistent across age-ATB cohorts than is the case with acute leukaemias. Cumulative curves for acute leukaemias are given in Fig.3, and for CGL in Fig.4.

Overall, the present analysis shows that there is firm evidence for what has been claimed previously: that radiation-induced leukaemias in the A-bomb survivor population have followed a characteristic latency pattern that distinguishes these leukaemias from those due to other causes.

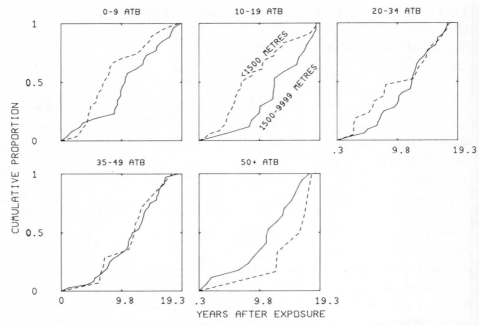

FIG.3.   *Cumulative proportions over time (date of onset) of acute leukaemia incidence in the leukaemia registries, 1946−64, by age ATB and exposure distance.*

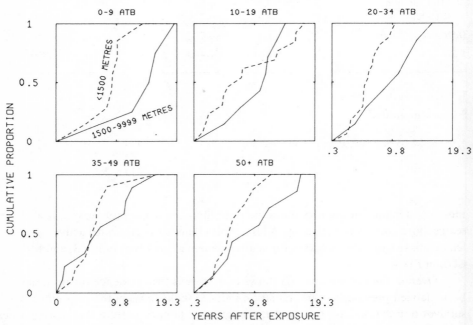

FIG.4.   *Cumulative proportions over time (date of onset) of chronic granulocytic leukaemia incidence in the leukaemia registries, 1946−64, by age ATB and exposure distance.*

Lung cancer

Although the evidence that lung cancer is a radiation effect among A-bomb survivors is strong at the death certificate level, the strength of the evidence is due to large numbers of deaths and not, as in the case of leukaemia, to high relative risks. The age-adjusted relative risk for survivors exposed to kerma doses of 100 rads or more, compared with the non-exposed and those exposed to less than 10 rads, is only 1.8 [4]. Lung cancer deaths have occurred mostly in the older survivors, and it is in these age groups that the radiogenic effect so far appears to have been greatest:

Age ATB	20–34	35–49	50+
Low-dose (No.)	33	170	101
High-dose (No.)	4	19	16
Relative risk	1.6 (p = 0.20)	1.5 (p = 0.05)	3.0 (p < 0.001)

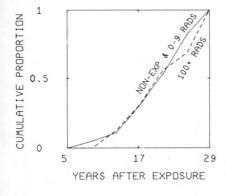

FIG.5. Cumulative proportions over time (date of death) of lung cancer mortality in the LSS sample, 1950–74, ages 50+ ATB, by radiation kerma.

Although it is not clear that the oldest cohort was more sensitive to the effects of radiation on lung tissue (the relative risks of the younger cohorts may change), it is evident from the relative risks that a plausible comparison of mostly radiogenic with mostly non-radiogenic lung cancers can be made only by using the cases occurring in survivors 50 or older ATB. This comparison, as shown in Fig.5, suggests that lung cancer deaths among high-dose members of this cohort and those among low-dose and non-exposed members have followed similar distributions over time. Since the mortality study tabulations present deaths only by four-year time intervals, no calculations have been made of average dates of death for the two exposure groups, but it is clear from the figure that they are very close.

TABLE III. FEMALE BREAST CANCER INCIDENCE IN THE
LSS SAMPLE, 1950–74,
ages 10–39 ATB, by age ATB and radiation dose to breast tissue

	Age ATB			
	10–19	20–29	30–39	Total
No. low-dose cases[a]	39	52	59	150
No. high-dose cases[b]	17	12	12	41
Relative risk	5.8	3.2	4.4	4.4[c]
Av. date of onset[d]				
Low-dose cases	23.7	20.8	18.2	20.7[c]
High-dose cases	23.8	20.6	19.7	21.2[c]
Difference (years)	− 0.1	0.2	− 1.5	− 0.5
± SD	± 1.2	± 1.9	± 1.6	± 0.9

[a]   Non-exposed and 0–9 rads breast tissue dose.

[b]   100+ rads breast tissue dose.

[c]   Age-standardized.

[d]   Years after the bombings.

*,** p $<$ 0.05 or p $<$ 0.01 in a two-tailed test.

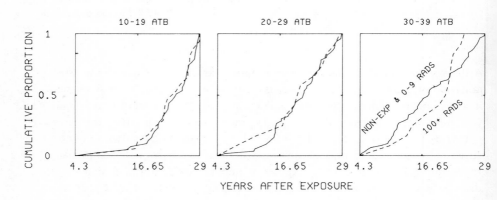

FIG. 6.   *Cumulative proportions over time (date of diagnosis) of female breast cancer incidence in the LSS sample, 1950–74, by age ATB and breast tissue dose.*

Breast cancer

Although breast cancer mortality among female A-bomb survivors is clearly related to radiation dose [4], this disease is best studied at the level of incidence. The most recent survey of breast cancer incidence in the LSS sample identified 360 cases diagnosed during the period 1950–74 [5]. The evidence for a radiation effect was strongest in the women who were 10–39 years-old ATB. Younger women had not yet, by 1974, had much breast cancer, there was no apparent high-dose excess in women 40–49 ATB, and the evidence for a radiation effect in older women was based on only a few high-dose cases. Numbers of high-dose (100+ rads to breast tissue) and low-dose (not-in-city and 0–9 rads) cases, relative risks and average dates at diagnosis are given in Table III. Unlike the average dates of onset in Tables I and II, the dates at diagnosis of breast cancer have no apparent dependence upon radiation dose, although they depend strongly on age ATB. That is, radiogenic breast cancers have not appeared earlier than other breast cancers in women of similar ages ATB. The cumulative curves in Fig.6 show this in greater detail.

The evidence provided by the breast cancer data is similar to that presented for lung cancer, but somewhat more impressive because the relative risks are higher. For these two cancers, the excess cases caused by radiation appear to have the same distribution over time as cancers due to other causes, contrasting markedly with the wave-like latency pattern of radiogenic leukaemias.

DISCUSSION

The preceding analysis supports the interpretation of Ichimaru and co-workers [3] that the latent periods of radiation-induced leukaemias correspond to a unimodal distribution conspicuously different from the usual distribution of naturally occurring leukaemias in a cohort followed over time. Radiogenic CGL incidence peaked within 5 to 10 years after exposure, regardless of age at exposure, whereas the incidence of radiogenic acute leukaemia tended to peak later, and less sharply, with increasing age at exposure. Radiation-induced cancers of the lung and female breast, on the other hand, had temporal distributions similar to those of naturally occurring cancers of the same sites. There appear to be at least two, and possibly more, fundamentally different patterns of latent-period distribution for cancers induced by a single exposure to ionizing radiation.

It is uncertain whether the latent-period distributions observed for radiogenic acute leukaemias in the various age cohorts represent a pattern distinct from those characteristic of CGL on the one hand and lung and breast cancer on the other, or a mixture of the two. Ichimaru and co-workers [3] observed that acute granulocytic leukaemia was notably infrequent, and acute lymphocytic leukaemia especially frequent, among the younger compared with the older survivors in the high-dose group. Unfortunately, the available numbers of cases were not large enough to allow separate comparisons by type of acute leukaemia in the present study.

The LSS sample permits the latent period to be studied in a way that is difficult or impossible with most other human data. One obvious advantage is that different exposure groups and age cohorts have been followed for exactly the same time span, so that there is no confounding due to changes in natural cancer rates over time. The ability to compare dose groups within age cohorts protects against possible confounding due to different sensitivity to radiation at different exposure ages, or due to age-dependencies of latent period. For example, the conclusion by Baral and co-workers [12] that the latent period of radiation-induced female breast cancer decreases with increasing dose appears, in the light of the present findings, to be due to an association in their series between radiation dose and age at exposure.

Some cancers seem especially difficult to study for the latent period. Thyroid cancer, for example, develops slowly, and the interval between exposure and detection probably depends more on the thoroughness of the search for cancer in exposed (and, for comparison purposes, in non-exposed) persons than on anything we might wish to call the latent period of the disease. For this reason, it is difficult to evaluate the observation by Maxon and co-workers [13] that the latent period of thyroid cancer occurring after external radiation in childhood has a lognormal distribution.

Inferences about the relationship between radiation dose and latent period are subject to other hazards besides the association of dose and age mentioned above with respect to the recent paper by Baral and co-workers [12]. If the cancer being studied is one that has a distinctly different latent period for radiogenic as opposed to naturally occurring cancers, the temporal distribution of cancers in a group exposed to an intermediate exposure level may be between the distributions corresponding to high- and low-dose groups simply because the proportion of radiogenic cancers is between the proportions in the two extreme groups. In experimental studies using dose levels and/or animal strains for which lifetime cancer incidence is extremely high, an association between dose and latent period may occur only because there is no other way for a dose-incidence relationship to be expressed. That is, if all the animals in a study eventually have cancer, but the high-dose animals have cancer earlier, this does not necessarily imply a relationship between dose and latent period for other dose levels and/or organisms for which the lifetime risk is only a few per cent. Finally, inferences about the latent period based on competing risk analyses are not necessarily applicable to 'latent period', in the sense of this discussion, because the Weibull model used in such analyses assumes that each animal, if it lives long enough, will eventually exhibit the cancer under study; a shortened 'latent period', therefore, is the only way increased incidence can be expressed under this model [14].

The cumulative curves in Figs 5 and 6 are consistent with a relative risk model of cancer incidence, in which the effect of a given dose of radiation is to multiply an individual's age-specific risk over the remaining lifespan (possibly excluding a minimal latent period) by a dose-dependent constant. An absolute risk model, on the other hand, assumes that for part of the exposed person's remaining lifetime, his risk is expressed as the sum of the natural age-specific risk and a constant, dose-dependent increment. The latent period data for cancers of the lung and female breast are, however, also consistent with an absolute risk model in which the dose-dependent increment does not apply until ages of substantial natural cancer risk are reached. The analytic method used in the present paper offers some hope of eventually deciding between the absolute and relative risk models, but only if it can be applied to substantially larger data sets.

An obvious inference about the different latent period distributions characterizing CGL on the one hand and breast and lung cancer on the other is that they correspond to different mechanisms of carcinogenesis. The expression of radiation carcinogenesis of the lung and the female breast follows the same pattern with respect to age at risk as that for non-radiogenic cancers of these organs. Radiogenic CGL, on the other hand, characteristically occurs soon after radiation exposure, regardless of age at exposure.

The two-mutation model proposed by Mole [15] and developed by Strong [16] would predict such a dichotomy of latent period distributions, provided that the radiation from the A-bombs caused only the first mutation necessary for lung and breast cancer (and which results from other causes in the development of non-radiogenic cancers of these organs), but caused the second mutation required for the development of CGL. This could happen if radiogenic CGL was confined to a susceptible subgroup, in whom the first mutation had already occurred, or if radiation caused the two necessary mutations to occur spontaneously. The behaviour of the leukaemia dose response functions for Hiroshima and Nagasaki is consistent with a linear dependence on neutron dose and on the square of gamma dose, suggesting that leukaemia may be associated with double-strand DNA breaks [17]. On the other hand, except for a statistically non-significant tendency for high-dose leukaemias to have a heavier proportion of CGL in Hiroshima than in Nagasaki, possibly because the substantial neutron component of dose may cause double-strand breaks to occur more frequently in Hiroshima, the data do not suggest that CGL is more likely than acute leukaemia to be the result of simultaneous double mutations. In fact, the average kerma associated with CGL is less than that associated with acute leukaemia, in each of the two cities.

The dose-response curves for Nagasaki and Hiroshima appear to be approximately linear with respect to female breast cancer, and the risk estimates for the two cities do not differ by much [5, 8]. This supports the theory that radiation causes a single mutation which may, if later events also occur, result in breast cancer. The dose-response curve for radiogenic lung cancer is less clear, perhaps because the disease is somewhat poorly diagnosed on death certificates [11]. In general, the contrast between radiogenic leukaemia and breast cancer, with respect both to dose response and latent period, supports the two-mutation model of carcinogenesis, but the contrast between CGL and acute leukaemia suggests that the model may be an oversimplification.

A practical implication of the results of the present study for epidemiological research is that it may be unwise to assume a wave-like latent period distribution for radiogenic cancers other than leukaemia. In dose-response analyses involving multiple exposures, it is clearly necessary to make some assumptions about latent period; the present results suggest that for some cancers, the most reasonable assumption about latent period is a particularly simple one, i.e. that a radiogenic cancer may occur at any time after the exposure (perhaps with a minimal latent period) at which there is a non-negligible age-specific risk of naturally occurring cancer of the irradiated organ.

REFERENCES

[1] LAND, C.E., McGREGOR, D.H., "Temporal distributions of risk after exposure", Proc. Third Int. Symposium on Detection and Prevention of Cancer, Part I: Prevention 1, Etiology, New York (1977) 831.

[2] BIZZOZERO, O.J., Jr., et al., Atomic Bomb Casualty Commission Technical Report 17−65, Hiroshima (1965)

[3] ICHIMARU, M., et al., Radiation Effects Research Foundation Technical Report 10−76, Hiroshima (1976).

[4] BEEBE, G.W., et al., Radiation Effects Research Foundation Technical Report 1−77, Hiroshima (1977).

[5] TOKUNAGA, M., et al., Radiation Effects Research Foundation Technical Report 17−77, Hiroshima (1977).

[6] BEEBE, G.W., USAGAWA, T., Atomic Bomb Casualty Commission Technical Report 12−68, Hiroshima (1968).

[7] MILTON, R.C., SHOHOJI, T., Atomic Bomb Casualty Commission Technical Report 1−68, Hiroshima (1968).

[8] McGREGOR, D.H., et al., J. Natl. Cancer Inst. 59 (1977) 799.

[9] MORIYAMA, I.M., OTAKE, M., Atomic Bomb Casualty Commission Technical Report 1−73, Hiroshima (1973).

[10] INTERNATIONAL COMMISSION ON RADIOLOGICAL PROTECTION AND MEASUREMENTS, Report 19, Washington, D.C. (1971).

[11] STEER, A., et al., Atomic Bomb Casualty Commission Technical Report 16−73 (1973).

[12] BARAL, E., et al., Cancer 40 (1977) 2905.

[13] MAXON, H.R., et al., Am. J. Med. 63 (1977) 967.

[14] PIKE, M.C., Biometrics 22 (1966) 142.

[15] MOLE, R.H., "Cancer production by chronic exposure to penetrating gamma irradiation",
      Natl. Cancer Inst. Monograph 14 (1964) 217.
[16] STRONG, L.C., "Theories of pathogenesis: mutation and cancer", Genetics of Human
      Cancer (MULVIHILL, J.J., MILLER, R.W., FRAUMENI, J.F., Jr., Eds), Raven Press,
      New York (1977) 401.
[17] ISHIMARU, T., et al., Radiation Effects Research Foundation Technical Report 14–77,
      Hiroshima (1977).

DISCUSSION

A.M. STEWART: You here invoked Mole's two-mutation model to account
for two observations: the short latent periods of leukaemias associated with
high-level radiation, and the fact that sensitivity to the cancer-induction effects
of radiation increases progressively with adult age. But the second effect could
be a host reaction similar to the one that allows all pathogens to be more
dangerous in old age than in the prime of life; and the first effect could be due
to direct damage of the immune system (by any cause including high-level
radiation) accelerating any cancer of this cell system by lowering the level of
immunological competence. According to this theory, reactions to low-level
radiation delivered at slow dose rates could be very different from reactions to
high-level radiation delivered at fast ones. Would you care to comment on
these suggestions?

C.E. LAND: The two-mutation theory is only one among several that are
consistent with the latent period data described in the present paper. You have
suggested another explanation that also seems plausible, at least at my
unsophisticated level of understanding. I don't believe, however, that the latent
period data necessarily suggest anything about the sensitivity to the carcinogenic
effects of radiation at different ages. For breast cancer induction, at least,
radiation sensitivity in the A-bomb survivors appeared to decrease with increasing
age at exposure, but regardless of age at exposure the incidence of radiogenic
breast cancers increased with increasing age at risk, similarly to the incidence
of non-radiogenic breast cancers. I suggest that your theory could be developed
further in relation to the differences between cancers observed among the
A-bomb survivors and other exposed groups on the one hand, and in the Hanford
plutonium workers on the other, and I am eager to learn more about it.

G.W. DOLPHIN: Is the incidence of radiogenic cancers of the breast affected
by marital status or number of children?

C.E. LAND: Nakamura, Kato and Wakabayashi, in an RERF technical
report now in the press, examined the McGregor series of breast cancer cases
(Journal of the National Cancer Institute, Sep. 1977) with respect to the usual
risk factors. They found that marital status and number of children, among
other factors, were related to breast cancer incidence, but the sample size was
too small to determine whether or not radiation interacted with other breast

cancer risk factors. They did determine that the apparent radiation effect was genuine and not an artifact due to a fortuitous association of radiation dose with other risk factors. Mr. Boice's paper at this symposium[1] also addresses this point.

G.W. DOLPHIN: Most naturally occurring lung cancers are caused by smoking. Are there differences in smoking habits between the high and low dose groups?

C.E. LAND: This question was investigated by Ishimaru and co-workers in a study of an autopsy series of lung cancer deaths in the Life Span Study sample (Cancer **36** 5 (1975) 1723). Smoking history was related to lung cancer mortality, but adjustment for smoking, age and other factors did not affect the relationship between radiation dose and lung cancer mortality. As in the breast cancer study just referred to, numbers were not sufficient to determine whether or not smoking interacted with radiation dose in causing lung cancer.

G.W. DOLPHIN: For cancers that increase with a power of 4 to 5 of age (A^4 or A^5) such as lung cancer, a several-stage model may be needed. For other malignancies, such as acute leukaemia, the variation of incidence with age is less marked. Hence a simple two-stage model may not be applicable to all types of malignancy.

C.E. LAND: I mentioned the two-mutation model only as an example of a model consistent with the observed latent period differences. I believe that two or more stages are probably necessary to explain the results with respect to breast and lung cancer, and that any model must treat CGL differently from cancers of the lung and breast. I'm sure that a more complex model will be needed for considering aspects other than latent period, as you have suggested.

Y. NISHIWAKI: You referred briefly to the possible difference in the mode of action of gamma and neutron radiation. I assume that this would be due to the difference in the LET of these two radiations. In the case of Nagasaki, the gamma contribution was much higher than the neutron in the low dose range compared with Hiroshima. What would be the relative contributions of the gamma and neutron radiation to the tissue dose in the dose range indicated in your paper?

C.E. LAND: According to the organ dose algorithms derived by a working group at Oak Ridge National Laboratories, and reported by Kerr[2], the relationships between kerma and breast tissue dose are as follows:

Breast tissue neutron rads = 0.56 × kerma neutron rads
Breast tissue gamma rads = 0.80 × kerma gamma rads + 0.045 × kerma neutron rads

---

[1]   BOICE, J.D., STONE, B.J., "Interaction between radiation and other breast cancer risk factors", these Proceedings **I**, IAEA-SM-224/713.

[2]   OAK RIDGE NATIONAL LABORATORIES, Report of Liaison Studies with the Atomic Bomb Casualty Commission, Hiroshima, Japan, Aug. 20–17 Sept., 1974, ORNL-TM-4830.

K.H. CHADWICK: Do you attach any significance to the fact that in some of the older group ATB the occurrence of the cancers in the irradiated group was later than in the control group?

C.E. LAND: I expect you are referring to the acute leukaemia results for the cohort 50 years old or older ATB in Table I and, especially, Table II. One possibility is that the types of acute leukaemia induced by radiation varied according to age at exposure, and that therefore the latent period comparison for acute leukaemia may confound age at exposure, radiation dose, and type of leukaemia. We did not subdivide according to type of acute leukaemia, because we thought the numbers would be too small, but I now believe that it would have been better if we had.

G.W. BARENDSEN: You have analysed latent periods for leukaemia, breast cancer and lung cancer. In general the latent period for any cancer consists of two parts: (1) a true 'latent period', during which a transformed cell is present but requires a second stimulus to start proliferation, and (2) a period during which proliferation from one or a few cells to a palpable mass of about 10^9 cells occurs. This second part is much longer in general for lung cancer and breast cancer than for leukaemia, because the solid cancers generally have an average cell number doubling time of $60-100$ days — which is considerably greater than that for many leukaemias. Because of this complexity of the latent period, it is difficult to draw conclusions about differences in basic mechanisms from differences between latent periods.

C.E. LAND: I don't believe that this comment has much bearing on the argument made in the paper — that the latent period distribution of radiogenic CGL does not depend on age at exposure, whereas those for radiogenic breast and lung cancers are highly age-dependent, and that this implies a difference in the carcinogenic mechanisms involved. That is, it is the age-dependence of radiogenic cancers of the lung and female breast versus the lack of such dependence for radiogenic CGL that suggests this difference. A difference in average latent period, without reference to age at exposure, would not suggest such a difference in basic mechanisms, as you correctly point out.

MORTALITY OF IN-UTERO CHILDREN EXPOSED TO THE A-BOMB AND OF OFFSPRING OF A-BOMB SURVIVORS

H. KATO
Radiation Effects Research Foundation,
Hiroshima,
Japan

Abstract

MORTALITY OF IN-UTERO CHILDREN EXPOSED TO THE A-BOMB AND OF OFFSPRING OF A-BOMB SURVIVORS.

A cohort-type follow-up study has been carried out by the Radiation Effects Research Foundation on the mortality of children exposed to A-bomb radiation while in utero. The mortality increased with tissue dose during the first year of life and did not increase during the following nine years, but an increase with dose was again suggested during 10–32 years of age. A detailed analysis of infant mortality revealed that the dose-associated excess in mortality among those under one year of age, especially within one month after birth, was attributable partly to the mechanical injury of the mother, but this does not provide the whole explanation. There was no increase of mortality from cancer including leukaemia with dose. As the number of cancer deaths is at present only five, further careful follow-up on this cohort is necessary to determine the state of radiation-induced cancer among this cohort. The continuing study on mortality rates among children born to A-bomb survivors has been updated to 1976. No clearly significant effect of parental exposure on survival of the offspring (average age 24 years) could be demonstrated either by a contingency χ^2-type of analysis or regression analysis.

1. MORTALITY OF IN-UTERO CHILDREN EXPOSED TO THE A-BOMB, 1945–76

Experimental evidence clearly indicates that ionizing radiation shortens the life span in animals. In man, in addition to the well-known increase in leukaemia attributed to radiation, a significant increase in mortality from other malignant neoplasms has also been observed among the A-bomb survivors [1]. The foetus would be expected to be especially sensitive to ionizing radiation. Earlier studies on the medical examination of children exposed in utero revealed an elevated prevalence of microcephaly with mental retardation [2], delay in growth and development [3] and suppression of antibody production [4] among those proximally exposed.

The Radiation Effects Research Foundation (formerly ABCC and JNIH) has been conducting a mortality study on a cohort of in-utero exposed children. The mortality experience for the period 1945—69 has already been reported [5].

This report is aimed at presenting a follow-up of the mortality experience in the same cohort for the subsequent seven years, and analysing the total 32 years' mortality experience (1945—76). The present analysis, moreover, is based on tissue dose estimates which only recently became available. This makes possible a more efficient study of the radiation effects than in the previous report which employed only tissue kerma in air of the mother (T-65 dose).

1.1. Method

1.1.1. Sample

All birth records for children born from the time of the A-bomb, 6 August in Hiroshima, 9 August in Nagasaki, to the end of May 1946 in both cities were collected. An extensive field survey was performed on all these subjects, 3992 in Hiroshima and 3728 in Nagasaki, to determine the mother's exposure status. The number of unknown cases was found to be less than 5%. A matched sample was drawn from children whose mother's exposure status was known. All subjects in the group exposed within 1500 m were included in the study sample and comparison subjects were selected from each of the following distance groups; 1500—1999 m, 2000—2999 m and 3000—3999 m and non-exposed matched as to city and sex, and as closely as possible on month of birth. The study sample thus selected totalled 1615 in Hiroshima and 329 in Nagasaki. A previous analysis [5] showed a difference between exposed and non-exposed mothers in the distributions of such concomitant variables as maternal age, birth order, parents' occupation and parents' education. In general, these differences were such as to inflate mortality rates in the exposed compared with the non-exposed, but there were no apparent differences in these variables among distance sub-divisions of the exposed group. In the analysis, therefore, the sample is limited to those whose mothers were exposed, 1073 in Hiroshima and 219 in Nagasaki.

Additional samples comprising children born outside the cities have been defined from the ABCC Master File and 1960 A-bomb Survivors Survey [5]. But as these auxiliary samples were completely defined only in about 1960, their use in the analysis of mortality began after 1960. The original sample size was increased by 25% as a result of this addition.

1.1.2. Ascertaining survival status

There has existed in Japan since the last quarter of the nineteenth century a system of compulsory family registration. The family record is termed the

Koseki, and the legal or permanent address of the family is the Honseki.
Accordingly, if the Honseki is known, the survival status of any individual can
be determined. The Koseki were checked for the entire sample in March 1977.
Causes of death were obtained from the Japanese vital statistics death schedules
kept at health centres throughout Japan.

1.1.3. Radiation dose

Recently the tissue dose of in-utero children was estimated from two different
sources; Oak Ridge National Laboratory (ORNL) in the United States of America
[6] and the Japanese National Institute for Radiological Sciences (NIRS) [7].

Although the method and parameters employed in the respective equations
are slightly different, the tissue doses obtained by the two methods are almost
identical and have good correlation with the T-65 dose, though they were decreased
to about 40%.

In the present analysis, the ORNL tissue doses were used for the sake of
convenience. The average T-65 dose and tissue dose of those exposed to 1 rad and
over are 90.2 rads and 34.4 rads respectively.

1.2. Results

1.2.1. Total mortality (all causes of death)

There were 203 deaths among 1293 subjects for the entire period 1945–76.
The mortality ratio increased linearly with both T-65 dose and tissue dose.

All subsequent analyses were made by both T-65 and tissue dose, but as the
results were similar in both instances, only the results based on tissue dose will
be presented hereafter.

The increase in mortality ratio with dose was observed in both Hiroshima
and Nagasaki.

1.2.2. Age at death

The mortality ratio in relation to dose was further observed by age at death;
under one month, 1–12 months, 1–9 years and 10–32 years as shown in Table I.
A linear increase of mortality ratio was observed in those under one year of age,
especially in those within one month after birth. No increase was observed at
1–9 years of age, but an increase was again suggested after ten years of age.

1.2.3. Trimester

The study subjects were divided into approximate trimesters of gestation at
time of exposure based on month of birth: I. February-May 1946; II. November

TABLE I. MORTALITY OF IN-UTERO EXPOSED CHILDREN BY AGE AT DEATH AND TISSUE DOSE

Age at death	Statistics	Total	Tissue dose (rad)					Test[a]	
			0	1–29	30–69	70+	Unk.	L	H
<1 month	Observed	38	21	7	2	8	0	++	++
	Observed/Expected		1.11	0.54	0.69	3.14	–		
	Sample	1293	675	443	86	65	24		
1–12 months	Observed	66	31	23	6	5	1	Sugg.	NS
	O/E		0.90	1.01	1.37	1.67	0.87		
	Sample	1255	654	436	84	57	24		
1–9 years	Observed	70	39	23	6	1	1	NS	NS
	O/E		1.03	0.96	1.36	0.39	0.73		
	Sample	1189	623	413	78	52	23		
10+ years	Observed	29	14	8	4	3	0	+	NS
	O/E		0.93	0.79	2.23	2.35	–		
	Sample	1119	584	390	72	51	22		

[a] L: Linear increase with dose (one-tailed).
H: Non-homogeneity of four known dose groups, regardless of pattern.
++: Significant at 1% level.
+: Significant at 5% level.
Sugg: Suggestive $0.10 > P > 0.05$.
NS: Not significant $P > 0.10$.

1945-January 1946; and III. August-October 1945. A significant increase in
mortality ratio with dose was observed only for the children who were exposed
in the third trimester.

1.2.4. Early infant mortality by injury of mother ATB

It has been pointed out that excess mortality among those under one year
of age may be attributable not to radiation per se, but to mechanical injuries
received by the mother at the time of the bombing. This is suggested especially
by the fact that the excess is observed only among children who were in their
third trimester.

As the tissue dose became available, a detailed analysis on infant mortality
was performed with due consideration given to this point. The increase with
dose was observed in groups both with or without mechanical injury. The excess
in early infant mortality seems to be observed only in children irradiated during
their third trimester, even in the group without mechanical injury. Therefore,
although mechanical injury does play a role, it fails to provide the whole explanation
for the excess in early infant deaths.

It is possible that exposure of the foetus during the early developmental
stage might have resulted in a higher rate of spontaneous abortion or stillbirth,
which may have caused the excess of early infant mortality among those irradiated
during their third trimester.

1.2.5. Concomitant variables

Concomitant variables such as birth order, birth weight and so on which
should affect mortality, especially infant mortality, were observed to see if they
were dissimilarly distributed among the comparison group. Analysis indicated
that all factors except birth weight were distributed homogeneously among the
five dose groups.

Therefore, these factors will not seriously affect the relationship between
mortality and radiation exposure.

1.2.6. Cause of death

The cause of death was not available for 55 of the total 203 deaths. These
55 deaths occurred almost exclusively within a year after birth, 1945–46, during
the immediate post-war period when death certificates were not available because
of confusion in the official vital statistics reporting system. Since the number of
deaths is so small, cause-specific mortality was analysed only for a few major
causes. Perinatal deaths increased with dose, which is consistent with the finding
that mortality for subjects under one year of age increased with dose. No increase

TABLE II. MORTALITY OF IN-UTERO EXPOSED CHILDREN BY CAUSE OF DEATH AND TISSUE DOSE

Cause of death	Statistics	Total	Tissue dose (rad)					Test[a]	
			0	1–29	30–69	70+	Unk.	L	H
Infection	Observed	59	35	18	3	2	1	NS	NS
	O/E		1.15	0.90	0.71	0.65	0.87		
	Sample	1293	675	443	86	65	24		
Neoplasm	Observed	5	2	2	1	0	0	NS	NS
	O/E		0.71	1.34	2.83	–	–		
Perinatal deaths	Observed	19	9	3	2	5	0	+	NS
	O/E		1.06	0.47	1.11	2.53	–		
Cause unknown	Observed	55	20	21	7	6	1	++	++
	O/E		0.67	1.10	2.24	2.91	1.14		

[a]   L: Linear increase with dose (one-tailed).

    H: Non-homogeneity of four known dose groups, regardless of pattern.

    ++:   Significant at 1% level.

    +:   Significant at 5% level.

    NS: Not significant $P > 0.10$.

in mortality with dose was observed for other causes of death, except for those
who died, for the most part in the first year, of unknown causes.

With respect to radiation-induced cancers, there were five deaths attributable
to malignant tumour; two leukaemia cases and one each with cancer of stomach,
liver and large intestine. There was no increase of death from cancer with dose
as shown in Table II. Nor was an excess in cancer death during the period 1960–76
observed among the total sample which was increased by 25% by the addition of
the two ancillary samples described earlier. However, it is still too early to conclude
that there is no excess in cancer deaths among the in-utero irradiated, because the
sample size is too small and the cohort has not reached the cancer age yet.
A considerably long period of follow-up will be required to clarify the effects
on this cohort.

2. MORTALITY OF OFFSPRING OF A-BOMB SURVIVORS, 1946–76

The extensive genetic studies of pregnancies terminating in 1948–53 [8]
and the final sex ratio study of births in 1954–62 [9] failed to show any genetic
effects of A-bomb radiation. Although there was no evidence of increased neonatal
or infant mortality in the early genetic study [8], some, but not all, experimental
findings continued to suggest that atomic radiation reduced the survival of F_1
progeny [10]. Accordingly an effort was made to determine the genetic effect
of atomic bomb radiation upon the death rate among children of atomic bomb
survivors. This report updates the results to 1976 from the previous report [10],
which covered the mortality experience during the period of 1946–69.

2.1. Method

2.1.1. Sample

The study sample of the genetic studies 1948–58 [8, 9], and birth records
for 1946–47 were used to select a new study sample [10] consisting of 53 000
children born from May 1946 through December 1958 to parents of known
exposure status in Hiroshima and Nagasaki, and grouped as follows:

Group 1: either or both parents <2000 m from the hypocentre at the
time of the bombings (ATB).
Group 2: neither parent <2000 m but either or both >2500 m from the
hypocentre ATB.
Group 3: both parents not in city ATB.

TABLE III. MORTALITY EXPERIENCE OF THE 25 GROUPS OF CHILDREN
OF A-BOMB SURVIVORS FOR BOTH HIROSHIMA AND NAGASAKI,
SEXES COMBINED

Mother		Father					
		100+rem	10−99	1−9	<1	NE	Total
100+rem	Observed	20	17	10	29	187	263
	Observed/Expected	0.86	1.42	1.33	0.86	0.99	0.99
	Subjects	323	169	110	510	2919	4031
10−99	Observed	18	63	20	59	248	408
	Observed/Expected	1.20	0.97	1.07	0.96	0.91	0.94
	Subjects	219	858	267	883	4130	6357
1−9	Observed	19	17	31	33	127	227
	Observed/Expected	1.51	0.94	1.00	0.87	0.95	0.97
	Subjects	181	258	414	568	2024	3445
<1	Observed	50	68	37	321	622	1098
	Observed/Expected	0.98	1.01	1.25	1.05	1.02	1.03
	Subjects	771	997	427	4266	9209	15 670
NE	Observed	73	70	37	202	1132	1514
	Observed/Expected	1.14	0.89	0.94	1.09	0.99	1.00
	Subjects	1026	1279	619	3036	17 262	23 222
Total	Observed	180	235	135	644	2316	3510
	Observed/Expected	1.08	0.98	1.07	1.03	0.98	1.00
	Subjects	2520	3561	1837	9263	35 544	52 725

$\chi^2 = 19.61$ d.f. = 24

Group 1 includes all eligible children, whereas groups 2 and 3 are matched by
age and sex with a final selection made randomly to yield groups equal in size
to Group 1. With samples of this size, to a close approximation, a 10% increase
in mortality in Group 1 could be detected with 95% probability at the 5% level
of significance in contrasting Group 1 with either Group 3 or 2.

In addition, an enumeration of children born after 1958 began in 1976 and
will be complete in about 1980. The mortality experience of about 2000 children
enumerated thus far was also analysed in this report.

2.1.2. Ascertainment of survival status

The method is the same as that described for the in-utero mortality study. Deaths occurring from birth to 1976 were ascertained, so that mortality during the average first 24 years of life could be determined.

2.1.3. Radiation dose

As described in detail elsewhere, the neutron component of the Hiroshima A-bomb was substantial, whereas that for Nagasaki was far less, consisting primarily of gamma radiation. On the basis of dose-response curves for acute radiation symptoms, in comparisons between Hiroshima and Nagasaki, the Relative Biological Effectiveness (RBE) of neutrons was estimated to be 4–5 [11]. The data for other mammals are not extensive, but Russell's appraisal [12] 'in general, for a given absorbed dose, neutrons prove to be far more mutagenic than X- and gamma rays, namely, of the order of 5 or 6 times both for oocytes and the rising part of the dose curve for spermatogonia' is consistent with this value. Accordingly, the exposure dose was calculated in rem on the assumption of an RBE of 5 for neutrons in relation to gamma radiation. The average parental dose for all parents of Group 1 children is estimated to be 117 rem; Group 2, 0 rem; and Group 3, 0 rem.

2.2. Results

There were 3510 deaths during the period 1946–76 among the total of 52 725 subjects. The exposure of each parent was subdivided into five classes of 100+ rem, 10–99 rem, 1–9 rem, <1 rem, and not exposed, and a χ^2 analysis was made of the 5 × 5 contingency table as shown in Table III. The expected numbers here were adjusted for differences in age, sex and city (Hiroshima, Nagasaki). As is evident from the χ^2 value of 19.61 on 24 degrees of freedom, variation in the contingency table was far from significant. The table also contains no suggestion that either the father's dose or the mother's dose, considered alone, influenced F_1 mortality. Analysis by cause of death for all natural causes, leukaemia, and all malignant tumours other than leukaemia produced similar results.

Among the 2028 children born after 1959 whose parents' exposure status is known, only 45 have died. As the number of deaths is so small, it is still too early to draw a conclusion, though it appears there is no difference in mortality by parental dose. Completion of enumeration of the sample born after 1959 is awaited.

As radiation dose estimates were available for individuals, a much more powerful statistical method, i.e. multiple regression analysis, was also employed. The method is particularly useful to control the effect of concomitant variables

TABLE IV. REGRESSION OF FACT OF DEATH ON YEAR OF BIRTH, SEX,
FATHER'S RADIATION DOSE, AND MOTHER'S RADIATION DOSE, AS
DETERMINED BY A STEPWISE REGRESSION PROCEDURE

Factor, in order of entry in the stepwise regression	Partial correlation coefficient	Percentage of variation explained[a] $100 \times R^2$*	Coefficient of regression
Year of birth	−0.08122	0.660	−0.00580 ± 0.000309**
Sex	0.02309	0.713	0.01147 ± 0.002164**
Father's dose	0.00729	0.718	0.000026 ± 0.000015
Mother's dose	−0.00184	0.718	−0.000006 ± 0.000013

 * R: multiple correlation coefficient.
** $P < 0.01$.

other than radiation dose. The results of stepwise regression analysis of the
relation between mortality in the children and the four variables of father's dose,
mother's dose, year of birth and sex of the children (Table IV), revealed that the
regression coefficient for mother's dose was far below the level of statistical
significance, but that the regression coefficient for father's dose was significant
at the 5% level. However, this regression coefficient became non-significant after
exclusion of the non-exposed groups. The non-exposed groups differ in many
respects, such as in parental age and birth order, from the exposed groups, and
these differences in general tend to make the mortality rates in the exposed groups
higher than in the control groups. Therefore, the regression coefficient for father's
dose derived from the analysis of the total sample must be regarded with considerable reserve. In any case, further follow-up studies and enlargement of the sample
seem called for.

The results are in agreement with most results from animal experiments
which have shown no clear evidence of dominant deleterious effects. These data
also agree with the results from other more limited studies of man, although the
numbers were so small and the dosage so low in these series that no real test of
hypothesis was involved.

These data were also used to calculate the gametic doubling dose for
mutations resulting in death during the first 24 years of life among liveborn
children conceived 0–13 years after parental exposure. The estimated doubling
dose does not differ significantly from the value previously reported [10].

REFERENCES

[1] BEEBE, G.W., KATO, H., LAND, C.E., Life Span Study Report 8, Mortality Experience of Atomic Bomb Survivors, Radiation Effects Research Foundation Technical Report 1−77 (1977).

[2] MILLER, R.W., BLOT, W.J., Small head size after in utero exposure to atomic radiation, Lancet i (1972) 785.

[3] WOOD, J.W., KEEHN, R.J., KAWAMOTO, S., JOHNSON, K.G., The growth and development of children exposed in utero to the atomic bombs in Hiroshima and Nagasaki, Atomic Bomb Casualty Commission Technical Report 11−66 (1966).

[4] KANAMITSU, M., MORITA, K., FINCH, S.C., KATO, H., ONISHI, S., Serologic response of atomic bomb survivors following Asian influenza vaccination, Jpn. J. Med. Sci. Biol. 19 (1966) 73.

[5] KATO, H., Mortality in children exposed to the A-bombs while in utero, 1945−1969, Am. J. Epidemiol. 93 (1971) 435.

[6] JONES, T.D., AUXIER, J.A., CHEKA, J.S., KERR, G.D., In vivo dose estimates for A-bomb survivors shielded by typical Japanese houses, Health Phys. 28 (1975) 367.

[7] HASHIZUME, T., MARUYAMA, T., NISHIZAWA, K., NISHIMURA, A., J. Radiat. Res. 14 (1973) 346.

[8] NEEL, J.V., SCHULL, W.J., The effect of exposure to the atomic bombs or pregnancy termination in Hiroshima and Nagasaki, Publication 461, National Academy of Sciences − National Research Council, Washington D.C. (1956).

[9] SCHULL, W.J., NEEL, J.V., HASHIZUME, A., Further observations on sex ratio among infants born to the survivors of the atomic bombs, Am. J. Hum. Genet. 18 (1966) 328.

[10] NEEL, J.V., KATO, H., SCHULL, W.J., Mortality in children of atomic bomb survivors and control, Genetics 76 (1974) 311.

[11] JABLON, S., FUJITA, S., FUKUSHIMA, K., ISHIMARU, T., AUXIER, J.A., RBE of neutrons in atomic bomb survivors: Hiroshima-Nagasaki, Atomic Bomb Casualty Commission Technical Report 12−70 (1970).

[12] RUSSELL, W.L., Factors that affect the radiation induction of mutations in the mouse, An. Acad. Bras. Cienc. 39 Suppl. (1967) 66.

DISCUSSION

K. NEUMEISTER: Do you have any new results from the Japanese study of biochemical-genetic effects in the F_1-generation after radiation exposure in utero?

H. KATO: A biochemical genetic study has been under way for the past two years at RERF on the F_1-generation of A-bomb survivors, but the results have not yet been analysed with respect to parents' exposure dose.

H.H. VOGEL: In rats, exposed whole-body to 50 rads of fission neutrons on the 18th day of gestation, there is a marked diminution in body weight at birth of young so irradiated in utero. After 150 rads to the mother, none of the young will live more than 48 hours.

Is there any comparable data in man for this decrease in body weight at birth?

H. KATO: Birth weight of in-utero exposed children decreases with dose in Hiroshima and Nagasaki.

A.M. STEWART: Mr. Mole has produced one explanation for the difference between the cancer experiences of A-bomb survivors exposed in utero and the Oxford survey findings for obstetric radiography. Our explanation is somewhat different and depends upon childhood cancers (especially leukaemia) lowering resistance to other causes of death (including trauma) before they are clinically recognizable. As a result of these early deaths a high risk of dying before or shortly after birth is necessarily associated with a low risk of dying from any cancers with in-utero origins. Hence we could fall into error by having expected numbers of leukaemia deaths of A-bomb survivors in national statistics — support for our theory is included in a paper on "Precancers and liability to other diseases" which is due to be published in the current number (March 1978) of the British Journal of Cancer.

H. KATO: It is conceivable that such a selection factor might affect the occurrence of cancer among A-bomb in-utero exposed groups. However, it is difficult to estimate the degree of influence of such a factor.

Y. NISHIWAKI: Mortality of in-utero children exposed to the A-bomb is an important subject of study. However, those who visited Hiroshima soon after A-bombing could have been subjected to a number of other possible noxious effects in addition to the radiation. Hospitals, laboratories, drug stores, chemists, pharmaceutical works, storehouses of chemicals, factories, etc., situated close to the hypocentre were all completely destroyed and various substances which could be mutagenic, carcinogenic or teratogenic must have been released. There was no medical care and no food in the region of high dose exposure and the drinking water was contaminated. There would have been various possibilities of infections. Mental stress would also have been much higher in the survivors closer to the hypocentre with higher estimated dose. All these effects would have been much smaller in the very low dose regions farther away from the hypocentre. In addition, there would be problems in accurately recording the position of the exposed persons at the time of atomic bombing. I think it is extremely important to keep all these factors in mind when analysing the atomic bomb effects in Hiroshima and Nagasaki.

H. KATO: We investigated whether concomitant variables such as birth order, birth weight, parents' age at birth and socio-economic status of the parents differ by dose comparison groups and found no variation except in birth weight, which decreases with radiation dose. I agree that the various possible effects you mentioned need to be allowed for when interpreting the results.

LATE RADIOBIOLOGICAL EFFECTS OF A-BOMBING IN JAPAN

A report on the international investigation carried out in July 1977

L.B. SZTANYIK
Frédéric Joliot-Curie National Research
  Institute for Radiology and Radiohygiene,
Budapest,
Hungary

Abstract

LATE RADIOBIOLOGICAL EFFECTS OF A-BOMBING IN JAPAN: A REPORT ON
THE INTERNATIONAL INVESTIGATION CARRIED OUT IN JULY 1977.
    On the occasion of the 32nd anniversary of the A-bombing in Japan, an international
investigation was held in Hiroshima and Nagasaki to review existing knowledge on the damage
and the after-effects of atomic bombing. The investigation was carried out by an international
team made up of Japanese and foreign scientists. A brief summary is given of the most
important statements and conclusions of the natural science group of the international team
with regard to the late biological effects of radiation on man. Particular attention is paid
to the effects of residual radiation which were somewhat disregarded in previous surveys.
The most carefully analysed late consequences are induction of leukaemia and other
malignancies, but cataract formation cannot be neglected either. Some of the possible
explanations why established long-term effects of radiation, such as increased mortality,
malignancies after exposure in utero, and genetic defects are absent among survivors, are
also mentioned.

1. INTRODUCTION

On the invitation of the International Peace Bureau, a team of about
40 scientists from 14 countries assembled in Japan in July 1977 to investigate
the damage and after-effects of atomic bombing. Participants in these investigations
were selected for their personal capacities and represented a broad spectrum of
specialities. The team visited research institutes and hospitals in Hiroshima and
Nagasaki, examined evidence, interviewed scientists, medical doctors, social
workers and survivors of the bombing. One of its major tasks was the revision in
joint discussions of documents on physical, biological, medical, genetic, social
and psychological effects of the A-bombs, which had been prepared by Japanese
experts and made available to the international team beforehand.

The investigations were carried out in two groups: a natural science group and a social science group. The documents produced as a result of these investigations give a fairly comprehensive description of knowledge on the short-term and long-term effects of the atomic bombs. They also call attention to facts overlooked or undervalued up to now, provide new information and reveal some serious gaps in our understanding of the long-term consequences, including the late somatic and genetic effects of ionizing radiation on man.

This report on the international investigation is restricted to a few important findings and conclusions with regard to late radiobiological effects, and is primarily based on two documents: the report of the natural science group entitled *The physical and medical effects of the Hiroshima and Nagasaki bombs,* and the summary report of the Commission I to the Symposium of NGOs on *Medical and genetic effects of atomic bombing in Hiroshima and Nagasaki,* and related publications [1, 2].

2.   THE EFFECTS OF RESIDUAL RADIATION

The importance of residual radiation in producing health impairment was regrettably overlooked during the early period following the A-bomb explosions. Only incomplete data can be found on the radioactivity induced by neutrons of the initial radiation in soil, building materials, iron and other metal constructions in the vicinity of the hypocentre. The same is also true for the radioactivity of areas where fission products and unfissioned bomb-explosives fell out.

Shortly after the detonation, thousands of people entered the affected areas in both cities for rescue work, in search of their relatives and to assist in removal of ruins. A paper by Hirose published in 1968 refers to about 37 000 people who entered Hiroshima City within the first week after the bombing [3]. Less reliable data are available concerning the number of entrants to the bombed area in Nagasaki City [4]. The total number of residents in the fall-out or 'black rain' areas in the two cities is assumed to be over 13 000 [5].

Only rough estimates have been made so far of the radiation doses that these people are likely to have received. The maximum possible cumulative doses of external irradiation in the bombed areas are thought to be about 100 rads in Hiroshima and 30 rads in Nagasaki [6]. People in the 'black rain' area could have been exposed to doses as high as 30 to 130 rads in Nagasaki and up to 50 rads in Hiroshima [7]. No attempt has been made to estimate radiation doses received by individuals from internally deposited radionuclides.

However, it was soon noted that some of the early entrants showed the acute radiation syndrome: bleeding, epilation, and even death occurred subsequently. In the Nishiyama District of Nagasaki, which had been protected by a hill from the instananeous effects of the explosion, but was heavily

TABLE I. INCIDENCE OF LEUKAEMIA AMONG ENTRANTS
TO HIROSHIMA (1950–67)

	Time of entry		
	6–9 August	10–13 August	14–20 August
Number of entrants[a]	25 798	11 001	7327
Leukaemia cases observed	45	8	1
Annual incidence of leukaemia ($\times 10^{-5}$)	9.7	4.0	0.8

[a] According to the 1960 National Census.

contaminated by fall-out afterwards, an abnormal increase in white blood cell
count of residents was reported. The WBC count of the 165 persons examined
reached a maximum average value of 18 500 250 days after exposure.

In addition to these acute effects, leukaemia cases began to appear after
1950 among the early entrants. Table I is taken from the paper of Hirose, which
refers to the incidence of leukaemia among the entrants to Hiroshima in the
18-year period 1950–67 [3]. Since the radioactivity was mostly short-lived,
those who entered the city after the third day received much smaller doses
than those who entered earlier. The annual leukaemia incidence among the
early entrants was indeed higher than the national average.

Two cases of chronic myelocytic leukaemia have also been detected among
the 200 inhabitants of the Nishiyama Valley. In such a small population, even
two cases suggest a high leukaemia incidence.

Increased incidence of malignant tumours of the salivary gland has also
been recorded between 1953–71 among the early entrants to Hiroshima
City [8].

If early entrants and residents of 'black rain' areas have been included in
the 0–9 rad and 10–49 rad groups of survivors, their additional exposure to
residual radiation may be an explanation why the excess incidence of certain
malignancies is higher in these groups than in the group of 50–99 rad.

3. LEUKAEMOGENESIS

Leukaemia is of special importance in the study of late radiobiological
effects, because it is the earliest of radiation-induced malignancies to manifest
itself. As can be seen in Fig.1, the incidence and mortality rate of leukaemia

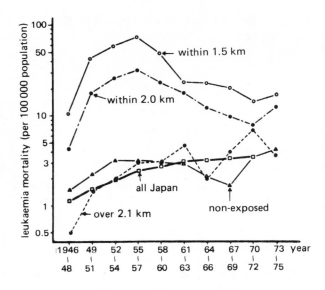

FIG.1.   Leukaemia mortality in Hiroshima by three-year intervals, 1946–75 [9].

increased fast among A-bomb survivors in the 1950s, reached a level of many times higher than that of non-exposed, then started to decrease slowly. But the level of the Japanese average has not yet been met.

Additional data were presented at the Symposium with regard to the leukaemogenic effect of radiation. According to these data, 298 cases of acute and chronic leukaemia were recorded up to 1975 among the inhabitants of Hiroshima who had been exposed to radiation with 5 km from the hypocentre. Of these, 221 had been irradiated within 2 km, confirming a dose-dependence [10].

It is known that the risk of leukaemia induction was higher in Hiroshima than in Nagasaki at every level of the T-65 dose. The dose-effect curve of Hiroshima cases seems linear and steeper than that of Nagasaki cases, which has a smaller initial slope, or suggests an apparent threshold of about 50 to 100 rads. This discrepancy is attributed to the high relative biological effectiveness of neutrons, significant constituents of the primary radiation in Hiroshima. Various RBE values have been suggested in the literature for the leukaemogenic effect of fast neutrons, but further analysis of data, and a comparison of tissue doses rather than air doses, are needed to achieve reasonable RBE values.

The suggestion that gamma rays have a threshold dose for leukaemogenic effect or are less efficient in small doses than higher ones, is open to doubt, especially in the light of what has been found about the incidence of leukaemia among early entrants.

Another intriguing question to be studied is why the generally more radiosensitive lymphoid cell system appears to be less susceptible to the leukaemogenic effect of radiation than the myeloid system.

4.   CARCINOGENESIS

Because of the long latent period of solid tumour induction, a definite conclusion cannot yet be drawn concerning the carcinogenic effect of A-bomb radiation. A significantly higher incidence of thyroid cancer in both sexes and a dose-dependent increase of breast cancer in females have been proved among those exposed to the initial radiation in both cities. The number of deaths from lung cancer has also been reported to be considerably higher among persons who were exposed to a dose of radiation in excess of 90 rads at an age of 35 years old or more, than the incidence of lung cancer in the general population (see Table II).

The occurrence of malignant tumours in salivary and prostate glands, bone tissue, digestive and other organs of survivors was reported to be higher than in the unexposed population, but no definite dose-relation could be established [11].

Since the average latency of these types of tumour seems to extend beyond 20 years, studies on tumour induction in A-bomb survivors should be continued. It has been suggested that a search should be made for thyroid tumours, both benign and malignant, among the people who lived in the fall-out areas or entered contaminated territory within the first few days after the bombing, and thus likely to have incorporated radioactive fission products.

5.   CATARACT

A typical late effect caused by the atomic bomb radiation is the development of cataract. A definite correlation between exposure distance (i.e. dose) and incidence of cataracts has been noted among the A-bomb survivors. The data confirm that cataract incidence was marked among those exposed within approximately 1.6 km of the hypocentre in Hiroshima and 1.8 km in Nagasaki.

According to the results of a survey made on atomic bomb survivors who visited the Hiroshima Red Cross Hospital in a period of almost 5 years between 1953 and 1958, cataracts were found in 68 of the 600 persons (11.3%) who had a history of acute radiation syndrome, and in 28 of the 501 persons (5.6%) who had not. In the same survey, cataracts were found in 55 of the 280 persons (19.6%) with a history of epilation, indicating that these two symptoms have a very strong correlation [12].

TABLE II. EXCESS MORTALITY FROM MALIGNANCIES IN HIROSHIMA AND NAGASAKI (1950–72)

Causes of death	Observed	Expected	Excess
Leukaemia	84	13.7	70.3
Other malignant neoplasms	1075	918.8	156.2
Breast	37	19.0	18.0
Respiratory organs	129	73.7	55.3
Digestive organs	678	652.4	25.6
Other organs	231	173.7	57.3
Benign and unspecified neoplasms	53	42.9	10.1
All neoplasms	1212	975.4	236.6

TABLE III. CATARACT INCIDENCE IN PERSONS EXPOSED IN HIROSHIMA DURING CHILDHOOD
12 years after the bombing

Exposure distance (m)	T-65D air-dose (rad)	Number of eyes examined	Number of cataracts found	Cataract incidence (%)
< 1000	> 450	18	10	55.6
1000–2000	2.5–450	156	21	13.5
> 2000	< 2.5	56	0	0
Total		230	31	13.5

TABLE IV. OVERALL MORTALITY IN HIROSHIMA AND NAGASAKI
of those exposed at > 10 rad

Causes of death	Observed	Expected	Excess
Leukaemia	84	14	70
Other malignancies	1075	919	156
Benign and unspecified neoplasms	53	43	10
All neoplasms	1212	976	236
Diseases except neoplasms	3970	4592	− 622
Total	5182	5568	− 386

To exclude cataracts due to age, a survey was made later in Hiroshima of 115 persons exposed to the bomb within 3 km of the hypocentre under the age of 5 years, i.e. junior and senior high school students of ages 12 to 18 at the time of examination [13]. The results are shown in Table III.

These data indicate that an exposure of eyes to high dose-rate radiation at a dose level of less than 100 rad can lead to the development of cataract. It is worth mentioning here that the ICRP believes that a total dose equivalent of 1500 rad would be below the threshold for the production of any lens opacification that would interfere with vision, when the lens is subjected to protracted irradiation with high or low LET radiation [14].

6.   SOME CURIOUS ANOMALIES

Whereas there are definite dose-related increases in the incidence of leukaemia, thyroid cancer, breast cancer, lung cancer and perhaps a number of additional malignancies, other well-known radiation effects are surprisingly absent among the A-bomb victims.

No significant genetic effects in children conceived by survivors after the explosion have been found so far, although the statistical material is sufficiently large for some end-points to be observed.

Another absent effect is any increase in the frequency of malignancies among children whose mothers were pregnant at the time of the A-bomb explosions. It has long been known that children exposed to diagnostic X-ray doses in utero are more prone to leukaemia and other malignancies [15].

Equally puzzling is the absence of an increase in overall mortality. Animal experiments show that whole-body exposure to a single dose of radiation results in a life-shortening proportional to dose. Studies on A-bomb survivors failed to prove any evidence of an increased mortality rate. In fact, there is a reduced mortality from causes other than neoplasms (see Table IV). This may be attributed to the circumstance that the survivors receive a better medical care than the rest of the population. Another possibility is that survivors constitute a selected population. They received injuries from blast and heat and radiation. The least resistant members of the population did not recover from these injuries and died in the early period. Rotblat even suggests that, if ability to survive is due to one's genetic make-up, then the survivors may also be a selected population from the genetical point of view [2].

REFERENCES

[1] BARNABY, F., New Sci. (London) 76 (1977) 472.
[2] ROTBLAT, J., New Sci. (London) 76 (1977) 475.

[3]   HIROSE, F., Acta Haematol. Jap. **31** (1968) 765.
[4]   ICHIMARU, M., Acta Haematol. Jap. **31** (1968) 772.
[5]   J. Radiat. Res. **16** Suppl. (1975) ii.
[6]   TAKESHITA, K., J. Radiat. Res. **16** Suppl. (1975) 24.
[7]   OKAJIMA, S., J. Radiat. Res. **16** Suppl. (1975) 35.
[8]   TAKEICHI, N., HIROSE, F., YAMAMOTO, H., Cancer **38** (1976) 2462.
[9]   OHKITA, T., Proc. Hiroshima Univ. RINMB. **16** (1976) 77.
[10] OHKITA, T., Personal communication.
[11] UNITED NATIONS, Sources and Effects of Ionizing Radiation, United Nations Scientific
      Committee on Effects of Atomic Radiation, Report to the General Assembly, UN,
      New York (1977) 361.
[12] MASUDA, Y., Acta Soc. Ophthal. Jap. **70** (1966) 1109.
[13] TODA, S., Folia Ophthal. Jap. **15** (1964) 96.
[14] INTERNATIONAL COMMISSION ON RADIOLOGICAL PROTECTION, Publication
      No. 26, Annals of the ICRP, **1** 3 (1977) 12.
[15] STEWART, A.M., KNEALE, G.W., Lancet ii (1970) 1185.

DISCUSSION

T. OHKITA: I should like to comment on the problem of early entrants. There have been cases where the biological damage from secondary radiation was reported to be very severe, but unfortunately there is not enough convincing and objective evidence available to resolve this question. In view of the circumstances prevailing soon after the Hiroshima atomic bomb and the end of World War II, it is not surprising that the biological importance of early entrants was not recognized. It is true that there are cases of leukaemia in persons who have a personal history of entering the hypocentre area soon after the explosion, but their detailed activity at that time is not necessarily defined on an individual basis. Identification of early entrants is based on the individual's reporting which must be supported by two or more witnesses. The precise number of early entrants is difficult to ascertain. According to surveys conducted in 1965 and 1975 it would seem that the figures from the 1960 census you referred to are under-estimates. The epidemiological findings of the early entrant population constitute valuable data in studying the effects of exposure to low doses of ionizing radiation. However, the exposure dose estimates have many factors and the individual differences in exposure dose are considered to be large. Therefore I do not think it would necessarily be appropriate to use this population for making a risk estimate of low dose irradiation.

L.B. SZTANYIK: I fully agree with you in that the lack of accurate data on the number of early entrants and their individual doses is understandable because of the circumstances that prevailed in both cities after the bombing. From the point of view of their scientific value, however, I consider it regrettable that these important data are missing, and that is what I have said in my presentation. It is also true that no attempt can be made to estimate the absolute risk of leukaemia induction among early entrants without knowing the individual dose values. That is the reason why only the relative risk has been determined by Hirose and quoted in my paper.

G.W. BEEBE: I find myself in complete agreement with Mr. Ohkita. The 'early entrants' are a most interesting group but (a) their dosimetry has always seemed elusive, and (b) they present both 'numerator' and 'denominator' uncertainties so that, overall, data on early entrants are not of the same quality as those on A-bomb survivors and should not be used to challenge the latter. In my report I did not say, nor do I believe, that non-neoplastic mortality has been more favourable than expectation among A-bomb survivors. I have shown that non-neoplastic mortality for 1950—74 does not increase significantly with dose in either city. I don't think there is any mystery here and I don't believe there is any mystery either in the failure of the first genetic study to show a genetic effect. That study of 70-odd thousand conceptions was quite powerful against a doubling of genetic defects, but much less powerful against smaller effects. The result does not mean and has not been taken to mean that there was no genetic effect, only that it was not so large as to be detectable in a sample of this size. All animal work suggests that radiation should cause genetic effects in man. Far from accepting the early genetic study of what now seem crude indicators of genetic damage as definitive, RERF investigators are proceeding with the new biochemical genetic study that Mr. Kato mentioned. It is to be hoped that the new study will at least help to put a narrower confidence band on estimates of the doubling dose for man.

L.B. SZTANYIK: With regard to the early entrants, my answer is the same as I have just given to Mr. Ohkita. Concerning mortality of A-bomb survivors, I have at hand the relevant data published by UNSCEAR in its 1977 Report. According to these, mortality in Hiroshima and Nagasaki from causes other than neoplasms has been about 600 less than expected on the basis of the Japanese average. Comparison of the mortality of those who were exposed to doses above 10 rads with the mortality of survivors exposed to doses less than 10 rads may be misleading if, for instance, early entrants and residents of fall-out areas are included in the 0—9 rads group. On the other hand, there is no disagreement between us in that the failure of the first genetic studies does not mean at all that radiation has no genetic effects in humans. This failure may be attributed to many factors, including the inadequate sensitivity of the methods used in these studies. Therefore, the natural science group is looking forward to seeing the results of the biochemical studies of genetic effects which were initiated by RERF not long before the international investigation.

G.W. DOLPHIN: I wish to support the comments made by the previous two speakers about the difficulty of interpreting the data on early entrants. The number of early entrants mentioned by the present author (25 798) comes from a paper by Hirose. The number was established in a census made by officials of Hiroshima City in 1960. The census was confined to this city district, so that an early entrant living in Tokyo, say, would not be included. Hence this number is an underestimate. Further, a bias was introduced when free medical treatment was extended to early entrants in 1958. This could have encouraged excess registration of leukaemias.

L.B. SZTANYIK: You are right that the number of early entrants given in Hirose's paper and referred to in my presentation can be an underestimate. However, the leukaemia cases reported as late consequences of residual radiation have been observed among this limited number of people. One may assume that in a larger exposed population group the number of leukaemia cases would also be higher. Provision of free medical care may well have led to an excess registration and introduced a bias in these studies. However, it should be taken into consideration that the fact of being registered as 'hibakusha', i.e. A-bomb victim, works in the opposite direction because of the social stigma.

R.A. CONARD: In view of the high incidence of thyroid tumours and hypothyroidism in the Marshallese exposed to fall-out it would seem likely that the Japanese exposed to the 'black rains' at Nishiyama valley would have been exposed to radio-iodines in the fall-out there. Have any studies of thyroid nodularity or hypofunction been undertaken or planned for these people?

L.B. SZTANYIK: As far as I know, no such studies have been performed. That is the reason why the international team has suggested studying the occurrence of benign and malignant tumours in the thyroids of people living in fall-out areas.

Y. NISHIWAKI: When the neutron-induced activity in sulphur used for insulation on electricity transmission lines was measured soon after A-bombing in Hiroshima, it was found to have a correlation with the distance. However, some of my colleagues noticed that the neutron flux or fluence did not seem to be uniform in all directions. Were directional differences in the effects of neutrons discussed at the international scientific meeting in Hiroshima, in which you participated?

L.B. SZTANYIK: No.

PREVALENCE OF LEUKAEMIA AND SALIVARY GLAND TUMOURS AMONG HIROSHIMA ATOMIC BOMB SURVIVORS

T. OHKITA, H. TAKAHASHI, N. TAKEICHI,
F. HIROSE
Research Institute for Nuclear
    Medicine and Biology,
Hiroshima University,
Hiroshima,
Japan

Abstract

PREVALENCE OF LEUKAEMIA AND SALIVARY GLAND TUMOURS AMONG
HIROSHIMA ATOMIC BOMB SURVIVORS.

As of 1975, 298 cases of leukaemia were recorded among members of the Hiroshima
population who were exposed within 5 km from the hypocentre. Of these, 221 were exposed
within 2 km of the hypocentre, corroborating a radiation dose-incidence relationship. Although
by 1961, the peak leukaemia prevalence among Hiroshima survivors appeared to have passed,
data in the five years from 1971 have shown that the leukaemia death rate of the survivors
exposed within 1.5 and/or 2 km from the hypocentre remains about 2 to 4 times higher than
for the non-exposed. A marked increase in chronic granulocytic leukaemia was observed among
proximally exposed survivors, especially in Hiroshima. This may have resulted from the relatively greater neutron component of the Hiroshima atomic bomb compared with that of
Nagasaki. Initially, chronic granulocytic leukaemia contributed substantially to the total
frequency of the disease, but after 1963 it made little contribution. The frequency of chronic
lymphocytic leukaemia was low through the term of observation. There were 73 cases of
salivary gland tumours histologically confirmed in Hiroshima between 1953 and 1971. Thirty-
one cases were atomic bomb survivors exposed within 5 km of the hypocentre. The incidence
of salivary gland tumours among the exposed individuals was significantly higher, 2.7 times
greater than that among non-exposed individuals for all tumours, and 10 times greater for
malignant tumours. The incidence increases with proximity to the hypocentre.

1. INTRODUCTION

The major potential hazard of ionizing radiation in humans is the induction
of cancer. Studies of every type of cancer in the population of atomic bomb
survivors are important not only for the survivors themselves but also for understanding the carcinogenic effects of ionizing radiation on man. In this report
the results are summarized of a survey on the prevalence of leukaemia and
salivary gland tumours among Hiroshima atomic bomb survivors.

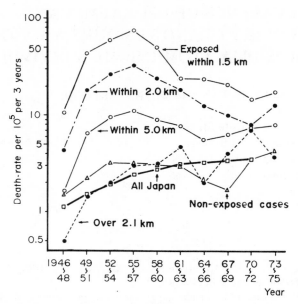

FIG.1. Death rate from leukaemia in Hiroshima City during the period 1946–75.

2.   LEUKAEMIA

Leukaemia was the first accepted neoplasm of the late atomic bomb disturbances, and during the past three decades numerous studies on this subject have
been reported [1–4]. In Hiroshima, epidemiological studies on leukaemia have
been continued by two groups. Studies at the Radiation Effects Research
Foundation (RERF) have focused almost entirely on a fixed cohort of about
109 000 survivors and their controls who were selected in 1950 for a mortality
study. Another study has been continued on the open city, unfixed population
by Japanese researchers, especially by workers at the Research Institute for
Nuclear Medicine and Biology of Hiroshima University. Both research groups
are co-operating closely with each other.

Figure 1 shows the crude leukaemia death rates for Hiroshima citizens from
1946 through 1975 by exposure distances from the hypocentre. Atomic bomb
survivors were defined as those directly exposed in the city at the time of the
bomb (within 5000 m from the hypocentre). The population of atomic bomb
survivors and that of non-exposed were based on census data obtained from the
National Census and the Atomic Bomb Survivors Actual State Surveys conducted
in 1950, 1960 and 1965. From 1971, the annual reports on atomic bomb survivors compiled by the Hiroshima City Office were also used. In 1975, those

TABLE I. LEUKAEMIA AMONG HIROSHIMA ATOMIC BOMB SURVIVORS,
BY TYPE AND DISTANCE FROM HYPOCENTRE, 1946–75
Cases observed inside and outside Hiroshima City are combined

Distance from hypocentre (m)	Total leukaemia	Acute form	Chronic form	Acute/Chronic
Within 2000	221	131	90	1.5
2000–5000	77	60	17	3.5
Total	298	191	107[a]	

[a] Only three cases with CLL have been detected.

exposed within 2000 m numbered about 39 000; those within 1500 m were
approximately 19 000. It is obvious from Fig. 1 that the high mortality among
the exposed was mainly due to the death rate of the proximally exposed survivors. According to the T-65D air dose values in Hiroshima, the radiation dose
at 1500 m was about 31.6 rad, consisting of 21.6 rad gamma and 10.1 rad
neutrons. At 2000 m, the dose was about 2.5 rad (1.9 rad gamma and 0.5 rad
neutrons). As Fig. 1 shows, the peak leukaemia prevalence among Hiroshima
survivors has passed, but even in recent years the death rate from leukaemia
among proximally exposed survivors remains higher than the mean death rate
of the non-exposed and for all Japan, as will be mentioned below.

As of 1975, there were 298 leukaemia cases among the Hiroshima population who were in the city at the time of the bomb, as shown in Table I. Two
hundred and twenty-one of these were survivors exposed within 2000 m of the
hypocentre. This is a clear manifestation of the strong correlation between
increasing leukaemia risk and decreasing distance from the hypocentre. Among
107 chronic cases, only three of chronic lymphocytic leukaemia have been
detected. Correlation of the ratio of acute and chronic leukaemia with exposure
distances is also shown in this table. Among those exposed within 2000 m of
the hypocentre there was a marked increase in chronic granulocytic leukaemia,
and the ratio of acute and chronic forms was 1 : 5, whereas almost the same ratio
as the average of all Japan, 3 : 5, was obtained among those exposed beyond
2000 m. Thus, chronic granulocytic leukaemia was the most prevalent leukaemia
among Hiroshima survivors. Figure 2 shows the number of leukaemia cases
observed annually among Hiroshima atomic bomb survivors exposed within
2000 m of the hypocentre. The largest number was observed between
1950 and 1953 with the peak in 1951. Since then, the number of cases
has generally declined with a wide fluctuation. It is also clear that the

OHKITA et al.

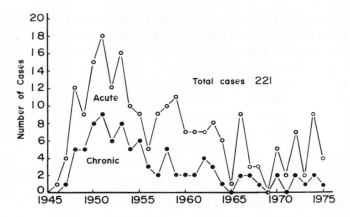

FIG.2. Number of leukaemia cases among Hiroshima survivors exposed within 2000 m of the hypocentre. Patients observed inside and outside Hiroshima City at the time of onset are combined.

TABLE II. LEUKAEMIA DEATHS BY SEX AMONG HIROSHIMA ATOMIC BOMB SURVIVORS EXPOSED WITHIN 2000 m OF THE HYPOCENTRE, 1971–75

Distance from hypocentre (m)	Sex	Number of deaths from leukaemia		O/E ratio
		Observed	Expected	
Within 1500	Male	8	2.3	3.5**
	Female	10	2.3	4.3**
Within 2000	Male	10	4.7	2.1*
	Female	13	4.7	2.8**

Significance: * $p < 0.1$
            ** $p < 0.05$

decline is more evident in the chronic forms. Nevertheless, we believe that the risk of developing leukaemia has not disappeared entirely. In the five years from 1971 to 1975, a total of 134 deaths from definite and probable leukaemia in Hiroshima was registered by our Institute, of whom 34 cases were in the city at the time of the bomb. Of these, 23 cases, consisting of 17 acute and six chronic forms, were exposed within 2000 m of the hypocentre. One of the six chronic cases was of the lymphocytic type, and this type of leukaemia is still rare. Eighteen of these 23 cases (78%) were older than 30 years at the time of the bomb (ATB).

With respect to the relation between the age ATB and latent period, it can be said for acute leukaemia that the latent period was shorter in those who were younger ATB and longer in those who were older ATB. For chronic leukaemia, the difference in latency by age was not clear and the risk of the disease persisted for about 15 years after exposure, then decreased subsequently regardless of the age ATB.

Table II shows a comparison of the observed and expected number of leukaemia cases during the period 1971 to 1975. The expected numbers were estimated by the death rate for leukaemia throughout Japan. It appears that even 25–30 years after the bomb, the risk of leukaemia among proximally exposed survivors is still significantly high, and has not returned to the mean of all Japan. As atomic bomb survivors have had regular blood examinations, it is possible that this population might yield a disproportionately larger number of leukaemia cases than the non-exposed population. The comparison of the death rate from leukaemia from 1971 to 1975 was also made between survivors exposed within and beyond 2000 m of the hypocentre. A significantly higher death rate was observed only for survivors exposed within 1500 m from the hypocentre (p < 0.01).

Using the confirmed cases of leukaemia occurring from 1950 to 1966 in the fixed cohort of atomic bomb survivors and controls, Ishimaru and co-workers found that the risk of leukaemia in Hiroshima was significantly elevated even in those exposed to less than 50 rads [3]. In the smaller Nagasaki series, however, a significant increase in risk could not be demonstrated among those exposed to low doses. According to Ichimaru and co-workers, the risk was greater in Hiroshima than in Nagasaki in every dose category, and there was no case of leukaemia in Nagasaki among high-dose subjects who received 100 or more rads, in a fixed cohort from July 1966 to the end of 1971, whereas the incidence was still above the normal expectation in Hiroshima [5]. On the basis of their data, the total number of leukaemia cases observed among persons born before the atomic bomb in both cities are essentially the same, if the atomic bomb survivors are ignored. For atomic bomb survivors, however, the two cities differ quite significantly regarding the number of leukaemia cases who received 1 or more rads. It is considered that the leukaemogenic effect may not be the same for gamma rays and for neutrons [1–3]. Therefore, it is important to analyse the data for the two cities separately, and careful surveillance of leukaemia should be continued for Hiroshima survivors.

3.   SALIVARY GLAND TUMOURS

Both benign and malignant salivary gland tumours have been considered rare. In 1970, during an investigation of head and neck disease among inpatients

TABLE III. HISTOLOGIC CLASSIFICATION OF SALIVARY GLAND
TUMOURS, HIROSHIMA, 1953–71

Tumour	Exposed[a] cases	Non-exposed cases
Malignant tumours	17	5
Benign tumours	14	25
Total	31	30
Malignant tumours (%)	54.8	16.7

[a] Survivors exposed to A-bomb within 5000 m of the hypocentre.

TABLE IV. INCIDENCE OF SALIVARY GLAND TUMOURS BY EXPOSURE
STATUS IN HIROSHIMA, 1953–71

	Exposed within 5000 m	Exposed within 2000 m	Non-exposed
All tumours			
Observed cases	31*	20*	30
Expected cases	15.6	4.8	30
Crude incidence[a]	2.1	2.9	0.7
Standardized incidence[b]	1.9	2.8	0.7
Malignant tumours			
Observed cases	17*	11*	5
Expected cases	5.1	0.8	5
Crude incidence[a]	1.1	1.6	0.1
Standardized incidence[b]	1.0	1.6	0.1
Benign tumours			
Observed cases	14**	9**	25
Expected cases	10	4	25
Crude incidence[a]	0.9	1.3	0.6
Standardized incidence[b]	0.9	0.8	0.5

[a] Crude incidence per 100 000 annually.
[b] Rates are standardized to the age distribution of the 1960 National Census in five-year
age groups.

Significant in exposed versus non-exposed   * $p < 0.001$
                                           ** $p < 0.05$

at our Institute, an increased prevalence of parotid gland tumours was noted
among atomic bomb survivors. Our preliminary survey in Hiroshima and Kure
City showed that there were 287 cases of salivary gland tumours from 1945 when
the atomic bomb was detonated to 1971 [6]. All available clinical records and
histologic specimens were reviewed to confirm the diagnosis. The salivary gland
tumours were classified according to the classification of Foote and Frazell.
Two hundred and eleven cases could be confirmed. For Hiroshima City alone,
there were 73 confirmed cases, of whom 31 cases were atomic bomb survivors
exposed within 5000 m of the hypocentre. Thirty-seven were non-exposed, of
whom 30 cases were born before and 7 after the bomb. Five additional cases
were not directly exposed to the bomb, but entered the hypocentre area within
2 weeks after the detonation, these people being termed early entrants. In this
report, cases seen among the early entrants and also those born after the atomic
bomb were excluded from analyses. Sixty-one cases observed in Hiroshima
during the 19 years from 1953 to 1971 have been tabulated in Table III by
exposure status and historical classification. Among the exposed cases, malignant
tumours comprised 54.8% of all identified tumours, in contrast with 16.7%
among the non-exposed. There were no distinguishing histologic aspects among
tumours in irradiated subjects that differed from those in non-exposed persons.

The mean annual crude incidence for the 61 cases in Hiroshima is shown
in Table IV. Standardized incidence, which was standardized to the age distribution of the 1960 National Census in 5-year age groups, is also shown. Among
the exposed cases within 5000 m of the hypocentre 31 cases were identified and
the average annual standardized incidence rate was 1.9 cases per 100 000, which
was 2.7 times greater than the rate of 0.7 for the 30 cases among the non-exposed.
This difference was highly significant ($p < 0.001$). When malignant tumours
alone were considered, the increased incidence among the exposed individuals
was even more apparent. The average annual incidence for the 17 cases among
the exposed was 1.0 per 100 000, which was 10 times greater than the incidence
of 0.1 per 100 000 for the five cases among the non-exposed ($p < 0.001$). No
significant difference was observed for benign tumours. When the cases exposed
within 2000 m of the hypocentre were separated, the average annual standardized
incidence was 2.8 per 100 000 for the 20 cases of this group, which was four
times greater than that among the non-exposed. For malignant tumours alone,
it was 16 times greater than that of the non-exposed.

To examine the effects of exposure distance, the incidence was tabulated
in Table V for three groups at increasing distance from the hypocentre: the proximally exposed (within 1500 m); the distally exposed (1501–5000 m); and the
non-exposed (5000 m). The average annual standardized incidence in the proximally exposed for all salivary gland tumours was 3.8 per 100 000. The standardized
incidence in the non-exposed was 0.7 per 100 000, and the incidence among the
distally exposed was 1.3 per 100 000, which was intermediate. Thus the incidence

TABLE V. INCIDENCE OF SALIVARY GLAND TUMOURS BY EXPOSURE
DISTANCE IN HIROSHIMA, 1953–71

| Group | Distance from hypocentre (m) | | | |
	0–1500	1501–5000	> 5000 (Non-exposed)	χ^2-test
All tumours				
Observed cases	14	17	30	
Expected cases	3.38	12.23	45.39	p < 0.001
Crude incidence[a]	4.3	1.5	0.7	
Standardized incidence[b]	3.8	1.3	0.7	
Malignant tumours				
Observed cases	7	10	5	
Expected cases	1.22	4.41	16.37	p < 0.001
Crude incidence[a]	2.2	0.9	0.1	
Standardized incidence[b]	2.2	0.7	0.1	
Benign tumours				
Observed cases	7	7	25	
Expected cases	2.16	7.82	29.02	p < 0.01
Crude incidence[a]	2.2	0.6	0.6	
Standardized incidence[b]	1.6	0.6	0.5	

[a] Crude incidence per 100 000 annually.
[b] Rates are standardized to the age distribution of the 1960 National Census in five-year
age groups.

TABLE VI. INCIDENCE[a] OF SALIVARY GLAND TUMOURS BY AGE ATB
AND EXPOSURE DISTANCE IN HIROSHIMA, 1953–71

| Exposure distance (m) | Age[a] | | | | | |
| | 0–19 | | 20–49 | | > 50 | |
	Cases	Incidence	Cases	Incidence	Cases	Incidence
0–1500	5	4.9	8	4.2	1	2.2
1501–5000	4	1.0	8	1.4	5	3.4
> 5000 (Non-exposed)	19	0.6	10	0.7	1	1.3

[a] Crude incidence per 100 000 annually.

among the proximally exposed was 5.4 times greater, and in the distally exposed it was 1.9 times greater, than that among the non-exposed. The increased incidence with proximity to the hypocentre was statistically significant ($p < 0.001$). For malignant tumours the incidence among the proximally exposed was 2.2 per 100 000 compared with 0.1 per 100 000 among the non-exposed. The incidence among the distally exposed was 0.7 per 100 000. Thus the incidence among the proximally exposed was 22 times greater, and in the distally exposed it was seven times greater, than that among the non-exposed. The increased incidence of malignant tumours with proximity of exposure was highly significant ($p < 0.001$). For benign tumours, the incidence was higher in the proximal and distal survivors than in the non-exposed. In this analysis the increased incidence of benign tumours was also statistically significant ($p < 0.01$).

Tumour incidence by age at the time of bomb (ATB) and exposure distance is shown in Table VI. Among those 0–19 years ATB and 20–49 years ATB, the incidence increased with proximity of exposure. In those older than 50 years ATB no trend was apparent, but the number of observed cases were small. Among those proximally exposed, incidence was highest in those 0–19 years ATB. In the distally exposed and in the non-exposed, an opposite trend was seen in those older than 50 years ATB.

The incidence of salivary gland tumours was examined by sex. In the non-exposed the incidence of all salivary gland tumours and malignant salivary gland tumours was higher in the female, but in the exposed the incidence tended to be higher in the male.

The foregoing has shown that in the atomic bomb survivors the incidence of salivary gland tumours was higher the closer the exposure distance from the hypocentre. This suggests that there is a positive correlation between exposure dose and the incidence of salivary gland tumours. In 1972 Belsky and co-workers presented a report on 22 cases of salivary gland tumours among about 109 000 members of the extended JNIH-ABCC Life Span Study sample of Hiroshima and Nagasaki [7]. They observed a significant relation between exposure dose and the incidence of salivary gland tumours, especially malignant salivary gland tumours. According to their report the relative risk of salivary gland tumours in those exposed to 90 rads or more was 5. Subsequently we made a re-analysis by adding eight cases that we collected to the cases reported by Belsky and co-workers, and presented a joint report stating that in those exposed to 300 rads or more the number of cases of all salivary gland tumours and malignant salivary gland tumours is significantly greater than the expected number ($p < 0.01$) [8].

Recently, it was evident from our experiments in rats that salivary gland tumours could develop by local X-irradiation of the salivary gland [9]. In these experiments, histological changes of the salivary gland were observed by lapse of time after X-irradiation. During the regenerating process in the salivary gland, varying degrees of atypism could be observed in the proliferating intercalated-like

TABLE VII. HISTOLOGICAL DIAGNOSIS OF SALIVARY GLANDS IN
AUTOPSY CASES

| | Exposed cases | | | | Non-exposed cases | | | |
	Male	Female			Male	Female		
No. of cases	12	9			13	15		
(Histological changes)	(6)	(2)			(3)	(1)		
	Sm[a] Sl[b]	Sm Sl			Sm Sl	Sm Sl		
Adenoma	3 1	0 0			0 1	1 0		
Ductal hyperplasia	2 2	1 1			1 1	0 0		
Total	5 3	1 1			1 2	1 0		

[a] Submaxillary gland
[b] Sublingual gland

ducts, and many kinds of tumours were induced. These findings suggest that
those with weak atypism will develop into adenoma, whereas those with strong
atypism will develop into atypical ductal hyperplasia and eventually transform
into malignant tumours. In order to know whether the histological changes
observed in the salivary gland of rats following X-ray irradiation can also be
observed in survivors, the salivary glands of autopsy cases of atomic bomb survivors
preserved in the Medical Records and Specimens Center of our Institute were subjected to scrutiny of the histological changes. Twenty-one cases comprising 12
males and nine females were selected. These cases were survivors who were
exposed to the atomic bomb in Hiroshima within 1500 m of the hypocentre at
the age of 19 or less, and who died within the 10-year period from 1958 to 1967
of causes of death excluding salivary gland diseases and who had no past history
of salivary gland diseases. As control we selected 28 autopsy cases preserved in
the same Center as non-exposed cases and composed of 13 males and 15 females
of the same age who also satisfied other conditions. When both sexes were combined, four tumorous changes (adenoma and ductal hyperplasia) were observed
in four cases out of 28 non-exposed, whereas among the 21 atomic bomb survivors eight cases were found to have 10 tumorous changes, as shown in Table VII.
Further studies are needed to confirm these results and to clarify whether the
histological changes such as ductal hyperplasia seen in the salivary glands of
survivors are prodromal histopathological changes relating to the transformation
into neoplasms. We are aware of the need for caution in drawing any conclusion

from such a small number of cases, but the frequency of tumorous changes of the salivary gland in heavily exposed Hiroshima survivors seems to be greater than that among non-exposed.

REFERENCES

[1]   WATANABE, S., "Cancer and leukaemia developing among atom-bomb survivors", Handbuch der allgemeinen Pathologie 6, Geschwülste I (ALTMANN, H.W., BÜCHNER, F., Eds.), Springer-Verlag, Berlin (1974) 461.

[2]   TOMONAGA, M., et al., Leukemia in atomic bomb survivors from 1946 to 1965 and some aspects of epidemiology of leukemia in Japan (in Japanese with English abstract), J. Kyushu Haemat. Soc. 17 (1967) 375.

[3]   ISHIMARU, T., et al., Leukemia in atomic bomb survivors, Hiroshima-Nagasaki, 1 October 1950 − 30 September 1966, Radiat. Res. 45 (1971) 216.

[4]   OHKITA, T., Leukemia in Hiroshima atomic bomb survivors from 1946 to 1975; A summary of the findings and recent trends (in Japanese with English abstract), Proc. Res. Inst. Nucl. Med. Biol., Hiroshima Univ. 16 (1976) 77.

[5]   ICHIMARU, M., et al., Incidence of Leukemia in Atomic Bomb Survivors, Hiroshima & Nagasaki 1950-71, by Radiation Dose, Years after Exposure, Age, and Type of Leukemia, Radiation Effects Research Foundation Technical Report 10-76 (1977).

[6]   TAKEICHI, N., et al., Parotid gland tumours observed in the Research Institute for Nuclear Medicine and Biology, Hiroshima University, Jpn. J. Cancer Clin. 22 (1976) 307 (in Japanese).

[7]   BELSKY, J.L., et al., Salivary Gland Tumors in Atomic Bomb Survivors, Hiroshima and Nagasaki, 1957-70, Atomic Bomb Casualty Commission Technical Report 15-71 (1971).

[8]   BELSKY, J.L., et al., Salivary Gland Neoplasms following Atomic Radiation, Additional Cases and Reanalysis of Combined Data in a Fixed Population, 1957-70, Atomic Bomb Casualty Commission Technical Report 23-72 (1972).

[9]   TAKEICHI, N., HIROSE, F., Salivary gland tumors with special reference to radiation exposure, Acta Pathol. Jpn. (in press).

DISCUSSION

D.J. MEWISSEN: Among atomic bomb survivors, the leukaemia incidence, expressed as a percentage of the original population at risk, exhibited a peak incidence followed by a decrease over an extended period of time. If leukaemia incidence were expressed in terms of the actual population at risk during successive one-year intervals, would the time-incidence curve still exhibit a peak or would it rather have an increasing or decreasing trend?

T. OHKITA: To establish the general trend, the leukaemia death-rate was plotted for successive three-year intervals. Clearly, it has a decreasing trend but is still above the normal expectation in Hiroshima.

LE SECRET D'HIROSHIMA

M. DELPLA
Electricité de France,
Paris,
France

Abstract—Résumé

THE SECRET OF HIROSHIMA.
Thanks to their organizational ability, United States and Japanese scientific investigators have assembled an unequalled collection of data. For maximum benefit to be derived from such a collection, it would also be necessary to reveal 'the secret of Hiroshima' since in this city where the radiation included a relatively high proportion of neutrons, much of the information of interest is in the low-dose range. An attempt is made to examine this range but with data which in part are highly uncertain. It was found that, as at Nagasaki and after radiotherapy of the vertebral column (although for much lower doses), irradiation could reduce the frequency of leukaemia. It was also found that the relative biological effectiveness (RBE) of the neutrons increases when the dose decreases: apparently it reaches 100 and perhaps even more in the range of doses exerting a predominantly protective effect. The latent period of leukaemia is extremely short but there should now be sufficient perspective to be able to examine with profit the findings relating to other types of tumours.

LE SECRET D'HIROSHIMA.
Parce qu'ils ont su s'organiser, des chercheurs américains et japonais ont accumulé une collection inégalable de données. Pour tirer le maximum d'une telle collection, encore faudrait-il lever «le secret d'Hiroshima». En effet, dans cette ville où le rayonnement a comporté une proportion relativement importante de neutrons, l'essentiel de l'information intéressante se trouve dans le domaine des faibles doses. L'auteur tente d'explorer ce domaine, mais avec des données en partie très incertaines. Il retrouve là, comme à Nagasaki et comme après radio-thérapie sur le rachis, mais pour des doses très inférieures, que l'irradiation pourrait diminuer la fréquence des leucémies. Il retrouve aussi que le facteur d'efficacité biologique relative (EBR) des neutrons augmente quand la dose diminue: il atteindrait 100, et peut-être bien davantage, dans le domaine des doses à effet protecteur dominant. Le temps de latence de la leucémie est l'un des plus courts, mais on doit avoir maintenant un recul suffisant pour explorer profitablement les résultats relatifs à d'autres tumeurs.

1. INTRODUCTION

Je reprends ici le sujet d'un travail antérieur sur l'effet leucémogène des rayonnements ionisants [1, 2] à l'aide de données extraites de la littérature; certains textes sont bien connus [3, 4], l'un d'eux est récent [5]; un autre m'a été aimablement communiqué avant sa publication [6].

Parce que les neutrons constituaient une proportion importante du rayonnement, et que leur facteur d'efficacité biologique relative (EBR) augmente quand la dose diminue, il faut qu'à Hiroshima les survivants les moins irradiés fassent l'objet d'une attention particulière.

Pour cela, faute de mieux, j'ai dû reconstituer des données manquantes, le plus souvent sans risque d'erreur grossière, mais pas toujours. Aussi l'intérêt essentiel de ce travail tient-il dans l'exposé d'une méthode; il ne saurait que dégager des tendances et non des résultats définitifs, même pour ce qui concerne la leucémie, affection maligne dont le temps de latence est l'un des plus courts, la seule considérée ici.

J'envisage plusieurs formes possibles pour la relation entre effet leucémogène et dose. Il n'y a pas de relation simple, même approchée; la plus fidèle me paraît être graphique; chaque forme clinique de leucémie donne un graphe particulier; je retrouve graphiquement que l'EBR des neutrons augmente sensiblement quand la dose diminue. En terminant je compare les conséquences que l'on pourrait inférer de tels graphes avec celles que l'on prévoit, par «prudence», à partir de relations linéaires, sans seuil de dose.

2. LES DONNEES

Les données portent sur l'irradiation et sur la pathologie.

2.1. L'irradiation

Ce sont les rayonnements émis au moment de l'éclair qui ont causé l'essentiel de l'irradiation des personnes, les atteignant dans l'organisme entier, durant moins de dix secondes.

Auxier et al. [7] ont déterminé la variation de la dose en fonction de la distance. Plus précisément, ils donnent le kerma pour les neutrons et pour les rayons γ dans un volume élémentaire équivalent à du tissu, placé dans l'air et ayant vue directe sur la source. La somme des kermas des neutrons et des rayons γ, exprimée en rad, mesure le kerma total à l'air. Les physiciens [8, 9] ont déterminé la valeur du kerma à l'air et aussi celle de la dose à l'intérieur de l'organisme, en tenant compte, au besoin, pour chaque personne, de la présence d'un écran protecteur (toit, mur, tranchée, etc.).

Les informations recueillies n'ont pas permis de tenir compte de l'irradiation due à la contamination radioactive, même dans la zone des retombées [10–12].

Environ 60 000 survivants de l'explosion à Hiroshima et 20 000 à Nagasaki ont pu être localisés et classés en fonction de l'irradiation subie. Tous les auteurs les répartissent de la même façon dans l'une et l'autre des deux villes (cinq, six ou sept classes). Ils donnent pour chaque classe la valeur moyenne du kerma à l'air, pour les neutrons, pour les rayons γ, et au total.

La dosimétrie a été établie par des mesures sur le terrain et par le calcul. Les résultats de ces derniers sont meilleurs pour Nagasaki (10% d'erreur possible) que pour Hiroshima (30% d'erreur possible) où la bombe qui a explosé est demeurée l'unique exemplaire de son type [7]. Malgré les précautions prises, il y a évidemment incertitude sur l'emplacement de chaque personne et sur l'effet protecteur d'écrans éventuels. Il semble, malgré tout, que les résultats soient cohérents dans chacune des deux villes et que l'on puisse même tirer des enseignements de leur comparaison.

Les formules de Jones, rapportées par Ishimaru [6], m'ont permis de passer du kerma à l'air à la dose moyenne absorbée dans la moelle osseuse; cependant la conversion n'était pas absolument indispensable pour ce travail aux données incertaines.

2.2. Les leucémies

La fréquence annuelle moyenne brute des leucémies, la seule calculable ici, s'obtient en faisant le quotient de leur nombre par l'effectif de la classe correspondante, exprimé en personnes·ans.

Quatre documents permettent de retrouver les données, mais non sans quelques difficultés. Ainsi les leucémies qui y sont étudiées sont celles qui, durant la période d'observation (qui n'est pas la même pour tous), ont été ou dénombrées, ou seulement diagnostiquées, ou encore seulement observées sur un mort. Jablon et Kato ont retenu ces dernières: 31 pour Nagasaki et 95 pour Hiroshima. Ichimaru et al. [5] donnent une liste avec, par ville, pour chaque cas: le sexe, la forme clinique de la leucémie, l'âge en août 1945 et lors du diagnostic, les valeurs du kerma à l'air, pour les neutrons, les rayons γ et au total; pour les morts, la cause principale du décès dans le code international (généralement, mais non toujours, 207, c'est-à-dire la leucémie).

Dans cette liste, arrêtée un an après celle des auteurs précédents, le nombre des morts atteints de leucémie, de 30 à Nagasaki, n'est que de 84 à Hiroshima. On peut penser que les diminutions proviennent de l'élimination d'erreurs de diagnostic. Cependant, ainsi modifiées par Ichimaru et al., les données paraissent moins cohérentes; en effet, la fréquence moyenne de ces morts serait, malgré le peu de neutrons, plus faible à Nagasaki qu'à Hiroshima de près de 10%.

2.3. Les données retenues ici

Le tableau I pour Hiroshima et le tableau II pour Nagasaki contiennent les données utilisées telles qu'elles ont pu être reconstituées.

La période d'observation s'étend du 1er octobre 1950 au 31 décembre 1971.

Il m'a paru logique de considérer les morts parce que le diagnostic de leucémie, parfois difficile, voire impossible à confirmer, peut, pour eux, faire l'objet de vérifications complémentaires.

TABLEAU I. LES MORTS AVEC LEUCEMIE A HIROSHIMA (1950–1971)

Limite inférieure de classe (rad)	0	1	5	10	20	50	100	200	400
Nombre de									
personnes (10^3)	30,0	8,8	5,0	6,0	4,8	2,7	1,7	1,0	0,5
personnes·ans (10^3)	570	169	96	115	91	52	33	20	10
leucémiques morts	19	2	4	4	13	6	10	15	11
Fréquence des morts									
(pour 10^6 personnes·ans)	33	12	42	35	140	120	310	760	1 140
Kerma moyen total (rad)									
air	0	1,5	7	15	31	70	140	280	530
moelle	0	0,7	3,7	7,4	16	36	70	140	260

TABLEAU II. LES MORTS AVEC LEUCEMIE A NAGASAKI (1950–1971)

Limite inférieure de classe (rad)	0	10	50	100	200	400
Nombre de						
personnes (10^3)	11,4	3,7	1,3	1,4	1,0	0,4
personnes·ans (10^3)	221	71	26	27	20	7
leucémiques morts	8[a]	2	0	4	8	7
Fréquence des morts						
(pour 10^6 personnes·ans)	36	28	0	150	400	950
Kerma moyen total (rad)						
air	4	21	71	144	270	530
moelle	2,2	12	39	79	150	280

[a] Défalcation faite de la leucémie lymphoïde chronique.

A cause des neutrons et de l'augmentation de l'EBR, j'ai augmenté le nombre des classes pour les survivants peu irradiés à Hiroshima; c'est possible: ils sont beaucoup plus nombreux qu'à Nagasaki et les différents auteurs ne les ont pas répartis de la même façon.

La figure 1 représente, sur les mêmes axes, pour chacune des deux villes, chaque classe avec en ordonnée la fréquence annuelle moyenne des morts atteints de leucémie par million de personnes, et en abscisse la valeur moyenne de la dose (en rad) dans la moelle osseuse. Pour chaque point la barre verticale a été calculée pour un intervalle de confiance de 95%.

2.4. Discussion des données retenues

Le seul cas de leucémie lymphoïde chronique rapporté dans leur liste par Ichimaru et al. se trouve dans la classe qui a reçu moins de un rad: il n'a pas été retenu; en effet, selon Court-Brown et Doll [13], cette forme clinique ne serait pas induite par l'irradiation, ce qui a été confirmé par les observations faites à Hiroshima et Nagasaki. Elle est exceptionnelle au Japon.

Faute de meilleure référence, suivant d'autres auteurs, j'ai pris la classe la moins irradiée comme témoin dans chacune des deux villes. Le tableau III rapporte l'essentiel des données des deux premières classes de chacun des

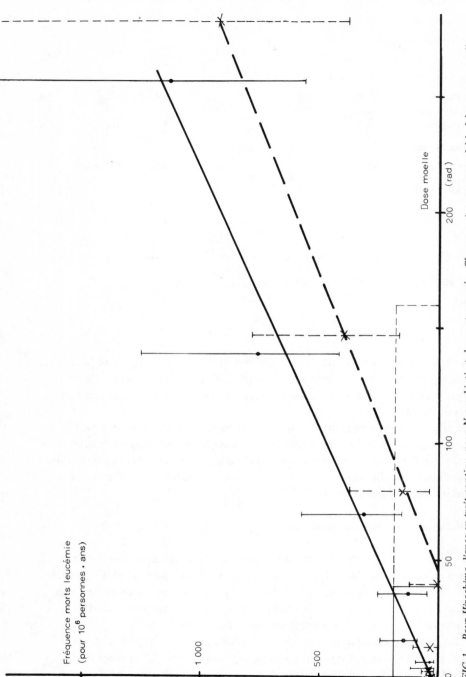

FIG.1. Pour Hiroshima, lignes en trait continu, pour Nagasaki, tirets longs et appuyés. Chaque point correspond à la fréquence annuelle moyenne des morts avec leucémie dénombrées dans l'une des classes des tableaux I et II; il se trouve sur la barre verticale qui représente l'intervalle de confiance à 95%. Pour Hiroshima, la droite a l'équation (1) indiquée dans le texte. Pour Nagasaki, la droite a été tirée par les

TABLEAU III.   RAPPEL DE DONNEES

	Hiroshima		Nagasaki	
Limite inférieure de classe (rad)	0	1	0	10
Effectif (10^3 personnes·ans)	570	169	221	71
Fréquence des morts (pour 10^6 personnes·ans)	33	12	36	28
Intervalle de confiance (95%)	20−52	1,4−43	16−71	3,3−100

TABLEAU IV.   DONNEES IMAGINEES POUR HIROSHIMA

Limite inférieure de classe (rad)	0	0,5	1
Nombre de personnes·ans (10^3) leucémiques morts	386 14	184 5	voir tableau I:
Fréquence des morts (pour 10^6 personnes·ans)	36[a]	27	données inchangées pour les autres classes
Kerma moyen total (rad) moelle	0[b]	0,3[b]	

[a] Même valeur que dans la classe de référence de Nagasaki.
[b] Valeur que les physiciens devraient préciser.

tableaux I et II (effectif et fréquence) et donne, en outre, l'intervalle de confiance
à 95% pour chacune de ces fréquences. Aucune ne diffère des trois autres de
façon statistiquement significative. Dans le tableau I et aussi dans le tableau II,
il faut atteindre la cinquième classe pour trouver une fréquence augmentée signi-
ficativement par rapport à celle de la première, avec 140 (l'intervalle de confiance
va de 75 à 240) à Hiroshima et avec 400 (de 170 à 800) à Nagasaki. Dans ces
classes, pour les personnes les moins irradiées le kerma total à l'air atteint au moins
20 rad à Hiroshima et au moins 200 rad à Nagasaki.

Il semble que l'on gagnerait encore de l'information en subdivisant en deux la classe de référence d'Hiroshima (tableaux I et III), ce qui a été fait dans le tableau IV. Pour cela j'ai supposé (sans justification, pour voir) que la fréquence des morts était exactement la même dans la nouvelle classe de référence que dans celle de Nagasaki (de 36); pour que l'effectif de l'autre classe demeure important, j'y ai laissé 386 000 personnes·ans, pour 14 leucémies. En l'absence d'information, il m'a fallu aussi imaginer les valeurs relatives à la dosimétrie.

Voyons maintenant, à l'aide des données publiées, complétées par des données retrouvées et, au besoin, imaginées, quelles formes pourrait prendre la relation entre l'effet leucémogène et la dose, et aussi ce que pourraient impliquer de telles relations.

3. RELATIONS ENTRE EFFET LEUCEMOGENE ET DOSE

En conservant le rad, unité de mesure utilisée dans les publications d'où proviennent les données, après avoir envisagé un certain nombre de formes de relation entre effet leucémogène et dose, je considérerai différentes formes cliniques; enfin, je calculerai l'EBR des neutrons.

3.1. Formules mathématiques

La forme linéaire est la plus simple. En représentant par $\underline{f}$ la fréquence moyenne annuelle des leucémies, calculée sur un million de personnes, et par $\underline{D}$ la valeur moyenne de la dose absorbée dans la moelle osseuse, exprimée en rad, compte tenu de l'intervalle de confiance de chaque point, l'équation de la droite de régression linéaire s'écrit

pour Hiroshima: $\underline{f} = 4,5\,\underline{D} + 20$ \hfill (1)

pour Nagasaki : $\underline{f} = 2,7\,\underline{D} - 10$ \hfill (2)

Chacune de ces droites a une pente positive, différente de zéro de façon statistiquement significative, en admettant un risque de première espèce égal à 5%.

Selon la première formule, la fréquence des leucémies spontanées dans la population d'Hiroshima paraît faible. Pour que la seconde formule soit admissible, il faut attribuer la valeur négative du terme constant aux erreurs de mesure, ou, ce qui n'est pas classique, admettre l'existence d'un seuil d'effet à quelques rad. Seule la droite de formule (1) est tracée sur la figure 1; l'autre droite, pour Nagasaki, passe simplement par les deux points les plus éloignés, ceux qui correspondent aux doses les plus élevées.

Les équations de régression quadratique pondérée, en dose totale, ou de régression linéaire pondérée séparant la dose due aux neutrons de celle des rayons γ et, *a fortiori,* les équations de régression quadratique pondérée qui séparent les neutrons et les rayons γ comportent des coefficients de la dose qui ne sont pas différents de zéro de façon statistiquement significative.

On se heurte donc à l'impossibilité de traduire la variation de l'effet leucémogène en fonction de la dose par des relations mathématiques statistiquement significatives autres que linéaires.

3.2. Des graphes

Abandonnant les formules mathématiques dans ce travail de prospection aux données incertaines, j'ai représenté graphiquement sur la figure 2 les données des tableaux I et IV pour Hiroshima, et celles du tableau II pour Nagasaki. Afin de mieux voir les détails que dans la figure 1, j'ai multiplié les échelles par 10, en ordonnées pour les deux villes et en abscisses pour Hiroshima. Les deux graphes, tracés à vue, d'abord confondus, par raison de simplicité[1], passent par un minimum; ils divergent ensuite pour, en croissant, tendre asymptotiquement vers chacune des droites qui, représentées entièrement dans la figure 1, ne le sont que très partiellement dans la figure 2.

Ces graphes ne représentent qu'à peu près les fonctions de dose réelles. Sachant bien qu'ils ne sont pas statistiquement différents des droites obtenues par régression pondérée, on peut tout de même remarquer que, selon eux, une irradiation de quelques rad à Hiroshima ou de quelques dizaines de rad à Nagasaki aurait diminué la fréquence des leucémies; au contraire, du moins à Hiroshima, selon la relation linéaire toute dose, pour aussi faible qu'elle ait été, aurait augmenté cette fréquence.

L'information, quoique beaucoup plus riche qu'à Nagasaki, se trouve pour Hiroshima reportée aux doses numériquement faibles; aussi ai-je pensé que les droites de formules (1) et (2) du paragraphe 3.1 pourraient bien n'être différentes que parce que la première dissimulerait «le secret d'Hiroshima».

Les fonctions à minimum ne retiennent pas l'attention des commentateurs des ⸍ormes de radioprotection qui, obstinément, ne s'en tiennent qu'à la possibilité d'effets délétères. Quant aux chercheurs, ils qualifient très généralement de «paradoxaux» les points qui pourraient faire penser à un minimum. Ne pas rejeter les fonctions à minimum présenterait cependant un double intérêt: l'intérêt scientifique de pouvoir, mieux que des droites, représenter l'effet observé sur toute l'étendue de la gamme des doses dans des conditions différentes d'irradiation,

---

[1] Cela revient à admettre qu'un même effet a été provoqué par une dose 10 fois plus grande à Nagasaki qu'à Hiroshima. En rapprochant les fréquences des morts avec leucémie des tableaux I et II, cela paraît excessif aux doses élevées, mais ne doit plus l'être aux doses faibles, en raison de l'augmentation de l'EBR des neutrons.

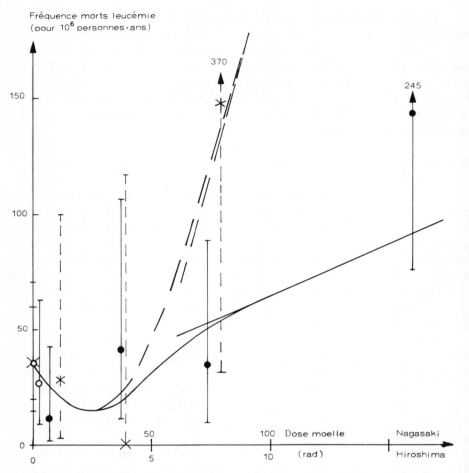

FIG.2. Représentation agrandie des points situés sur la figure 1, à l'intérieur des petits rectangles, en trait continu pour Hiroshima, en tirets pour Nagasaki. Toutefois, pour Hiroshima, on a substitué à la classe de référence du tableau I les deux sous-classes définies au tableau IV; elles sont représentées par les deux ronds vides. Tracés à main levée, les graphes rejoignent asymptotiquement les droites qui, représentées entièrement sur la figure 1, ne le sont que très partiellement ici.

après radiothérapie sur le rachis [13], à Nagasaki et, on peut maintenant le supposer à Hiroshima; l'intérêt pratique de libérer de leur inquiétude — plus ou moins ressentie — les utilisateurs de sources de rayonnements ionisants à des fins médicales ou industrielles et aussi, sans doute, les autorités responsables de la réglementation sur l'emploi de telles sources. Il est vrai que l'on peut craindre, en retour, de dangereux abus. Mais c'est aux autorités, non aux hommes de science, qu'il appartient de faire les règlements et de veiller à leur application.

3.3. Graphes et formes cliniques de la leucémie

Dans les tableaux I et II on peut, dans chaque classe, répartir les personnes mortes en état de leucémie en sous-classes. Comme Mole [14], j'ai distingué trois formes aiguës (granulocytaire, lymphocytaire et « autres ») et une forme chronique (granulocytaire).

Une telle subdivision augmente encore la longueur de l'intervalle de confiance de chaque point. En vue de gagner de l'information j'ai retenu ici tous les cas utilisables, morts et vivants, après et avant 1950 [5]. Il n'est malgré tout possible que de dégager des tendances; je m'y suis efforcé, sur la figure 3, pour chacune des quatre sous-classes d'Hiroshima, et pour une seule à Nagasaki en raison de l'insuffisance du nombre des cas dans les autres sous-classes. La séparation des formes cliniques accentue les variations dont les graphes de la figure 2 ne représentent que la résultante. La fréquence de la forme chronique (granulocytaire) augmenterait à peu près proportionnellement à la dose. Pour les formes aiguës non granulocytaires, le seuil d'action (action délétère) serait de plusieurs rad à Hiroshima. Les personnes qui n'ont reçu que quelques rad à Hiroshima, ou que quelques dizaines de rad à Nagasaki, seraient protégées contre l'apparition de leucémies granulocytaires spontanées: à Hiroshima, on n'en trouve aucun cas dans les trois classes comprises entre 1 et 20 rad à l'air (avec 20 000 personnes, soit plus de 400 000 personnes·ans); à Nagasaki, on n'en trouve aucun cas dans les deux classes comprises entre 10 et 100 rad (avec 5 000 personnes, soit plus de 100 000 personnes·ans); par contre de fortes doses augmenteraient considérablement la fréquence de cette forme clinique, qui atteint 600 à Nagasaki dans la classe la plus irradiée. A Hiroshima, autant que l'on puisse en juger, dans la classe qui a été le plus fortement irradiée les fréquences ne croîtraient pas par rapport à la précédente, peut-être à cause des neutrons.

3.4. Graphes et EBR des neutrons

D'après Poston et al., dont Rossi et Kellerer [15] ont rapporté et confirmé la remarque, l'EBR des neutrons augmenterait quand la dose diminue. On sait que, par ailleurs, la valeur de cet EBR varie avec l'énergie des neutrons; cependant, comme on peut le vérifier sur les graphes de la publication d'Auxier et al. [7], l'atténuation des neutrons dans l'air ayant été à peu près la même à Hiroshima et à Nagasaki, ils formaient des spectres assez semblables lorsqu'ils atteignirent des survivants.

Soit, pour un groupe de ces survivants, $\underline{n}$ la dose moyenne de neutrons et $\underline{g}$ celle de rayons γ, avec l'indice $\underline{H}$ ou $\underline{N}$, suivant la ville (Hiroshima on Nagasaki). Sur la figure 2, pour une valeur de la fréquence on trouve deux points d'abscisses

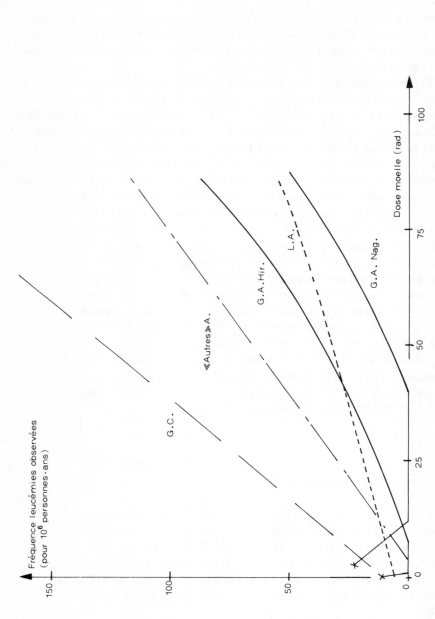

FIG.3. Schéma des tendances de variation de la fréquence des formes cliniques de la leucémie. Seule la forme granulocytaire aiguë a pu être représentée pour Nagasaki (G.A. Nag.). Pour Hiroshima, on trouve sur la droite de la figure, successivement, de bas en haut, les formes lymphocytaire aiguë (L.A.), granulocytaire aiguë (G.A. Hir.), autres formes aiguës groupées («Autres» A.), granulocytaire chronique (G.C.).

$\underline{n}_H + \underline{g}_H$ sur un graphe, et $\underline{n}_N + \underline{g}_N$ sur l'autre.[2] Pour un même effet, c'est-à-dire une même fréquence des morts avec leucémie, ces doses, différentes parce qu'elles sont exprimées en rad, doivent devenir égales quand on les convertit en équivalents de dose exprimés en rem.

Soit $(\underline{EBR})_{\underline{n}_H}$ et $(\underline{EBR})_{\underline{n}_N}$ les valeurs de l'EBR qui correspondent respectivement aux doses $\underline{n}_H$ et $\underline{n}_N$; on écrit:

$$\underline{n}_H(\underline{EBR})_{\underline{n}_H} + \underline{g}_H = \underline{n}_N(\underline{EBR})_{\underline{n}_N} + \underline{g}_N \tag{3}$$

Pour cela, il faut admettre que les rayonnements ne différaient que par la proportion des neutrons; que les erreurs sur la dosimétrie individuelle se compensent statistiquement dans chaque ville et que les erreurs systématiques ne créent pas d'importantes différences entre villes; que les personnes ont été réparties comme par tirage au sort entre les classes des tableaux I et II. De telles conditions ne sont, bien sûr, remplies qu'approximativement.

J'ai pris les valeurs de $\underline{n}_H + \underline{g}_H$ et de $\underline{n}_N + \underline{g}_N$ d'une part sur les graphes de la figure 2, d'autre part sur ceux qui, à la figure 3, représentent la variation de fréquence de la leucémie granulocytaire aiguë (G.A.) à Hiroshima et à Nagasaki. La publication d'Auxier et al. [7] donne, ou permet de retrouver à peu près, la valeur du rapport $\underline{n}/\underline{g}$ tant que les doses ne sont pas très faibles. Si l'on considère le produit $\underline{n}_N(\underline{EBR})_{\underline{n}_N}$ comme négligeable aux faibles valeurs de $\underline{n}_N$, on peut ramener l'équation (3) à une seule inconnue et calculer l'EBR à la dose $\underline{n}_N$. De fait, cette approximation est grossière, mais on peut améliorer les résultats par itération. L'amélioration serait bien meilleure si les physiciens donnaient le rapport $\underline{n}/\underline{g}$ et la dosimétrie individuelle pour des doses beaucoup plus faibles allant, par exemple, jusqu'à 0,5 rad à l'air pour $\underline{n} + \underline{g}$, et même en deçà à Hiroshima (tableau IV).

D'après les graphes de la figure 2 et ceux de la figure 3 pour la leucémie granulocytaire aiguë, l'EBR, d'environ 100 pour des doses de neutrons voisines du rad, serait voisin de 10 pour une vingtaine de rad; lorsque je m'aventure vers les très faibles doses, en extrapolant pour $\underline{n}/\underline{g}$ vers une dizaine de mrad de neutrons, je trouve un EBR qui dépasse 300. La droite d'équation (1) pour Hiroshima, rapprochée de celle qui correspond aux deux dernières classes du tableau II pour Nagasaki, me donne un EBR voisin de 5 pour 100 rad de neutrons.

Ces valeurs que je trouve ne détonnent pas auprès de celles que Rossi et Kellerer ont pu tirer de la littérature; ces dernières sont relatives à des effets délétères, ou considérés comme tels, et à un matériel biologique qui va de la graine de maïs à la mamelle de rate. Ici il s'agit de personnes, et de leucémies inhibées ou provoquées suivant la dose. J'en arrive à me demander si l'attention des chercheurs ne serait pas, à tort, obstinément polarisée sur les effets délétères.

---

[2] Il faut prendre les abscisses des deux points situés du même côté du minimum.

3.5. Importance pratique des relations entre effet et dose

Court-Brown et Doll [13] ont proposé en 1957, comme hypothèse de travail, d'admettre que, dans une population qui a été irradiée, l'augmentation de la fréquence des leucémies soit considérée comme proportionnelle à la dose moyenne reçue dans la moelle osseuse des personnes. Cela paraissait bien plausible, par analogie. En effet, à cette époque on croyait bien savoir pourquoi l'augmentation de fréquence des mutants dans la progéniture de parents irradiés (première génération) ne pouvait qu'être proportionnelle à la dose administrée aux gonades, quel qu'ait été le mode d'irradiation.

Les conceptions s'affirmant, actuellement, pour juger de l'acceptabilité des normes de radioprotection ou, plus précisément, de celle des doses à ne pas dépasser pour l'irradiation des personnes, on calcule des *dommages prévisionnels*. Les calculs reposent sur l'hypothèse de proportionnalité entre le nombre de victimes attribuées à l'irradiation et la *dose collective*. Ces victimes mourraient cancéreuses, ou seraient handicapées par des anomalies génétiquement transmissibles.

De tels maux frapperaient au hasard des personnes dans leur chair et sur leur descendance, simplement parce qu'elles ont été irradiées, sans le vouloir, souvent sans même le savoir. Ce serait atroce, inquiétant, bouleversant, révoltant.

Il est vrai que les calculs majorent l'importance des dommages sanitaires; cependant les commentateurs des normes de radioprotection ne croient pas pouvoir prendre le risque de rassurer à tort les responsables de l'irradiation de personnes [16, 17]. On peut craindre que, ce faisant, ils ne bloquent toute possibilité de communication avec l'ensemble des utilisateurs — actifs, ou passifs — de ces normes. En effet, les autorités exigent des précautions de plus en plus coûteuses en sûreté nucléaire et en radioprotection sans, pour autant, parvenir à rassurer, à se rassurer. Par ailleurs, les crédits leur font bien cruellement défaut, particulièrement pour la prévention sanitaire [1].

Une bonne prévention repose sur des prévisions correctes. En pratique, dans l'ensemble des modifications du milieu susceptibles de nuire à la santé, et parmi les relations quantitatives envisageables entre ces modifications et leurs effets, des choix s'imposent. Souhaitons que, pour le bilan des «coûts» et des «bénéfices», l'évaluation des coûts sanitaires ne demeure plus longtemps encore majorée systématiquement, par «prudence».

4. CONCLUSION

Parce que des chercheurs américains et japonais ont, très vite, su coordonner leurs efforts, et grâce à la compréhension des survivants des bombes atomiques malgré leurs souffrances, une collection inégalable de données, sans cesse améliorée, a pu être constituée.

Il serait dommage de ne pas s'efforcer d'exploiter plus à fond une telle collection, non seulement pour l'effet leucémogène, mais aussi pour d'autres effets, car le recul doit être maintenant suffisant pour bien des tumeurs solides, bénignes ou malignes. Il conviendrait sans doute de demander aux physiciens de préciser au mieux la dosimétrie des survivants qui, à Hiroshima, se trouvaient à un endroit exposé à moins de un rad.

Une différence fondamentale sépare les résultats de cette étude des conclusions classiques. Il est vrai que je n'ai pu que m'efforcer de dégager des tendances. Tout de même, les tendances observées corroborent les résultats de certaines expérimentations qui, elles aussi, ont donné des graphes à minimum.

Ensemble complexe qui vit, et qui se reproduit, un organisme vivant ne saurait être assimilé à une juxtaposition de cellules, ou, encore moins, de «cibles». Une formule linéaire ne représente qu'une approche, d'autant meilleure que l'intervalle d'interpolation est plus étroit; malgré sa grande simplicité on ne devrait jamais l'extrapoler. Dégager des relations entre effet et dose autres que linéaires ou, à défaut, tout un faisceau de tendances ferait bien progresser nos connaissances en radiopathologie et, partant, aiderait à mieux délimiter les nécessités de la radioprotection et celles de la prévention sanitaire en général.

REMERCIEMENTS

L'auteur remercie A. Baumerder, du Service Informatique et mathématiques appliquées, de la Direction des études et recherches d'Electricité de France, pour l'aide qu'il lui a apportée, en particulier dans le domaine des interprétations statistiques.

REFERENCES

[1] DELPLA, M., «L'environnement des centrales nucléaires», Biological and Environmental Effects of Low-Level Radiation (C.R. Coll. Chicago, 1975) II, AIEA, Vienne (1976) 333–350.

[2] DELPLA, M., «Evaluation de risques somatiques à faibles doses», Ibid., p. 351–359.

[3] JABLON, S., KATO, H., Mortality Among A-Bomb Survivors, 1950–70, ABCC Technical Report 10–71.

[4] ISHIMARU, T., HOSHINO, T., ICHIMARU, M., OKADA, H., TOMIYASU, T., TSUCHIMOTO, T., YAMAMOTO, T., Leukemia in atomic bomb survivors, Hiroshima and Nagasaki, 1 October 1950 – 3 September 1966, Radiat. Res. 45 (1971) 216–233.

[5] ICHIMARU, M., ISHIMARU, T., BELSKY, J.L., Incidence of Leukemia in Atomic Bomb Survivors, Hiroshima & Nagasaki 1950–71, Technical Report RERF 10–76.

[6] ISHIMARU, T., Communication personnelle, 19 mai 1977.

[7] AUXIER, J.A., CHEKA, J.S., HAYWOOD, F.F., JONES, T.D., THORNGATE, J.H., Free-field radiation-dose distributions from the Hiroshima and Nagasaki bombings, Health Phys. 12 (1966) 425–429.

[8] AUXIER, J.A., Physical dose estimates for A-bomb survivors, Studies at Oak Ridge, USA, J. Radiat. Res., Suppl. (1975) 1—11.
[9] HASHISUME, T., MARUYAMA, T., Physical dose estimates for A-bomb survivors, Studies at Chiba, Japan, ibid. (1975) 12—23.
[10] TAKESHITA, H., Dose estimation from residual and fallout radioactivity, ibid. (1975) 24—31.
[11] OKAJIMA, S., ibid. (1975) 35—41.
[12] OKAJIMA, S., TAKESHITA, K., ANTOKU, S., SHIOMI, T., RUSSELL, W., FUJITA, S., YOSHINAGA, H., NERIISHI, S., KAWAMOTO, S., NORIMURA, T., Effects of the Radioactive Fallout of the Nagasaki Atomic Bomb, ABCC Technical Report 12—75.
[13] COURT BROWN, W.M., DOLL, R., Leukaemia and Aplastic Anaemia in Patients Irradiated for Ankylosing Spondylitis, H.M.S.O., Londres (1957).
[14] MOLE, R.H., Ionizing radiation as a carcinogen: practical questions and academic pursuits, Br. J. Radiol. 48 (1975) 157—170.
[15] ROSSI, H.H., KELLERER, A.M., The validity of risk estimates of leukemia incidence based on Japanese data, Radiat. Res. 58 (1974) 131—140.
[16] NCRP, Report No. 43, Washington (1975).
[17] ICRP, Publication 26, Pergamon Press, Oxford (1977).

DISCUSSION

G.W. BARENDSEN: In view of the limitations inherent in the data obtained from studies of atomic bomb survivors, it is possible to devise a large number of hypotheses that are not incompatible with the data. However, we should recognize that some restrictions or boundary conditions must be taken into account which limit the types of hypotheses that can be considered sensible. One of the restrictions is imposed by microdosimetric parameters based directly on simple physical laws. At very small doses microdosimetric data imply that only a fraction of the cells in an irradiated biological system will be traversed by an ionizing particle. If the suggestion is made that such low doses, which especially with neutrons result in energy deposition in, for instance, only one per cent of cells, nevertheless prevent leukaemias from developing, then this hypothesis would imply that ionizing particles can selectively eliminate cells that carry already malignant genetic information. In view of the fact that this is highly improbable, your conclusion that low doses of ionizing radiation have a protective effect is difficult to accept.

M. DELPLA: Your comment gives me an opportunity to enlarge somewhat on this subject. You are saying that, according to microdosimetric data, in particular for neutrons, a low dose reaches a very small proportion of cells, and you find this incompatible with my hypothesis that small doses could 'add a negative risk'. You are in fact likening the human body to a juxtaposition of cells or 'isolated targets'. I feel it preferable to regard a body formed of cells grouped into tissues and vascularized and nerved organs, not as a collection of elementary units but as an active and reactive whole, and it does not seem unreasonable to suppose that a 'moderate degree of agression' would, all things considered, be beneficial to such a system.

Y. NISHIWAKI: It has been reported that the effects at Hiroshima appear to be higher than those at Nagasaki in the low-dose range. This is ascribed to a higher contribution of neutrons at Hiroshima, compared with Nagasaki. If my memory is correct, there was a plant producing poison gases such as yperite (sulphur mustard) and chlorine situated on an island called Kuno-shima about 70 km east of Hiroshima and about 5–6 km off the coast in the Seto Inland Sea. (The name of the island may be Okhuno-shima today.) The area was a good fishing ground. The place was chosen on the basis of the meteorological conditions, to ensure that any possible exposure of the densely populated Hiroshima area by the effluent from this facility would be minimal. However, in view of the violent disturbance of the local meteorological conditions by the atomic explosion, I think that it is important to keep in mind the possibility of other factors apart from radiation being responsible for the effects observed, when we discuss the consequences of atomic bombing. The condensation cloud and rain after the explosion might have accelerated the precipitation of the gas effluent and the various chemicals evaporated in the hypocentre area, in addition to the deposition of radioactive debris.

THYROID HYPOFUNCTION APPEARING AS A DELAYED MANIFESTATION OF ACCIDENTAL EXPOSURE TO RADIOACTIVE FALL-OUT IN A MARSHALLESE POPULATION*

P.R. LARSEN
Thyroid Unit,
Department of Medicine,
Peter Bent Brigham Hospital,
Boston,
Massachusetts

R.A. CONARD, K. KNUDSEN
Brookhaven National Laboratory,
Upton,
New York

J. ROBBINS, J. WOLFF, J.E. RALL
National Institute of Arthritis, Metabolism
    and Digestive Diseases,
Bethesda,
Maryland

B. DOBYNS
Department of Surgery,
Case-Western Reserve University,
Cleveland,
Ohio,
United States of America

Abstract

THYROID HYPOFUNCTION APPEARING AS A DELAYED MANIFESTATION OF
ACCIDENTAL EXPOSURE TO RADIOACTIVE FALL-OUT IN A MARSHALLESE
POPULATION.
    The increased incidence of thyroid nodularity and carcinoma appearing as a late effect
after exposure of the human thyroid to ionizing radiation is well recognized. Despite the
high prevalence of thyroid nodularity in Marshallese inadvertently exposed to fall-out in 1954,

* This work has been carried out under contract EY-76-C-02-0016 with the United
States Department of Energy.

only two subjects, both about one year of age at exposure, have been found to have primary hypothyroidism. The recent availability of sophisticated immunoassay techniques for thyroxine (T_4) and thyrotropin (TSH) has allowed more thorough thyroid evaluation of the exposed population who do not have known thyroid abnormalities (43 Rongelap people). Initially, prophylactic T_4 was discontinued for two months in a sample group of exposed subjects and 10 U of bovine TSH were given intramuscularly. Plasma T_4 was measured before and 24 hours after TSH. The mean increment in T_4 was 2.4 ± 1.2 μg/dl (mean $\pm$ SD) in the exposed group, significantly less than the value of 4.2 ± 1.3 μg/dl in controls. This suggested a decrease in thyroid reserve in exposed subjects. Accordingly, prophylactic T_4 treatment was discontinued for two months, and basal plasma T_4 and TSH, as well as the increment in TSH after Thyrotropin Releasing Hormone (TRH) was measured. The upper limit of the normal basal plasma TSH was 3 μU/ml and of the TRH-induced TSH response was 22 μU/ml in control Marshallese subjects. Four of 43 Rongelapese had abnormally high basal TSH and TRH-induced TSH release on two such tests as opposed to only two of 214 controls. Plasma T_4 concentrations were low, or low-normal in these individuals. These results indicate the presence of early thyroid dysfunction. Several other subjects have shown at least one abnormal finding but have not had the required number of tests to meet the established criteria. In three-quarters of these subjects the estimated thyroid exposure dose was <400 rads. Hypothyroidism has been previously noted after therapeutic doses of ^{131}I for hyperthyroidism, but not in individuals exposed to the relatively low levels of thyroidal radiation (<400 rads) estimated for these individuals.

BACKGROUND

This report concerns late radiation effects on the thyroid in a population in the Marshall Islands inadvertently exposed to fall-out. The accident occurred on 1 March 1954, during the United States atomic testing programme when an unexpected shift of winds, following detonation of a thermonuclear device at Bikini, caused radioactive fall-out to be deposited on several inhabited islands to the east. Evacuation of exposed persons was accomplished by two days. The following were estimated whole-body gamma doses in the Marshallese on three atolls: Rongelap (64 people), 175 rads; Ailingnae (18 people), 69 rads; and Utirik (158 people), 14 rads. (There were also 28 American servicemen on the island of Rongerik who received about the same exposure as the Ailingnae group.)

Acute effects of gamma exposure were noted in the Rongelap and Ailingnae groups, but not in the Utirik group. These consisted of early, transient anorexia, nausea and vomiting in a number of people followed by depression of white blood cells and platelets to about half normal levels. Fortunately the haematological depression was not great enough to result in detectable clinical signs of infection or bleeding. No specific therapy was necessary and no deaths occurred, and blood cells returned to near normal levels by one year. In addition, in the Rongelap and Ailingnae groups, beginning about two weeks post exposure, radiation burns ('beta' burns) and spotty epilation of the head developed where fall-out material had been deposited on the skin. These burns were largely superficial and healed within several weeks with normal regrowth of hair. Slight scarring remained in some cases but no development of skin malignancy has been noted in subsequent years. Another source of exposure in all the island groups came from internal absorption of radionuclides from inhalation and ingestion of contaminated food and water. Radiochemical urinalyses run during the first few weeks showed the following estimated body burdens (μCi) of the principal radionuclides in the Rongelap population at one day post exposure: ^{89}Sr 1.6–2.2; ^{140}Ba 0.34–2.7; rare earth group 0–1.2; ^{131}I (in thyroid gland) 6.4–11.2; ^{103}Ru 0–0.013; ^{45}Ca 0–0.019; and fissile material 0–0.016 (μg). No acute symptoms were noted from this internal absorption of radionuclides, and by six months urinalyses indicated they were virtually completely eliminated. Nevertheless, the early exposure to radioiodines resulted in serious injury to the thyroid glands with late effects to be described below. The thyroid dose was estimated to be considerably higher in the children because of the smaller size of the thyroid glands. In the Rongelap people the thyroid dose from gamma radiation and radioiodines (principally ^{131}I, ^{132}I, ^{133}I and ^{135}I) was estimated to be about 335 rads in the adults whereas in small children the doses ranged up to 700–1400 rads. The thyroid doses in the Ailingnae and Utirik groups were extrapolated from the Rongelap estimates assuming the ratio of whole body gamma and iodine doses were the same as in the Rongelap people.

Following the initial studies, annual examinations and, more recently, quarterly examinations of the exposed people, as well as an unexposed control Marshallese population, have been carried out, and results of these examinations have been published [1–4].

In the first ten years after the accident few findings were noted that could be related to radiation exposure. An increase in miscarriages and stillbirths in the exposed Rongelap women was thought to be possibly related to exposure.

During the second decade, however, serious late effects developed related primarily to the thyroid gland. In addition a Rongelap man who had been exposed at one year of age, died of acute myelogenous leukaemia which was likely related to radiation exposure [3].

Before thyroid abnormalities became apparent, it was noted that about five children exposed at less than five years of age showed some degree of growth retardation [4]. In two boys growth retardation was marked and frank myxoedema developed. Thyroid hypofunction related to thyroid injury later became apparent with more sophisticated techniques for determining thyroxine levels. It was not detected early in the children by PBI determinations because of masking of true thyroxine levels by unusually high levels of iodoprotein, later found to be characteristic of the Marshallese people [5].

Nodules of the thyroid gland began to appear in Rongelap children and to a lesser extent in adults beginning about nine years post exposure. These nodules have continued to appear over the subsequent 15 years, and virtually all of these

LARSEN et al.

TABLE I. THYROID LESIONS IN MARSHALLESE, SEPTEMBER 1977

Group	Age at exposure	Est. thyroid dose[a] (rads)	% Subjects[b] with thyroid lesions	No. subjects with surgery	% Subjects[b] with malignant lesion
Rongelap exposed (175 rads)	<10	810–1150	89.5 (17/19)	15	5.3 (1/19)
	10–18[c]	335–810	25.0 (3/12)	2	8.3 (1/12)
	>18	335	12.1 (4/33)[d]	4	6.1 (2/33)
	All	556[e]	37.5 (24/64)	21	6.3 (4/64)
Ailingnae exposed (69 rads)	<10	275–450	33.3 (2/6)	1[f]	
	10–18	190	0.0 (0/1)	0	
	>18	135	36.4 (4/11)	3	
	All	217[e]	33.3 (6/18)	4	
In utero exposed		175+?	33.3 (1/3)	1	
		69+?	0.0 (0/1)	0	
Rong. + Ail.	All	135–153	36.0 (31/86)	26	4.7 (4/86)
Utirik exposed (14 rads)	<10	60–95	1.7 (1/58)	1	1.7 (1/58)
	10–18	27–60	14.3 (3/21)	2	4.8 (1/21)
	>18	30	7.6 (6/79)	5	1.3 (1/79)
	All	50[e]	6.3 (10/158)	8	1.9 (3/158)
Rong. + Ail. + Utirik	All	30–1150	16.8 (41/244)	34	2.9 (7/244)

a   Dose from ^{131}I, ^{132}I, ^{135}I and ^{135}I plus gamma; mean dose extrapolated from calculations for adults and three-year-olds.
b   Based on number of people exposed, excluding those in utero (number of cases/total number in group).
c   The thyroid is considered to be fully developed by about age 18.
d   One additional case of adenoma, found at autopsy, not included here.
e   Weighted mean dose.
f   Pathologists differed as to whether this lesion was malignant: it was scored as benign.

have been resected surgically. The incidence of thyroid nodularities and estimated thyroid doses in the various age groups exposed to fall-out are depicted in Table I. It is apparent that more than two-thirds of those individuals in the combined Rongelap and Ailingnae groups, who were under the age of ten at the time of exposure, and over 15% of those exposed over the age of ten have developed thyroid lesions. Four Rongelap children were exposed in utero. One of these, a boy exposed at 22–24 weeks gestation (at which time the thyroid was functional), had benign nodules of the thyroid removed at age 20. A much smaller proportion of the Utirik group of either age has developed thyroid abnormalities. The occurrence of three thyroid cancers in the exposed Utirik population (compared with four in the Rongelap group) appears to implicate radiation exposure in the aetiology, but the high incidence is puzzling since it is greater than would be predicted based on Rongelap and Japanese data, and there does not appear to be any increase in benign thyroid tumours in that group compared with the much greater prevalence in the Rongelap group.

The high incidence of thyroid nodularity in the irradiated subjects is in agreement with previous data linking irradiation of the gland with subsequent development of thyroid nodules or carcinoma [6]. Since ^{131}I is considered much less tumorigenic for thyroid tumours than X-rays, it is rather surprising that, in view of the large contribution of radioiodines to the thyroid dose in the Marshallese, the risk factor (risk/rad) is comparable with that noted following X-ray exposure. This may be related to the presence of more potent short-lived isotopes of iodine present in fall-out which accounted for two to three times the dose from ^{131}I.

Aside from the two subjects with frank hypothyroidism, there has been an increasing suspicion of possible hypothyroidism in other cases. The evidence supporting this conclusion is summarized in Table II. The two boys who developed myxoedema had received an estimated thyroid dose of 1150 rads. In addition at least five of the Rongelap population, who had appropriate testing before surgery, had either hypothyroidism or decreased thyroid reserve [7]. In addition a number of subjects with sub-total thyroidectomy have shown elevation in serum TSH concentrations and reduction in serum T_4 when their thyroid replacement schedule was not rigorously adhered to. This is significant since in general subtotal, thyroidectomy or lobectomy is not associated with frank hypothyroidism, since the remaining thyroid lobe may often hypertrophy to supply the needed thyroid hormone requirements of the individual. All the subjects so tested and listed in Table II were irradiated at a young age, and therefore received thyroidal dosage of about 800–1150 rads. Because of the suspicion of possible hypothyroidism in individuals to even lower calculated doses, a series of studies of thyroid reserve in previously unoperated exposed Marshallese was initiated in 1974, and the following report summarizes the data obtained in this study up to the present time.

TABLE II.   PRIOR EVIDENCE OF THYROID HYPOFUNCTION AND CALCULATED THYROID EXPOSURE

Description	Subject identification number	Thyroid estimated dose (rads)
1. Two subjects with frank hypothyroidism ~10 years after exposure	3	1150
	5	1150
2. Five subjects with hypothyroidism or decreased thyroid reserve pre-operatively	2	810–1150
	20	810–1150
	33	810–1150
	42	810–1150
	65	810–1150
3. Three subjects with impaired thyroid function following subtotal thyroidectomy	17	810–1150
	21	810–1150
	69	810–1150

TABLE III.   RESULTS OF TSH STIMULATION TESTS IN EXPOSED RONGELAP SUBJECTS AND CONTROLS
Mean ± SD

	Mean serum T_4 prior to TSH (10 U 1M) (μg/dl)	Mean serum T_4 increment 24 h after TSH (μg/dl)
Controls	6.0 ± 1.7	4.2 ± 1.3
Exposed Rongelapese (n = 26)	6.6 ± 1.7	2.4 ± 1.2

METHODS

Studies were performed during the annual or semi-annual visits of the Brookhaven medical team to the Marshall Islands. Subjects were instructed to discontinue thyroid medication for two months before the studies of thyroid function which are described below. Occasionally, this instruction was not followed. However, the nature of the tests performed was such that this circumstance would result in an underestimation (rather than an overestimation) of the frequency of abnormalities in thyroid function.

Plasma was separated by allowing the red cells to sediment and was frozen within eight hours after obtaining the specimen. Serum Thyroid Stimulating Hormone (TSH) and thyroxine (T_4) were measured as previously described [8]. The normal range for serum TSH in our laboratory is from <0.05 to 3 μU/ml in the United States population (mean 2.0 μU/ml). Thyrotropin Releasing Hormone (TRH) stimulation tests were performed by infusion of 500 μg of TRH intravenously, plasma samples were obtained at 0 and at 20 minutes after the infusion. TSH stimulation tests were performed by administration of ten units of bovine TSH intramuscularly with plasma obtained for T_4 determinations before injection and 24 hours later. The normal range for serum T_4 concentrations is 5–10 μg/dl. Estimation of the free fraction of T_4 was obtained by a T_3 charcoal uptake method developed in our laboratory (TBG Index). Twenty-five μl of plasma are incubated in 1 ml of glycine acetate buffer, pH 8.6, containing ^{125}I T_3. Dextran-coated charcoal is added at 4°C with subsequent centrifugation to sediment the charcoal. The fraction of the total ^{125}I T_3 bound to charcoal is determined and this result is normalized to the results of simultaneously assayed quality control samples containing normal quantities of T_4 and thyroxine-binding globulin (TBG). The normal range for the test is 0.85–1.10. The TBG Index increases parallel to the free fraction of the serum T_4 and T_3 and is therefore elevated in hyperthyroidism or TBG deficiency.

RESULTS

TSH stimulation tests

To determine whether or not there was impaired thyroid reserve in the exposed subjects, TSH stimulation tests were carried out using an increase in serum T_4 as the response endpoint. In normal subjects in the United States of America, the mean increment in plasma T_4 was 4.7 ± 1 μg/dl (mean $\pm$ SD) in 13 subjects following injection of 10 U of TSH. In Table III are shown data for the Marshall Islands population. The control subjects who had not been exposed to radiation were given TSH, and the mean increment in T_4 was 4.2 ± 1.3 (SD) not statistically different from the results in the United States population. However, in 24 exposed Rongelap subjects, a mean increment of only 2.4 ± 1.2 μg/dl was obtained, which was significantly less ($p < 0.001$) than in the control subjects.

TABLE IV. BASELINE SERUM TSH CONCENTRATIONS AND RESPONSE TO 500 μg THYROTROPIN RELEASING HORMONE (TRH) IN CONTROL MARSHALLESE SUBJECTS
Mean ± SD

		μU/ml
Basal TSH	Mean ± SD	2.0 ± 0.73
	Range	0.5 − 3.0
TSH 20 min after TRH		11.5 ± 4.5
	Range	4.7 − 20

TABLE V. CRITERIA FOR THE DIAGNOSIS OF BIOCHEMICAL THYROID DYSFUNCTION

1. Basal plasma TSH	> 5 μU/ml	on two occasions
or		
2. a. Basal plasma TSH	> 3 μU/ml	on two occasions
b. Plasma TSH after TRH	> 22 μU/ml	

TABLE VI. FREQUENCY OF AT LEAST A SINGLE ELEVATED BASAL SERUM TSH CONCENTRATION IN THE MARSHALLESE POPULATION

	Number tested	Number > 3.0 μU/ml	%
Control unexposed	115	11	10
Utirik exposed (Thyroid dose < 95 rads)	99	12	12
Rongelap and Ailingnae exposed (Subjects without surgery and excluding Nos 3 & 5)	43	11	26

Basal serum TSH concentrations and response to TRH

Since the most sensitive index of impaired thyroid function is an elevation
in serum TSH which occurs through the hypothalamic-pituitary-thyroid feedback
axis, serum TSH concentrations and their response to TRH were measured in
both the control and the exposed Rongelap population. In primary hypothyroidism,
the response of the pituitary to TRH is excessively great [8]. Mean basal TSH
was 2 μU/ml in 25 non-exposed euthyroid Marshallese, and the range was from
undetectable (<0.05 μU/ml) to 3 μU/ml (Table IV). Serum TSH 20 minutes
following TRH was increased in all control subjects. The mean increment was
11.5 ± 4.5 (SD) with a range of from 4.7 to 20 μU/ml. These results are not
significantly different from those previously reported in other populations [9].

On the basis of these studies, criteria were established for classification of
patients as having biochemical evidence of impaired thyroid function. These
criteria are summarized in Table V, and include either two basal TSH determinations greater than 5 μU/ml (>4 standard deviations above the mean) or basal
plasma TSH >3 μU/ml (but <5 μU/ml) and plasma TSH after TRH >22 μU/ml.
Consistent observations in these ranges were required on two occasions to meet
the criteria for biochemical evidence of thyroid dysfunction. While serum T_4
concentration is an important determinant in the thyroid status of the individual,
previous studies have indicated that evidence of impaired thyroid function can
be elicited by these tests before serum T_4 concentrations have fallen below the
normal range [10]. Therefore, the serum T_4 concentration was not used as a
criterion in establishing the diagnosis of impaired thyroid function.

In Table VI is shown the frequency of at least a single elevated basal TSH
concentration in various Marshallese populations. In a control group of 115
who were not exposed to radiation, 11 subjects or 10% of the population had
a serum TSH greater than 3 μU/ml. In ten of these, serum TSH was only
minimally elevated (4.0 μU/ml or less); the remaining value was 6.1 μU/ml. None
of these patients had detectable clinical hypothyroidism or thyroid enlargement,
but serum T_4 concentrations were generally in the low normal range.

In the exposed Utirik population, 12 of 99 subjects tested had at least one
basal serum TSH greater than 3 μU/ml, though none of these was in excess of
5 μU/ml. The incidence of elevated TSH in this population is not significantly
different from that of the unexposed group. In the Rongelap and Ailingnae
population, 11 of 43 subjects were found to have at least a single elevated basal
serum TSH greater than 3 μU/ml, and in two cases serum TSH was in excess of
7 μU/ml, and in two cases serum TSH was in excess of 7 μU/ml. This is a
significantly higher prevalence than in the other two groups pooled (p <0.05).
In Fig. 1 are shown the responses to TRH of the four individuals who met the
criteria given in Table V. The normal basal TSH and response to TRH are shown
in the shaded bars. In these four individuals, the basal serum TSH was elevated,

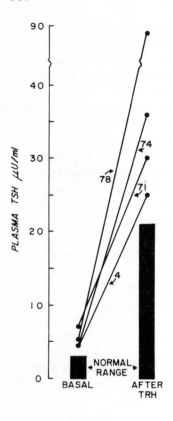

FIG.1.   *Basal plasma TSH and TRH-stimulated TSH in euthyroid Marshallese and in four exposed subjects with biochemical evidence of impaired thyroid function. Plasma was obtained 20 min after infusion of 500 μg TRH.   The upper limits of the normal range are indicated by the shaded bars.*

TABLE VII.   CHARACTERISTICS OF MARSHALLESE WITH BIOCHEMICAL EVIDENCE OF THYROID DYSFUNCTION

Subject	Age at exposure	Estimated thyroid dose (rads)	Serum T_4 (μg/dl)	TBGI units	T_4 Increment 24 h p TSH (μg/dl)
Normal values			5−10.2	0.85−1.10	1.6−6.8
74	16	335−810	5.8	0.97	0.8
71	28	335	5.2	0.98	N.T.[a]
78	37	335	6.1	0.82	0.8
4	38	335	7.4	0.79	0.9

[a]   Not tested.

and the TSH response to TRH was also significantly increased, indicating the presence of impaired thyroid function.

Characteristics of Marshallese with biochemical evidence of thyroid dysfunction

In Table VII are presented the results of other studies in the four individuals with biochemical evidence of impaired thyroid function. At present, these are the only individuals who have fulfilled the criteria described in Table V, though several other subjects have shown at least one abnormal finding but have not had the required number of tests to meet the established criteria. The age at exposure varied from 16 to 38 years and the estimated thyroid dose was thought in three or four to be less than 400 rads. Serum T_4 concentrations in all four subjects are in the low normal range when considered in the light of their estimated serum Thyroxine-Binding Globulin (TBG). Subjects 74 and 71 have approximately normal serum TBG concentrations, whereas subjects 78 and 4 apparently have a modestly elevated serum TBG. In the last column of Table VII are shown results of the TSH stimulation tests of these subjects performed in 1974. In all three, the serum T_4 response to TSH was impaired, suggesting decreased thyroid reserve.

DISCUSSION

An association of thyroid nodularity and cancer with prior radiation of the thyroid gland, particularly in younger patients, is well recognized and the association has recently been reviewed [11]. In addition, it has been recognized that radiation to the thyroid delivered in the course of treatment of patients with thyroid dysfunction is associated with hypothyroidism in a significant fraction of the patients (as high as 50%) at the higher dosage levels [12]. The lowest dosage considered in previous studies of this type has been approximately 3400 rads estimated dose to the thyroid which was associated with a 6% probability of hypothyroidism within one year and a 13% probability in 13 years [13].

There are few data available in the literature relative to the possibility of hypothyroidism following ^{131}I dosages of less than 2500 rads. Preliminary results of Hamilton and Thompkins indicated that eight of 443 subjects (1.8%) subsequently became hypothyroid after diagnostic ^{131}I tests at less than 16 years [13]. A summary of these preliminary data has been presented. None of 146 subjects with an estimated thyroid absorbed dose of 30 rads developed hypothyroidism, but three of 146 subjects receiving 31 to 80 rads estimated thyroid dose had this condition [14]. Of 151 subjects with an estimated dose range of 81−1900 rads, five hypothyroid patients were found with an incidence of hypothyroidism of 0.23% yearly.

The present studies suggest that there is a significant risk of development of impaired thyroid function many years following estimated thyroid doses of less than 500 rads from the mixture of radioiodines present in fall-out from nuclear detonations. In the Rongelap and Ailingnae groups, the effect has apparently not been significantly severe as to result in clinically evident hypothyroidism, but by currently accepted criteria there is evidence of impaired thyroid reserve in these subjects. If left untreated, it would be expected that thyroid function would continue to decrease in such subjects to the point of clinical hypothyroidism. The data in Table VI also indicate that the frequency of an elevated serum TSH, the earliest biochemical evidence of impaired thyroid function, is also significantly more common in the exposed Rongelap population than in the control-unexposed group. There are several other exposed Rongelap individuals in whom results of basal TSH and at least one TRH test have suggested the possibility that they may also have evidence of impaired thyroid function. These individuals are currently undergoing repeated testing to determine whether or not this preliminary evidence of thyroid dysfunction can be confirmed.

In summary, these data indicate that in addition to thyroid nodularity, a well-recognized manifestation of exposure of the thyroid to radioactive iodine or external radiation, biochemical evidence of thyroid dysfunction can appear as long as 25 years after thyroid doses as low as 350 rads.

ACKNOWLEDGEMENTS

This work was supported in part by the Department of Energy.

P.R. Larsen is an investigator, Howard Hughes Medical Institute.

We are grateful to S.T. Bigos for allowing us to review Ref. [11] before its publication.

REFERENCES

[1] CONARD, R.A., et al., "Summary of thyroid findings in Marshallese 22 years after exposure to radioactive fallout", Radiation-Associated Thyroid Carcinoma (DE GROOT, J., Ed.), Grune & Stratton, New York (1977) 241.

[2] CONARD, R.A., et al., A Twenty Year Review of Medical Findings in a Marshallese Population accidentally exposed to Radioactive Fallout, Rep. BNL 50424, Brookhaven National Laboratory, Upton, New York (Sep. 1975).

[3] CONARD, R.A., Acute myelogenous leukemia following fallout radiation exposure, J.Am. Med. Assoc. 232 (1975) 1356.

[4] SUTOW, W.W., CONARD, R.A., "The effects of fallout radiation on Marshallese children", Radiation Biology of the Fetal and Juvenile Mammal (Proc. 9th Ann. Hanford Biology Symp. Richland, 1969) (1969) 661.

[5] RALL, J.E., CONARD, R.A., Elevation of the serum protein-bound iodine level in inhabitants of the Marshall Islands, Am. J. Med. 40 (1966) 883.

[6]   HEMPELMANN, L.H., HALL, W.J., PHILLIPS, M., COOPER, R.A., AMES, W.R.,
      Neoplasms in persons treated with X-rays in infancy; Fourth survey in 20 years,
      J. Natl. Cancer Inst. **55** (1975) 519.
[7]   ROBBINS, J., RALL, J.E., CONARD, R.A., Late effects of radioactive iodine in fallout,
      Combined Clinical Staff Conference at the National Institutes of Health, Ann. Intern.
      Med. **66** (1967) 1214.
[8]   LARSEN, P.R., "Radioimmunoassay of thyroxine, triiodothyronine, and thyrotropin
      in human serum", Manual of Clinical Immunology (ROSE, N.R., FRIEDMAN, H., Eds),
      American Society for Microbiology, Washington (1976) 222.
[9]   SABERI, M., UTIGER, R.D., Augmentation of thyrotropin responses to thyrotropin
      releasing hormone following small decreases in serum thyroid hormone concentrations,
      J. Clin. Endocrinol. Metab. **40** (1975) 435.
[10] SAWIN, C.T., HERSHMAN, J.M., The TSH response to thyrotropin-releasing hormone
      (TRH) in young adult men: intra-individual variation and relation to basal serum TSH
      and thyroid hormones, J. Clin. Endocrinol. Metab. **42** (1976) 809.
[11] BIGOS, S.T., RIDGWAY, E.C., KOURIDES, I.A., MALOOF, F., The spectrum of
      pituitary alterations with mild and severe thyroid impairment., J. Clin. Endocrinol.
      Metab. (in press).
[12] MAXON, H.R., THOMAS, S.R., SAENGER, E.L., BUNCHER, C.R., KEREIAKES, J.G.,
      Ionizing irradiation and the induction of clinically significant disease in the human
      thyroid gland., Am. J. Med. **63** (1977) 967.
[13] BECKER, D.V., MC CONAHEY, W.M., DOBYNS, B.M., "The results of the thyrotoxicosis
      therapy followup study", Further Advances in Thyroid Research **1** (FELLINGER, K.,
      HOFER, R., Eds), Gistel G. et Cie, Vienna (1971) 603.
[14] UNITED STATES NUCLEAR REGULATORY COMMISSION, Reactor Safety Study,
      An Assessment of Accident Risks in U.S. Commercial Nuclear Power Plants, Appendix VI,
      Calculations of Reactor Accident Consequences, Rep. WASH 1400, NUREG-75/014,
      U.S. Nuclear Regulatory Commission, Washington (1975); Protection of the thyroid
      gland in the event of releases of radioiodine; Recommendations of the National
      Council on Radiation Protection and Measurements, NCRP Rep. No. 55, Washington
      (1977).

DISCUSSION

M. DELPLA: I wonder what reliance can be placed in the doses you
report, because I do not believe that 1000 rads, or even 1500, would have been
enough to suppress the hormonal activity of the thyroid gland of two children
contaminated when they were one year old. In fact, to obtain such a result,
doctors have to administer a dose of ^{131}I giving at least 100 000 rad. It is true
that this applies to adults, but all the same the dose difference appears considerable.

R.A. CONARD: There are uncertainties in the thyroid dose estimates in
the Marshallese, particularly in the children. I agree it would seem likely that
the two boys who developed myxoedema received higher doses than those
estimated to produce atrophy of the thyroid gland.

K. SHIMAOKA: The normal human thyroid is radioresistant as far as
thyroid function is concerned; patients with head and neck tumours treated by

radiation alone seldom develop hypothyroidism. However, there are two
populations of patients who may develop hypothyroidism following external
radiation therapy: those with head and neck tumours who received radiation
therapy following surgical manipulation, and those with malignant lymphoma
treated with radiation therapy after lymphoangiography. Since hypothyroidism
is usually associated with high doses of radiation to the thyroid, how do you
account for your findings with low doses?

   R.A. CONARD: In our studies we are using very sensitive tests for thyroid
function, and our findings indicate only biochemical or subclinical hypothyroidism
at present. If these sensitive tests were used in other cases following external
irradiation, perhaps such effects might be demonstrable.

   Y. NISHIWAKI: I also conducted an analysis in Japan of the highly
radioactive fall-out on the Japanese fishing boat that was engaged in fishing
about 80—90 miles east of Bikini at the time of the thermonuclear test conducted
early in the morning of 1 March 1954, and which returned to Japan in the middle
of the same month. According to the statements of some of the crew, a few
hours after the thermonuclear detonation in Bikini the whitish dust began to
fall on the boat so heavily that for a period they could hardly bear to open their
eyes and mouths. It continued to fall for several hours. Some of the crew
apparently tasted it, to see what it was, without knowing that it was highly
radioactive. Owing to the difficulty of dose estimation without more accurate
information on the initial condition, the radioactive fall-out conditions on the
boat were experimentally reproduced by M. Miyoshi, the chief physician in
charge of treatment of the exposed crew at the Tokyo University Hospital,
using pulverized coral reef. This experiment was carried out in the presence of
the crew as witnesses of the actual amount of ash which had fallen on the boat.
This amount was then estimated to be about $3.38-8.52$ mg/cm^2. The radioactivity
of the ash was estimated by extrapolation to be about 1 Ci/g at the time it fell
on the boat. Taking into consideration various possible exposure conditions
of the crew during the voyage, the probable gamma dose was estimated to be
in the range 170—600 rad. The degree of uncertainty was far greater for the
internal dose. The long-lived radionuclides detected in organs such as the liver
many weeks later could not be considered the only sources of internal exposure.
Depending on the assumed degree of initial incorporation of short-lived radionuclides, a wide range of estimates was possible: for the liver, a few rads to a
few tens of thousands of rads, the probable dose range being $10-10^4$ rads; and
for bone and bone marrow, a few rads to about 60 rads. If we assume a non-
uniformity factor of five for bone, the dose estimation could be five times
higher. I am pleased to see that the thyroid doses you estimated in your report
correspond more or less to our estimates in order of magnitude. However, I
assume there would be some uncertainty in this type of dose estimation. What
level of accuracy do you assign to your dose estimation? Did you also observe

other radiation syndromes such as radiodermatitis, epilation, decrease of leucocytes, decrease of spermatozoa, etc. in the exposed Marshallese?

R.A. CONARD: The thyroid doses in the Marshallese were based primarily on radio-iodine measurements in urine 15 days after exposure. Uncertainties included length of time of the fall-out, relative absorption from inhalation versus ingestion, etc. Therefore the doses are subject to error. The gamma doses received should be more accurate, as they are in agreement with the values estimated from the degree of haematological changes observed.

The skin lesions, epilation and haematological effects in the Marshallese were similar to those reported by your group for the Japanese fishermen and have been described elsewhere. We were not able to do sperm counts on the Marshallese. No doubt there must have been some degree of relative sterility soon after exposure, though in subsequent years fertility does not appear to have been impaired.

HUMAN STUDIES:
LATE EFFECTS DUE TO
MEDICAL EXPOSURE
Session 3 and Session 5, Part 1

FINDINGS IN CHILDREN AFTER RADIATION EXPOSURE IN UTERO FROM X-RAY EXAMINATION OF MOTHERS
Results from children studied after one to seven years

K. NEUMEISTER
Nuclear Safety and Radiation Protection Board
   of the German Democratic Republic,
Berlin,
German Democratic Republic

Abstract

FINDINGS IN CHILDREN AFTER RADIATION EXPOSURE IN UTERO FROM X-RAY
EXAMINATION OF MOTHERS: RESULTS FROM CHILDREN STUDIED AFTER ONE TO
SEVEN YEARS.

The biological-medical consequences of radiation exposures to low radiation doses in early
pregnancy due to X-ray diagnostics have been the subject of numerous, mostly casuistic scientific
investigations. So far there has been no uniform agreement on the conclusions. The dose range
between 1.5 and 10 rem is mostly discussed with respect to inducing deformations, functional
disturbances, disturbances of mental development, induction of carcinomas and leukaemias,
and an increase in morbidity and genetic damages. In the Nuclear Safety and Radiation Protection Board of the German Democratic Republic, a Central Advisory Centre headed by the author
has been established to cover the problems of interruption or maintenance of pregnancy after
radiation exposures in early pregnancy. So far more than 120 cases have been assessed. For
the assessment, a detailed case history covering the occupation, family history and personal
details of both parents was compiled, special attention being paid to hereditary diseases, deformations in the family and noxae that could also induce foetal damages (diseases, drugs, tobacco,
etc.). The time of conception and foetal radiation exposure were determined as exactly as
possible. Finally the foetal dose was measured at the phantom or calculated. In eight cases
pregnancy was interrupted (foetal dose above 10 rem). Pathomorphological examination of
foetal material showed developmental disturbances. Embryological examinations are in progress.
In co-operation with the Paediatric Clinic of the Leipzig Karl-Marx University (S. Wässer) a
systematic checking programme was developed, in which all children are subjected to paediatric
and laboratory examinations at fixed intervals up to their tenth year. It has thus become
possible to follow up scientifically almost all cases of radiation exposure in utero in the German
Democratic Republic. In this way evidence on damage within a dose range below 10 rem will
be obtained. Also, if there are health disturbances, all necessary medical measures can be
immediately and centrally taken without loss of time. The present results are obtained from
children examined between one and seven years after radiation exposure in utero. In four cases,
there were deviations from the norm in terms of deformations that could be surgically corrected.
Noteworthy was a reduction in birth weight compared with the norm in 37% of cases, retarded
bone development (carporadiogram) in 37% of cases and pronounced proneness to infection
in 74% of cases. In addition, biochemical-genetic and cytogenetic examinations were made
of 19 children who did not exhibit any deviations from the norm and represent the basic
material for the future F_1 generation. The extensive programme represents an attempt to
study systematically the problems of radiation exposure in utero and its consequences on a
national scale, and at the same time to arrange for suitable measures to be taken to prevent
such events.

The chief subjects of interest concerning radiobiological effects on the human foetus are (a) genetic effects, (b) somatic effects, and (c) somatic-stochastic effects (induction or favouring of malignant neoplasms, general increase in morbidity and mortality, etc.). As is well known, at the stage of blastogenesis (pre-implantation period), irradiations of the foetus with appropriate doses induce mainly prenatal foetal death with subsequent absorption, at the stage of embryogenesis (the main period of organ formation), mainly anomalies in the skeleton or organs, and at the stage of the foetal period (growth period) growth inhibitions or only histologically or functionally detectable disturbances. Apart from various malformations in the skeletal system and organs, damage to the central nervous system has in particular been described. In our own investigations retardations of physical development, and particularly a delayed development of the electrocorticogram and other central nervous functions could be proved in rats irradiated with 200 R on the 19th day of gestation [1].

The period from the 7th to 36th day after conception is considered to be a particularly radiosensitive phase of the human foetus [2, 3]. Within the first three weeks of pregnancy, foetal death is to be expected after irradiation with sufficiently high doses; between the 20th and 42nd day malformations are to be expected [4, 5]. Damage to the human foetus has been repeatedly described. A survey by Schaaf [6] covered 107 cases up to 1963, almost exclusively after therapeutic radiation exposures. A more recent survey has been given by Roedler-Vogelsang [7]. Literature on animal tests shows that the same radiation doses are effective to a different extent on different days of pregnancy, that the effects are dependent on irradiation dose and dose rate, and that no threshold dose can be detected. In animal tests, part of the damage during embryogenesis proved to be repairable.

Jacobsen [8] demonstrated in 3150 mouse foetuses that already doses of 5 R on the 8th day of gestation (corresponding to the 20th day of pregnancy in man) induce malformations, and he did not exclude an extrapolation of these results to human conditions. Rugh [9] described an 11% increase in the mortality and absorption rate in mice at irradiations with 5 R on the first day of gestation. In spite of the problem of extrapolating such values to human conditions, it has to be concluded that careful consideration, case by case, should be given to the interruption of pregnancy at foetal radiation exposure to low doses.

The extrapolation of the numerous results in test animals to human conditions is extraordinarily difficult and possible only with great reservation. The findings made in investigations of human beings are more interesting. Beside the problems already mentioned of the induction of malformations after exposure to sufficiently high radiation doses, problems of radiation-induced carcinoma and leukaemia in children exposed to radiation in utero and problems of genetic changes in the subsequent F_1 and F_2 generations have been discussed in the last few years. Based on epidemiological studies of the last 20 years, a hazard of the

TABLE I.   LEUKAEMIA IN CHILDREN AFTER EXPOSURE IN UTERO
TO DIAGNOSTIC X-RAYS

Reference	Leukaemia group			Control group			Relative risk
	Total	Exposed	%	Total	Exposed	%	
[10]	78	21	26.9	306	56	18.3	1.64
[11]	251	69	27.5	251	58	23.1	1.26
[12]	304	47	15.5	7242	770	10.6	1.55
[13]	313	27	8.6	854	54	6.3	1.40
[15]	2947	458	15.5	6347	645	10.2	1.61

order of 1.6 to 2.0 compared with controls (see also Table I) was reported for
radiation-induced carcinoma and leukaemia in children after exposure to small
radiation doses (X-ray diagnostics) in utero [10−15]. These results did not pass
unchallenged [3]. Furthermore, an increase in infantile mortality (without classification of causes) by a factor of 1.86 was found [16, 17]. In the Japanese
children exposed to the atom bomb explosion in utero, a striking increase in the
mortality rate could be proved only at high radiation doses for the first 10 years
of life [18].

Highly detailed epidemiological studies have been undertaken by the group
of Meyer [19]. They cover 1458 women, who were exposed to irradiation with
small doses in utero through X-ray diagnostic examination of their mothers.
Their further development and the subsequent F_1 generation were followed up
from the epidemiological aspect but without clinical or genetic investigations.
In comparison with carefully selected controls, there were significantly more
pregnancies in the women irradiated in utero, and the more markedly so, the
younger the women observed. The authors try to explain their findings by the
assumption that ionizing radiation at an especially critical time in prenatal life
damages some oocytes, but at the same time stimulates the development of
undamaged oocytes so that after menarche there could be more conceptive
oocytes than in controls. Increased disturbances in health could not be clearly
proved statistically in this group of persons. Such epidemiological studies are
difficult to perform and, as a result, dependent on numerous factors of influence.

The working group of Oppenheim [20] tried to supply evidence in a similar
study (939 persons) with comparable radiation exposure in utero, although at
the end of pregnancy (X-ray examination of the pelvis), that is, in a phase of
lower foetal radiosensitivity. However, no increase in radiation-induced diseases
could be found in these persons exposed in utero. Contradictory results of other
authors were explained by errors in selection.

Nokkentved [21] followed up the development of 152 children who had been exposed to an irradiation of between 0.2 and 7.1 R in the first four months of their foetal life. In comparison with the malformation rate in the entire population of Denmark and with non-irradiated siblings, no increase in anomalies or developmental disturbances could be detected in these children. Only a lower birth weight was noted. Of course, no discussion of dose-effect relations was possible, since there were no dose estimations for the single cases.

Thus the biological-medical effects of radiation exposures to small doses in early pregnancy (occupational radiation exposure, exposures from X-ray diagnostics, nuclear-medical or radiotherapeutic measures) have been the subject of various investigations. So far there have been no agreed conclusions. In the centre of discussions is the dose range between 1.5 to 10 R with regard to inducing malformations, functional disturbances, carcinoma formation, increase in morbidity and genetic damage.

In the German Democratic Republic, an advisory centre for problems of interruption or continuation of pregnancy after radiation exposures in early pregnancy or preconceptional gonad exposure of a parent has been introduced under the author's management by the Nuclear Safety and Radiation Protection Board in Berlin. From this work (120 cases so far) more than 70 expert opinions on radiation exposure in utero will be analysed below. Out of these, 37 cases date back to the period from 1970 to 1975 before this advisory centre had been opened [22].

For the purpose of assessment, a detailed case history regarding occupation, family and life-history was drawn up for both marriage partners, particular attention being paid to hereditary diseases, malformations in the family and to noxae that could also possibly damage the foetus (diseases, drugs, tobacco, alcohol, etc.). The time of conception and foetal radiation exposure were determined as exactly as possible. Finally the foetal dose was calculated or measured in a phantom [23–27].

FINDINGS

In 23 cases (examinations after the 6th week) a pregnancy should have been considered possible. The indications for X-ray examinations had been carefully made in almost all cases. Possibilities of gonad protection, however, were not always made use of.

The individual determination of the foetal dose shows that, depending on the X-ray set-up, physical-technical conditions of X-ray photographing or screening and individual constitution, highly different exposures result (Table II). The highest foetal dosages were determined for the examination methods where the foetus lay in the useful beam (gastro-intestinal tract, intravenous pyelography, hysterosalpingography, cholesystography).

TABLE II. FOETAL DOSES AT RADIATION EXPOSURES IN EARLY PREGNANCY

56 cases up to 15 January 1977

Type of radiation exposure	Number of examinations [a]	Foetal dose
Thorax	7	0.1 − 0.2 R
Lumbar spine	9	0.2 − 1.2 R
Pelvis	6	0.2 − 0.5 R
Tract of stomach and intestine	13	0.1 − 18 R(!)
Colon contrastive agent	1	2.5 R
Cholecystogram	13	0.2 − 6 R
iv pyelogram	9	1 − 8 R
Pelvis − leg arteriogram	1	1 R
Leg venogram	2	1 R
Aortogram	1	3.5 R
Hysterosalpingogram	3	1.2 − 8.6 R
Isotope nephrogram (^{131}I-hippurate/^{197}Hg-neohydrine)	1	1 − 7 R (?)
Telecobalt therapy in case of lymphogranulomatosis	1	20 R
Occupational exposure (X-ray diagnostics)	3	1 R

[a] In some cases there were combinations of several X-ray examinations.

Results interesting from the clinical point of view are listed in Table III. In addition it should be mentioned that an interruption of pregnancy has been made in eight cases so far. In three of these cases the interruption had been applied for by the patient against our recommendation, although there were only very small foetal exposures. In addition, there were three cases of spontaneous abortion.

In one case of an interruption applied for by us (see Table III) (a patient with a typically high foetal exposure at gall-bladder and kidney X-ray examination), a pathological-anatomic investigation of the foetus was possible. Its result showed an underdeveloped foetus without macroscopically detectable malformations (foetal exposure in the 16th week = growth period: about 11 R).

TABLE III. MEDICAL OPINIONS ON RADIATION EXPOSURE IN EARLY PREGNANCY

Name	Age Female	Male	Anamnesis	Foetal date	Radiation exposure Type	Dose	Interruption	Special features	Pathological-anatomical findings/age of foetus at this time
H.P.	27	33	Without findings	2nd week	iv pyelogram	5 R	No	Myelomeningocele lumbosacralis	–
J.L.	27	29	Without findings	4th–6th week	Cholecystogram	1 R	No	Talipes calcaneus	–
J.H.	19	18	Without findings	8th week	X-ray of stomach	1 R	Yes (application of patient)	–	No examination
C.U.	22	28	Without findings	6th week	Right ankle joint	0.1 R	Yes (application of patient)	–	No examination
J.W.	16	24	Without findings	16th week	Thorax, cholecystogram iv pyelogram	10.2 R	Yes	Small, slender woman	Male foetus: 230 g, 20.5 cm, no internal and external malformations (6th month) = underdeveloped foetus
K.L.	32	36	Without findings	7th week	Cholecystogram, X-ray of stomach	18 R	Yes	Unfavourable examination conditions	Embryotomy no examination
M.B.	21	23	Without findings	1st week	Telecobalt therapy at lymphogranulo-	20 R	Yes	–	No examination

TABLE IV.   FINDINGS IN CHILDREN AFTER RADIATION EXPOSURE
IN UTERO

Foetal exposure	No.	Decreased weight/size at birth [a]	Carporadiogram: lower limit of reference	Malformations	High proneness to infection
1 R	13	4 (0.31)	4 (0.31)	3 (0.23)	10 (0.77)
2 R	2	1 (0.50)	2 (1.0)	–	1 (0.50)
3 R	2	1 (0.50)	–	–	1 (0.50)
5 R	1	1	1	1	1
7 R	1	–	–	–	1
Total	19	7 (0.37)	7 (0.37)	4 (0.21)	14 (0.74)

[a] <3000 g/<49 cm/birth date $\pm$ 10 d around the date calculated; decrease by $\overline{x} = 300$ g (100–600 g); shortening by $\overline{x} = 2$ cm.

Four cases of foetal radiation exposure by nuclear-medical diagnostics did not
exhibit any special characteristics. There were four cases of occupational radiation
exposure during early pregnancy. In one of these cases disciplinary measures had
to be taken.

RE-EXAMINATIONS

The conditions resulting from radiation exposures of the human foetus in
early pregnancy have been the subject of separate investigations.

A survey of recent literature and a detailed presentation of problems can be
found in Neumeister [28–30]. In this study, first examinations made by the
author on children after radiation exposure in utero, based on a questionnaire,
were reported. In co-operation with the paediatric clinic of the Leipzig Karl-Marx
University (S. Wässer), a systematic re-examination programme has been drawn
up in the meantime, subjecting all children up to their 10th year of life to
paediatric and laboratory examinations at set intervals. It thus becomes possible to
follow up scientifically almost all cases of in-utero radiation exposure in the
German Democratic Republic. In this way evidence should be obtained on the
above-mentioned problems of damage within the dose range below 10 rem, and in
addition all necessary medical measures can be taken immediately and centrally
in case of health disturbances.

TABLE V. SPECIAL FINDINGS IN CHILDREN AFTER EXPOSURE IN UTERO

Name/ dose/ date	Brothers/ sisters	Process of pregnancy/ date of birth	Weight/ size at birth	Fully developed at birth	Sex/age at time examination	Malformations/ other findings	Diseases, chronic disturbances	Physical and mental development	Carporadiogram	Haemogram
R.R., 0.5 R, 3rd week	No	Normal/ − 10 d	2960 g, 52 cm	Yes	♀ 1 y 5 m	Talipes calcaneus	Prone to infection	Normal	Normal	Without findings
J.L., 1 R, 4th–6th week	No	Normal/ + 10 d	3350 g, 52 cm	Yes	♀ 1 y 7 m	Talipes calcaneus	Prone to infection	Normal	Normal	Without findings
G.H., 1 R, 7th week	No	Normal/ + 10 d	3490 g, 51 cm	Yes	♂ 1 y	Talipes calcaneus et valgus	No	Normal	Lower limit of reference	Without findings
H.P., 5 R, 2nd week	No	Premature birth/ − 7 d	2460 g, 47 cm	No	♀ 1 y 8 m	Myelomeningocele lumbosacralis, talipes calcaneus, struma	No	Under- developed (− 10 cm)	Lower limit of reference	Without findings

The extensive programme is an attempt to study systematically the problems of radiation exposure in utero and its effects on a national scale and, at the same time, to organize corresponding measures to avoid such events.

Within the framework of this systematic after-care programme, at first 19 children between 10 months and $7\frac{1}{2}$ years of age were subjected to a single extensive re-examination in a pilot study [31]. The findings deviating from normal ones are listed in Table IV. The results are as follows: The process of pregnancy was normal. At the time of birth there were signs of full development. Deviations in birth date lay within the range of physiological variations. Within the examination period, the children's physical and mental development was normal (for exceptions see Table V). There were no chronic health disturbances. The blood count was normal (pre-leukaemia diagnostics). There were no differences in comparison with siblings. In seven out of 19 cases the birth weight was below 3000 g. In this pilot study, the date of gestation could not be taken into consideration. The influence of smoking was excluded, as well as that of other noxae. In the carporadiogram, seven out of 19 children showed a bone development at the lower limit of the norm. In 14 out of 19 cases there was a high proneness to infections. Four out of 19 children had malformations or other deviations from the norm. These findings could be observed also at foetal exposures around 1 R in the 1st to 6th week (see Table IV).

Because of the small number of cases studied so far it is too early to comment on the question whether they exhibit radiation-induced effects, although the effects observed, mostly, however, in casuistic reports after higher doses, have been repeatedly described in literature as induced by radiation [30].

We wish to make this reservation, for the time being, also in assessing the malformations found (Table V). In case No.4, of course, there was an exposure to 5 R, but the time of irradiation does not correspond with that of the differentiation of the respective organ. All changes observed (malformations, postural anomalies) could be surgically corrected.

The paediatric examinations of the 19 children were supplemented by cytogenetic and biochemical-genetic investigations. Thus additional information at the cellular level was obtained in order to be better able to determine and assess responses to small-dose irradiation.

Chromosomal investigations of lymphocytes (banding technique) showed the following results (Table VI): Essential deviations from the norm could not be determined. The investigation of biochemical-genetic markers implied the following consequences: (1) Registration of basis material for long-term observation of these children and their offspring; (2) Exclusion of any influence on markers by irradiation in the first weeks of foetal development (complex of problems: heredity and environmental influences).

TABLE VI. CYTOGENETIC FINDINGS IN CHILDREN AFTER EXPOSURE IN UTERO

Specimen	Number of examined metaphases	Number of cells with 46 chromosomes	Status of chromosomes	Chromatid breaks and gaps	Fragments	Other chromosome aberrations
1	100	89	46, XX	0	0	0
3	100	89	46, XX	0	0	0
4	100	95	46, XY	2	0	0
5	100	93	46, XY	1	1	1
6	100	91	46, XY	1	0	0
7	100	91	46, XY	0	1	0
8	100	87	46, XX	2	0	0
9	100	88	46, XY	0	0	0
10	100	90	46, XX	0	0	0
11	100	90	46, XY	4	0	0
13	100	92	46, XY	1	0	0
14	50	47	46, XY	0	1	0
15	100	8	47, XX, + 21	2	0	0
16	100	94	46, XX	0	0	0
17	100	91	46, XX	0	0	0
18	100	95	46, XX	0	0	0
19	100	90	46, XX	0	0	0
20	50	48	46, XY	0	0	0

TABLE VII. BIOCHEMICAL-GENETICAL MARKERS EXAMINED

Enzyme markers:	Acid erythrocyte phosphatase (AEP)
	Adenylate kinase (AK)
	Phosphoglucomutase (PGM_1)
	Adenosine desaminase (ADA)
	Glutamate-pyruvate transaminase (GPT)
	Esterase D (EsD)
System of blood groups:	ABO, MN, S, P, Rh, K
Serum groups:	Gm, Hp, Inv, Tf, C3, Gc
HLA-System	
Electrophoretic positions of haemoglobin and albumin	

Twenty-one markers were studied (Table VII). The genetic enzyme markers were determined for the following enzymes:

(1) Acid erythrocyte phosphatase (AEP)
(2) Adenylate kinase (AK)
(3) Phosphoglucomutase (PGM_1)
(4) Adenosine desaminase (ADA)
(5) Glutamate-pyruvate transaminase (GPT)
(6) Esterase D (EsD)

The findings are listed below.

(1) Out of the 6 different phenotypes of this enzyme occurring in European populations (A, BA, B, CA, CB and C), in the children examined were found:
      type A,   11%
      type AB, 32%
      type B,   42%
      type BC, 15%
(2) Type 1 prevailed with 95%.
(3) 14 children were of type PGM_1 1, 74%, and
    5 children were of type PGM_1 2−1, 26%.
(4) Type 2−1, 26%; type 1, 74%.
(5) The two phenotypes 2−1, 2 and 1 occurred in normal distribution.
(6) Type 1 prevailed with 74%, the remaining 26% being represented by type 2−1.

The following blood groups were studied:

(1) ABO system
(2) MN system

TABLE VIII.   DISTRIBUTION OF ENZYME MARKERS

Enzyme markers	Phenotypes	Observed types	Distribution
AEP	A, BA, B, CA BC, C	A, AB, B, BC	A = 11% AB = 32% B = 42% BC = 15%
AK	1; 2−1; 2; 3−1	1; 2−1	1 = 95% 2−1 = 5%
PGM$_1$	1; 2−1; 2	1; 2−1; 2	1 = 74% 2−1 = 26%
ADA	1; 2−1; 2	1; 2−1	1 = 74% 2−1 = 26%
GPT	1; 2−1; 2	1; 2−1; 2	1 = 42% 2−1 = 26% 2 = 32%
EsD	1; 2−1; 2	1; 2−1	1 = 74% 2−1 = 26%

In the German population the frequency of these factors is distributed as follows: M = 30%, MN = 50%, N = 20%. The distribution in the children examined was: M = 29%, MN = 29%, N = 42%.

(3)   S system
(4)   P system
(5)   Rh factor
(6)   Kell system (K) = 2 children exhibited the Kell factor (K+) = 8%, 92% were K

The following serum groups were determined:

(1)   Gm factors
(2)   Haptoglobin variants: The children examined were of the type Hp 1−1, 4%, of the type 2−2, 29%, and of the type 2−1, 67%.
(3)   Inv system
(4)   Transferring groups: In Central European populations the C type occurs with 94 to 96%; this was confirmed by the present study (100% C type).

(5) C3 group: This group belongs to the immunologically important complementary system and lies within the beta globulin range. Of the children
studied 5% were of the F type, 20% of the FS type and 75% of the S type.
(6) Gc proteins: Gc 1—1 was represented with 50%, Gc 2—1 with 45% and Gc 2—2
with 5%.

In the investigation of haemoglobin and albumin both markers had the
normal electrophoretic position in all samples. The study of the HLA (human
leucocyte locus A) system showed normal distribution.

The distribution of especially interesting enzyme markers in percentages
is shown in Table VIII.

The results of the biochemical-genetic investigations can be summarized as
follows: Quality and type of marker types determined correspond to the normal
distribution in the European population. No deviations from normal can be
detected. Thus the basis material has been obtained, and the potential changes
according to the second consequence mentioned above, did not occur. It is
probable that damage in the genetic control system (occurrence of unexpected
homozygotes due to deletion of a gene site) cannot be unambiguously excluded
without studying all relatives. These studies will be made in selected cases
(malformations).

A summary assessment of the results reported in literature so far shows that
damage to the human foetus at a sufficiently high dose has been proved. In the
range of small radiation doses as usual during X-ray diagnostics and nuclear-medical
measures the proof of the type and extent of radiation damage to the human
foetus cannot yet be considered as concluded, but epidemiological studies and so on
indicate an increased hazard of carcinoma and leukaemia as well as an increased
morbidity and mortality. In addition there are the main radiogenetic considerations calling for an avoidance of any radiation exposure of gonads, the gonads in
prenatal life being especially radiosensitive.

CONCLUSIONS

The following conclusions can be drawn:

(1) According to our investigations, radiation exposures in early pregnancy from
X-ray diagnostics almost always lead to foetal doses which, according to the
present state of knowledge about the occurrence of malformations, do not
make an interruption necessary. The considerable individual differences in
foetal doses at comparable exposures, however, make it necessary to calculate
exactly foetal exposure in every case and to make a decision accordingly.

(2)   As literature on animal tests unanimously rejects a so-called threshold dose
      for foetal damage after irradiation in early pregnancy, and epidemiological
      studies in man indicate an increased carcinoma and leukaemia hazard, it is
      definitely necessary, however, to avoid radiation exposures in early
      pregnancy. More attention should be paid to the rule of X-ray examinations
      of the female abdomen only within the first 10 days after menstruation in
      order to avoid irradiations of unknown pregnancies.

(3)   Present findings enable us to recommend as before an interruption at foetal
      exposure of above 10 R. At lower radiation exposures an interruption
      should be advised in case of additional noxae [22, 28–30].

(4)   The results of cytogenetic and biochemical-genetic investigations also suggest
      this recommendation.

(5)   The studies are being continued. It is intended to examine regularly if possibl
      all children in the German Democratic Republic for several years after radia-
      tion exposure in utero to obtain further information on whether it is necessar
      to change the value of 10 R (problems of carcinoma induction, increase in
      morbidity, etc.).

(6)   Within the framework of further education in radiation protection of
      physicians in the German Democratic Republic, special seminars on the
      problems of radiation exposure in pregnancy have been introduced by the
      Nuclear Safety and Radiation Protection Board in favour of improved
      prophylactic work.

ACKNOWLEDGEMENTS

We wish to thank S. Wässer, L. Brüning, H. Baumann, G. Geserick, G. Radam,
H. Strauch, H. Waltz, S. Hähnel and C. Niemiec for their assistance.

REFERENCES

[1]   KLINGENBERG, F., PICKENHAIN, L., NEUMEISTER, K., Acta Biol. Med. Ger. **19**
      (1967) 503.
[2]   FRITZ-NIGGLI, H., Strahlenbiologie, Georg Thieme Verlag, Stuttgart (1959).
[3]   STIEVE, F.E., Roentgen-Bl. **29** (1976) 465.
[4]   RUGH, R., Am. J. Roentgenol., Radium Ther. Nucl. Med. **89** (1963) 182.
[5]   RUGH, R., WOHLFROMM, M., Radiat. Res. **26** (1965) 493.
[6]   SCHAAF, H.O., Strahlenembryopathie, Dissertation, University of Bonn, 1966.
[7]   ROEDLER-VOGELSANG, T., STH-Bericht 10/1977.
[8]   JACOBSEN, L., Low Dose X-Irradiation and Teratogenesis, Verlag Munksgaard,
      Copenhagen (1968).
[9]   RUGH, R., GRUPP, E., J. Exp. Zool. **141** (1959) 571.
[10] FORD, D.D., PATHERSON, J.C., TREUTING, W.L., J. Natl. Cancer Inst. **22** (1959) 1093.
[11] POLHEMUS, D.W., KOCH, R., Pediatrics **23** (1959) 453.
[12] MACMAHON, B., J. Natl. Cancer Inst. **28** (1962) 1173.

[13] GRAHAM, S., LEVIN, M.L., LILIENFELD, A.M., SCHUMANN, L.M., GIBSON, R.,
      DOWD, J.E., HEMPELMANN, L., Natl. Cancer Inst. Monogr. **19** (1966) 347.
[14] STEWART, A., WEBB, J., HEWITT, D., Br.Med. J. i (1958) 1495.
[15] STEWART, A., KNEALE, G.W., Lancet i (1968) 104.
[16] LILIENFELD, A.M., Yale J. Biol. Med. **39** (1966) 143.
[17] DIAMOND, E.L., SCHWERLER, H., LILIENFELD, A.M., Am. J. Epidemiol. **97** (1973)
      283.
[18] KATO, H., Am. J. Epidemiol. **93** (1971) 435.
[19] MEYER, M.B., TONASCIA, J.A., MERZ, T., "Long-term effects of prenatal X ray on
      development and fertility of human females", Biological and Environmental Effects of
      Low-Level Radiation **II** (Proc. Symp. Chicago, 1975), IAEA, Vienna (1976) 273.
[20] OPPENHEIM, B.E., GRIEM, M.L., MEIER, P., "An investigation of effects of prenatal
      exposure to diagnostic X rays", Biological and Environmental Effects of Low-Level
      Radiation **II** (Proc. Symp. Chicago, 1975), IAEA, Vienna (1976) 249.
[21] NOKKENTVED, K., Effects of Diagnostic Radiation Upon the Human Fetus, Verlag
      Munksgaard, Copenhagen (1968).
[22] NEUMEISTER, K., TIETZE, B., GURSKY, S., Dtsch. Gesundheitsw. **27** (1972) 549.
[23] BRÜNING, L., Erprobung einer indirekten Methode zur Ermittlung der Gonadendosis
      bei röntgendiagnostischen Untersuchungen, Forschungsbericht Staatliches Amt für
      Atomsicherheit und Strahlenschutz der DDR Berlin (1969).
[24] GURSKY, S., Messung der Strahlenbelastung des Patienten bei röntgen-diagnostischen
      Untersuchungen mittels großflächiger Ionisationskammer, Dissertation B, Technische
      Hochschule Ilmenau, 1973.
[25] HELLER, M.B., TERDMAN, J.F., PASTERNACK, B.S., Br. J. Radiol. **39** (1966) 686.
[26] JACKSON, W., Br. J. Radiol. **40** (1967) 301.
[27] JACKSON, W., Br. J. Radiol. **42** (1969) 231.
[28] NEUMEISTER, K., "Problems arising from effects of low radiation doses in early
      pregnancy", Biological and Environmental Effects of Low-Level Radiation **II** (Proc.
      Symp. Chicago, 1975), IAEA, Vienna (1976) 261.
[29] NEUMEISTER, K., Med. Akt. **2** (1976) 490.
[30] NEUMEISTER, K., Report SAAS-203, Staatliches Amt für Atomsicherheit und Strahlen-
      schutz der DDR (1976).
[31] NEUMEISTER, K., WÄSSER, S., Proc. IVth International Congress of International
      Radiation Protection Association, Paris **3** (1977) 895.

DISCUSSION

V. VOLF: You recommend an interruption of pregnancy when the foetal
radiation exposure exceeds 10 rads. How accurate are the estimates of the foetal
radiation doses?

K. NEUMEISTER: Estimation of the foetal radiation dose is very difficult.
In some cases there might be an error of about 50%, while in others the estimates
are very accurate.

Y.J. KIM: I have two questions. First, according to Table VI showing your
cytogenetic findings, you examined 100 metaphases in most cases, yet the number
of cells with 46 chromosomes, chromatid breaks and other chromosome aberrations analysed do not come to 100. Could you please explain the reason for this?

Second, in your enzyme studies you found that the percentage of PGM_1 hetero-zygote was 26%. What is the percentage in a normal population?

K. NEUMEISTER: I am sorry that I cannot answer these questions at the moment, as these are only preliminary results. The investigations are still going on.

R.E. LINNEMANN: I would take issue with your 'ten-day' rule. I believe that if a woman of childbearing age needs an X-ray, it should be obtained, no matter the time of menses. If she doesn't need an X-ray, she shouldn't have one. Sometimes waiting to take an X-ray until the first ten days following start of menses may mean that you deliver the radiation during the most sensitive period of gestation — organogenesis — if the woman turns out to be pregnant. Also we don't know the leukaemogenic effect of radiation delivered to the ova just before conception.

K. NEUMEISTER: The ten-day rule is necessary. It is a protection for unknown pregnancy (after the tenth day). I'm afraid I dont' share your opinion. Leukaemogenic effects of radiation to the ova just before conception are not described in the literature.

M. DELPLA: You have attributed the pathology observed to irradiation. In fact, for such a conclusion to be valid, you would need to have compared the irradiated group with a control group and to have formed these two groups by selecting people at random from the population. Since this was not apparently done, I should have preferred to see a note of reservation in your conclusions.

PROBLEMS OF MALIGNOMA INDUCTION FOLLOWING RADIATION EXPOSURE OF THE THYROID

K. NEUMEISTER
Nuclear Safety and Radiation Protection
    Board of the German Democratic Republic,
Berlin

H.J. CORRENS
Nuclear Medicine Clinic of the
    Humboldt University,
Berlin,
German Democratic Republic

Abstract

PROBLEMS OF MALIGNOMA INDUCTION FOLLOWING RADIATION EXPOSURE
OF THE THYROID.
    Since the 1950s, reports have been published again and again in literature on the
radiation induction of malignomas in the thyroid. Most of these publications represent
exclusively casuistic studies and in many cases it is not possible, because dose effect analyses
are missing, to compare the results of the various working groups. The epidemiological
studies made so far cannot be considered as completed. Therefore uniform conclusions and
recommendations cannot be drawn from the literature. This also holds true for the problems
of how far an especially high radiosensitivity with respect to radiation-induced malignomas
can be assumed for the thyroid or these frequent occurrences can be considered as accidental.
Within the framework of recent systematic investigations on problems of radiocarcinogenesis
following diagnostic or therapeutic application of ionizing radiation in the German Democratic
Republic, an analysis was made of the problem of the radiation induction of malignomas
in the thyroid. More than 300 cases of thyroid carcinomas from nuclear medicine and
radiological institutions in the universities of Berlin, Jena and Greifswald have been analysed
so far. From all cases, the present state of analysis yields 13 malignomas of the thyroid with
radiation exposures in anamnesis with a latent period of up to 47 years. The examinations of
this group were completed by January 1978. Pathomorphological and clinical analysis showed
in these cases mainly carcinomas. The clinical development did not differ from the well-known
development of this type of tumour. The examinations are continuing with the aim of obtaining
reliable dose-effect relations and working out recommendations for radiation-protection
medicine and for therapy with ionizing radiation.

EARLIER INVESTIGATIONS

Results of animal tests indicate that almost all tissues can be stimulated to malignant growth by ionizing radiation. Radiation-induced thyroid carcinomas were registered among the survivors of the atom-bomb explosions in Hiroshima and Nagasaki but also among the population of the Marshall Islands who, by the explosion of an atom bomb in 1954, were exposed to an increased fall-out of ^{131}I and a number of short-lived iodine isotopes ([133]I, [132]I, [135]I). This survey also covers the thyroid carcinomas occurring in patients subjected to radiotherapeutic measures in their childhood. In the cases described, the indication for radiotherapy was given by a hyperplasia of the thymus gland or an infection of *tinea capitis*.

The assessed hazard that may be inferred from the given examination results has been reported by UNSCEAR [1] to be 50 to 150×10^{-6} rad^{-1} within an observation period of an average 25 years after radiation exposure. An exception in this respect is the relatively low rate of thyroid carcinoma among the survivors of Hiroshima and Nagasaki. In 1974 Parker and co-workers [2] published the results of their hazard calculations for this group of persons. The authors assessed the hazard to be 37×10^{-6} rad^{-1} (observation period: $13-26$ years). The potential causes given by the authors for the low hazard are as follows:
(1) Incomplete registration of thyroid tumours in autopsy; and (2) the high rate of thyroid carcinomas in the control population. The control population consisted of persons who were not present in the two cities during the atomic explosion and of persons who were exposed to a radiation of below 1 rad. For the entire Japanese population, however, a value has been determined which lies below that of the control population. UNSCEAR [1] assesses, however, that these two reasons do not suffice to exclude other causal connections.

In their analyses, Parker and co-workers [2] and Hempelmann and co-workers [3] measured a 2.3-times higher induction rate per dose unit absorbed in women compared with that in men. UNSCEAR [1] assesses the hazard for women to be higher by the factor 2 to 2.5 than that for men. The investigations of Wood and co-workers [4] also confirmed this fact but with the qualification that this sex-dependent hazard could not be proved for persons who were younger than 20 years at the time of increased radiation exposure. This suggests a connection with endocrine processes and does not directly contradict the results mentioned above. In their investigations on the Marshall Islands, Conard and co-workers [5] measured a frequency of 5.4 (2.5 to 10.2)% for women and one of 0.0 (0.0 to 2.7)% for men.

The results of analogous studies on carcinoma induction with respect to age-specific induction rates suggest similar attention has been given to these special problems. In Japan Parker and co-workers [2] found a 4.1 ± 2.1-times higher rate for persons who were younger than 10 years at the time of the atomic explosion than for the group of persons who were older than 20 years. This study covered both men and women. In these problems, however, there is a factor of uncertainty resulting from indications that the latency for tumour induction is prolonged with reaching adult age. On the other hand, some of the persons will die of other causes before a carcinoma can develop. A final answer to this question will be possible only in the future, depending on later investigations. Deviating results with respect to the age-specific induction rate were found in re-examinations on the Marshall Islands. For persons exposed to radioactive iodine at childhood, Conard and co-workers [5] found a hazard of 80 (15 to 260) $\times 10^{-6}$ rad^{-1} compared with that of 180 (80 to 740) $\times 10^{-6}$ rad^{-1} for persons who were older than 17 years at the time of fall-out (observation period: 21 years). In this case the hazard for children is only about 0.4-fold compared with that for adults. This fact is interpreted by Conard as follows: The smaller size of the critical organ in children led to an increased radiation exposure at the same fall-out concentrations. Decreased thyroid functions indicate an increased mortification rate of thyroid cells, which involves a smaller risk of malignant degenerations. On the other hand, it should of course be pointed out in this case that the therapy applied in such cases — among others by means of hormonal treatment — may have suppressed the development of thyroid carcinomas.

Colman and co-workers [6] made extensive re-observations on 1200 persons who, between 1938 and 1955, had been subjected to radiotherapy in the region of the tonsils or nasopharynx because of inflammatory diseases (doses: 50 to 1500 rads — 80% of cases) or because of other indications in the head-neck region. Significant changes in the thyroid region were found by nuclear-medical examinations in 288 cases, i.e. in 24.2%. Out of these, 186 were subjected to surgical treatment. In 61 cases (5.1%) thyroid carcinomas were found. By means of back calculations, radiation exposure could be determined for the individual cases. A correlation was found between the frequency of thyroid changes and the dose applied. In surgically treated patients the frequency of thyroid carcinomas was 8.6 (± 1.2) % in those who had been exposed to a radiation of 700 to 750 rads. In patients exposed to 1300 to 1500 rads the frequency of carcinomas rose to 19.4 (± 6.1) %. The hazard of thyroid carcinomas derived from these values for a mean dose of 783 rads (50 to 1500 rads) and a mean observation period of about 28 years (19 to 35 years) was 3.7×10^{-6} rad^{-1} a^{-1}.

Among a group of 10 902 persons who had been exposed to irradiations of head and neck because of *tinea capitis* during childhood, Modan and co-workers [7] registered a total of 12 thyroid carcinomas. The observation period after exposure lay between 12 and 24 years. In a control group also consisting of 10 902 persons of the same age, sex, native country and date of immigration into Israel, only two thyroid carcinomas were found. The skin of the head of children suffering from *tinea capitis* had been exposed in five fields to 350 to 400 rads each on different days. Detailed measurements at a phantom

TABLE I. LIST OF CASES STUDIED

No.	Name	Sex	Radiation exposure	Assessed dose in thyroid (approximate) (rads)	Age at radiation exposure	Age at tumour detection	Diagnosis
1	R, HJ	M	X- and radium irradiation for fibrosarcoma of epipharynx	3000	13	49	Thyroid carcinoma
2	R, E	F	X- and radium irradiation for haemangioma at the neck	2000–3000	1	30	Follicular carcinoma
3	Q, H	F	X-irradiation for neck-lymph-node tuberculosis	500–600	3	42	Thyroid carcinoma; in 1957 and 1962 plate-epithelial carcinoma of the skin in irradiated region
4	G, C	M	X-irradiation for laryngeal carcinoma	3000	58	84	Thyroid carcinoma
5	D, R	F	X-irradiation for neck-lymph-node tuberculosis	500–600	35	56	Follicular carcinoma
6	B, A	F	X-irradiation for struma	1600	19	36	Papillary carcinoma
7	B, Ag	F	X-irradiation for struma	1700	30	73	Hürthlezell tumour
8	T, J	F	X-irradiation for neck-lymph-node tuberculosis	600	7	54	Thyroid carcinoma (follicular-papillar)
9	M, M	F	X-irradiation for thyroid carcinoma	3000	39	53	Adenoma with metastases in the lungs
10	J, M	F	X-irradiation for haemangioma at the neck	3000	2	9	Adenoma of the thyroid with metastases

No.	Name	Sex	Radiation exposure	Assessed dose in thyroid (approximate) (rads)	Age at radiation exposure	Age at tumour detection	Diagnosis
11	P, N	F	X-irradiation for hyperthyreosis	900	31	48	Follicular carcinoma with metastases in the bones
12	A, N	F	X-irradiation for haemangioma at the neck	2000–3000	3	18	Intravasated thyroid carcinoma
13	D, N	F	X-irradiation for hyperthyreosis	1500	28	44	Follicular carcinoma with metastases in the bones

made by Werner and co-workers [8] showed, for this type of therapy, a thyroid dose of about 6.2 to 7.4 rads. The respective induction rate derived by Modan and co-workers [7] was 140 ($\pm$ 50) $\times$ 10^{-6} rad^{-1}. Harley and co-workers [9] also made assessments of the dose affecting the thyroid and pituitary gland and other organs of the head in children subjected to X-ray epilation because of *tinea capitis.* The dose measurements were performed by means of a child's-head phantom and thermoluminescence dose meters. For the conventional performance of this radiotherapy, a dose at the thyroid of about 6 $\pm$ 2 rads was estimated. This value agrees well with the dose assessment made earlier by Werner and co-workers [8]. Harley and co-workers [9] analysed neoplasm formation in the thyroid gland for various results given in the literature, and came to the conclusion that neoplasm formation in the thyroid after irradiation in childhood can be described by a linear dose-effect curve.

Hempelmann and co-workers [3] made re-examinations in persons who had been subjected to irradiation in early childhood because of hyperplasia of the thymus gland. The authors derived a hazard of 100 ($\pm$ 50) $\times$ 10^{-6} rad^{-1} within a latency of 20 years.

THE PRESENT STUDY

During recent systematic investigations in the German Democratic Republic on problems of radiocarcinogenesis after diagnostic and therapeutic irradiation [10], a preliminary analysis of the problem of radiation-induced malignomas of the thyroid gland was made.

Whereas most publications to date proceed from radiation exposure in the thyroid region and register the number of thyroid carcinomas developed, we studied potential radiation exposure in the neck region of 302 patients (224 women (74%) and 78 men (26%)) who were hospitalized for diagnostics or therapy of a thyroid carcinoma in the radiological and nuclear medicine facilities of the Berlin, Jena and Greifswald Universities. In 13 of these cases (4.4%) a radiation exposure to higher doses (about 500 to 3000 rads) for various indications could be proved. An exact retrospective determination of the dose was hardly possible in most cases, since some of them were older cases in which exact values had not been given and dosages had been determined only by time or MED. The material has been set out in Table I. Average latency was 22.1 years, the shortest one 7, the longest 47 years. The average exposure age of our patients lay around 20.7 years. The youngest patient was 1 year at the time of radiation exposure, the oldest patient was 58 years of age. Seven patients were below 20 years at the time of exposure, 5 cases were above 20. Sex distribution was 2 men: 11 women (15%:85%). This corresponds to the sex distribution of all patients.

Eleven patients were subjected to conventional X-ray therapy, 2 cases to an additional radium therapy. The original diseases which indicated radiotherapy were 1 fibrosarcoma of the epipharynx, 3 haemangiomas in the neck region, 1 laryngeal carcinoma, 2 hyperthyreoses, 3 neck-lymph-node tuberculoses, 1 thyroid carcinoma and 2 euthyreotic strumae. In the case of thyroid carcinoma, there was a 14-year interval between the first and second carcinoma, so that in our view this might be not a relapse but a potential radiation effect.

As far as histological findings could be made within this study there were 2 cases of metastasising adenomas, 1 of a follicular-papillar, 4 follicular, 1 papillar carcinoma and 1 Hürthlezell tumour.

The clinical history of the cases was not different from the well-known history of this type of tumour formation.

Analysing the cases described it can be stated that there was a pre-exposure to ionizing radiation in 4.4% of the cases. Thus a radiation induction of thyroid carcinomas in our patients is difficult to prove since, according to Creutzig and Hundeshagen [11], a spontaneous prevalence of thyroid carcinomas of 2 to 5% has to be assumed in a non-struma-endemic region. In 1977 these authors found 6 cases (2.5%) among 204 patients suffering from thyroid carcinomas, in which there had been a previous radioiodine therapy because of hyperthyreosis at an interval of up to 10 years. They do not claim a radiation induction in these cases. It should be noted, however, that our patients and those of Creutzig and Hundeshagen [11] are persons selected for their fitness for therapy, particularly with respect to treatment with radioiodine. This restricts the epidemiological evidence of the two studies. Therefore radiation induction cannot be clearly excluded either in the 13 thyroid carcinomas of our patients described since in all cases — in contrast to the above-cited literature — there were high previous radiation exposures of the thyroid due to therapeutic measures. The studies will therefore be continued taking in other clinics in the German Democratic Republic in order to obtain more reliable evidence.

Finally, a summary based on our study and with certain reservations and allowing for the small number of cases at the present state of the research programme, can be made as follows:

(1) We were unable to observe any accumulation of radiation-induced thyroid carcinomas.

(2) The cases studied by us with high radiation exposure in the past are historical examples of radiotherapy which are hardly of any practical relevance today.

(3) On the basis of our material, we cannot comment on the problem of radiation-induced thyroid carcinomas after high-dose radioiodine therapy, but it may be stated in agreement with Creutzig and Hundeshagen that, because of the relatively short re-observation periods reached so far, the latencies of tumour development have not yet been exceeded.

(4) In comparison with the results of the extensive studies in Japan and on the
     Marshall Islands, we did not find any accumulation of thyroid carcinomas
     in the women among our radiation-exposed patients, not even if allowance
     is made for age, and we could not find any preference for a certain age
     group, e.g. of children, in studying the age of exposure. Considering our
     small number of cases these statements can be made only with the greatest
     reservation and regarded as provisional.

(5) Although we stressed the fact of relatively high radiation exposure in the
     history of our 13 cases, because of which radiation-induced tumours cannot
     be clearly excluded − this agrees with the dose-dependent frequency of
     carcinoma induction (range: about 700−1500 rads) described by Colman
     and co-workers − on the other hand, it should be considered that the high
     doses applied in our cases could have decreased the potential induction
     of malignant diseases by cell killing in the thyroid tissue. This idea is
     corroborated by the findings of Conard and co-workers [5]. The inter-
     pretation of our findings should be definitely suspended for the time being.

The programme is being continued in order to obtain the necessary evidence.
Results on a national scale will be reported in due course. It would also be
valuable for control investigations to be carried out at clinics in other countries.

REFERENCES

[1] UNITED NATIONS, Sources and Effects of Ionising Radiation, United Nations
     Scientific Committee on the Effects of Atomic Radiation, Report to the General
     Assembly (1977).
[2] PARKER, L.N., BELSKY, J.L., YAMAMOTO, T., KAWAMOTO, S., KEEHN, M.,
     Ann. Intern. Med. 80 (1974) 600.
[3] HEMPELMANN, L.H., PIFER, J.W., BURKE, G.J., TERRY, R., AMES, W.R., J. Natl.
     Cancer Inst. 38 (1967) 317.
[4] WOOD, W.J., TAMASAKI, H., NERIISHI, S., SATO, T., SHELDON, W.F., ARCHER, P.G.
     Am. J. Epidemiol. 89 (1969) 4.
[5] CONARD, R.A., DOBYNS, B.M., SUTOW, W.W., J. Am. Med. Assoc. 214 (1970) 316.
[6] COLMAN, M., SIMPSON, L.R., PATTERSON, L.K., COHEN, L., "Thyroid cancer
     associated with radiation exposure", Biological and Environmental Effects of Low-Level
     Radiation (Proc. Symp. Chicago, 1975) 2, IAEA, Vienna (1976) 285.
[7] MODAN, B., BAIDATZ, D., MART, H., STEINITZ, R., LEVIN, S.G., Lancet i
     (1974) 277.
[8] WERNER, A., MODAN, B., DAVODOFF, D., Phys. Med. Biol. 13 (1968) 247.
[9] HARLEY, N.H., ALBERT, R.E., SHORE, R.B., PASTERNACK, B.S., Phys. Med. Biol.
     21 (1976) 631.
[10] NEUMEISTER, K., Dtsch. Gesundheitsw. 32 (1977) 1793.
[11] CREUTZIG, H., HUNDESHAGEN, H., Med. Klin. (Muenchen) 72 (1977) 855.

DISCUSSION

I. SCHMITZ-FEUERHAKE: I should like to recommend you to listen to our presentation [1] on radiation-induced thyroid cancer. From the data in the literature it is not surprising that you did not find an accumulation of thyroid carcinomas above 1000 rads. I refer to the study by Dobyns and co-workers in the United States of America (1974) dealing with about 34 600 cases (see Ref.[9] of paper SM-224/712).

K. NEUMEISTER: Colman et al. (Ref.[6] in my paper) found an increasing incidence of radiation-induced thyroid cancer in cases with a radiation exposure of more than 1000 rads.

G.W. DOLPHIN: In Publication 26 of ICRP it is assumed that most radiation-induced thyroid cancers are curable and that the patient survives for a normal life span. There is good evidence to support this assumption in young persons but there is less evidence for survival of older patients with thyroid cancer. Have the older patients in this survey survived after treatment for their cancer?

K. NEUMEISTER: Yes, they survived after treatment. There is no difference between these and other cases of thyroid cancer not resulting from radiation.

K. SHIMAOKA: Induction of thyroid carcinoma by external irradiation to the head and neck areas has been well established. In the United States of America there were shown to be 25 new thyroid cancers per million yearly in the 1940s. More recently the incidence has been shown to be 38 per million yearly. Most of us believe the increase is largely due to the frequent treatment given to the head and neck areas by radiologists in the 1940s and 1950s. The practice of radiologists varies from country to country. I should be interested to know whether the incidence of thyroid cancer has increased in your country.

K. NEUMEISTER: There is no increase in thyroid cancer in the German Democratic Republic.

---

[1] SCHMITZ-FEUERHAKE, I., MUSCHOL, E., BÄTJER, K., SCHÄFER, R., "Risk estimation of radiation-induced thyroid cancer in adults", these Proceedings 1, IAEA-SM-224/712.

EFECTOS BIOLOGICOS TARDIOS DE LA RADIOTERAPIA EN 500 PACIENTES TRATADAS POR CANCER DEL CUELLO UTERINO

A. RADA
Servicio de Radioterapia,
Instituto del Cáncer,
Guayaquil,
Ecuador

Abstract—Resumen

DELAYED BIOLOGICAL EFFECTS OF RADIOTHERAPY IN 500 PATIENTS TREATED FOR CERVICAL CANCER.

The incidence of cancer of the uterine cervix is high in Ecuador, accounting for 45% of all cancer cases and 60% of cancer cases in women. This study considers the delayed biological effects of radiotherapy in 500 patients out of 3200 treated between 1957 and 1972. In spite of the large number of patients treated, it was possible to follow up only 500 cases because a large proportion were in stage IV of the disease and many did not return for clinical check-up. Therefore a report is made on a study of 500 cases, considering a survival of at least five years. The study shows what were the delayed biological effects of radiation treatment and also the frequency and chronology of the appearance of lesions. The following sequelae are studied: severe sclerosis of the skin and subcutaneous cell tissue, whether or not followed by necrosis; chronic oedema of the lower extremities which is conducive to the recurring phenomena of infection in those organs; damage to the pelvic girdle; coxo-femoral osteo-arthrosis and necrosis of the femur head; fracture of the neck of the femur and the pubis; serious lesions in the bladder and in the rectosigmoid; radiation cancer. The patients in question were treated regularly and always by the same technique; it is therefore possible to know the relation between these lesions and the following factors: tumour dose administered; radiation quality; mode of treatment (radiation therapy, alone or associated, before or after surgery); age of the patients treated.

EFECTOS BIOLOGICOS TARDIOS DE LA RADIOTERAPIA EN 500 PACIENTES TRATADAS POR CANCER DEL CUELLO UTERINO.

La incidencia del cáncer de localización en el cuello uterino es notable en Ecuador; representa el 45% de todos los casos de cáncer y el 60% de los casos de cáncer en la mujer. Este estudio considera precisamente los efectos biológicos tardíos de la radioterapia en 500 pacientes, de 3200 casos tratados entre 1957 y 1972. A pesar del gran número de pacientes tratadas, solamente se han podido seguir 500 casos, debido al gran porcentaje que se halla en el estadio IV de la enfermedad, y a que muchas no han vuelto a la consulta para control clínico. Se presenta pues un estudio de 500 casos, considerando por lo menos una sobrevida de cinco años, estudio que va a demostrar cuáles han sido los efectos biológicos tardíos del tratamiento con radiaciones, así como la frecuencia y la cronología de la aparición de las lesiones. Se estudian las siguientes secuelas: esclerosis severa de la piel y del tejido celular subcutáneo, seguida o no de necrosis; edema crónico de las extremidades inferiores, lo que

favorece fenómenos infecciosos a repetición a ese nivel; daños en la cintura pelviana;
osteoartrosis coxo-femoral y necrosis de la cabeza del fémur; fractura del cuello del fémur
y del pubis; lesiones graves en la vejiga y en el recto-sigmoide; radiocáncer. Se trata de
pacientes que han seguido el tratamiento regularmente, y siempre con la misma técnica;
se podrá pues conocer cuál ha sido la relación de estas lesiones con los factores siguientes:
dosis tumor administrada; calidad de la radiación; modalidad del tratamiento (radioterapia
sola o asociada antes o después de la cirugía); edad de las pacientes tratadas.

INTRODUCCION

Hasta 1969, el Instituto del Cáncer de Guayaquil contaba solamente con
radioterapia convencional de 250 kV; a partir de esa fecha, cuenta con una bomba
de cobalto de 4500 $R \cdot h^{-1} \cdot m^{-1}$. Para nuestro estudio hemos seleccionado
319 pacientes tratadas por medio de 250 kV, y 178 por medio de ^{60}Co; pre-
sentamos además tres pacientes que han sido tratadas por una asociación de
radio y cirugía. Hemos considerado al menos una sobrevida de cinco años,
pensando que es necesario disponer de ese tiempo para estudiar los efectos
biológicos tardíos de la radioterapia.

Solo a partir de 1957 la radioterapia ha sido realizada con la misma técnica,
con algunas variaciones en lo que concierne a la dosis total y al fraccionamiento.
Estando las secuelas en relación directa con la técnica usada, es necesario describir
brevemente la que nosotros hemos empleado: para la radioterapia convencional
hemos empleado cuatro campos; uno anterior, otro posterior, y dos, derecho
e izquierdo, a través de la escotadura ciática (fig.1). Para el ^{60}Co hemos empleado
también cuatro campos, uno anterior, otro posterior, y dos laterales, derecho
e izquierdo (fig.2). En ambos casos hemos protegido la línea media con un bloque
de plomo de 4 cm de espesor y 4 cm de ancho al final del tratamiento, con el
fin de proteger la región ya irradiada por el radio.

Con los 250 kV, la dosis tumor administrada se sitúa entre 3800 y 4200 rad
en el centro de la pelvis, y de 4100 a 4600 rad a 5 cm de la línea media. Con
el ^{60}Co, entre 4600 y 5400 rad en el centro de la pelvis, y de 5500 a 6200 rad
a 5 cm de la línea media.

Para el radio seguimos una técnica vecina de la de Regaud, o sea una sonda
intrauterina con tres tubos de 10 mg de Ra cada uno, y un colpostato con dos
tubos de 10 mg de Ra cada uno. A veces no es posible colocar la sonda intrauterina y se ha colocado solamente un colpostato con dos o tres tubos de 10 mg
de Ra cada uno. En todo caso, la dosis administrada oscila entre 5000 y
6500 rad a nivel del cuello uterino, y 1250 a 1600 rad a 5 cm de la línea media;
la cara posterior de la vejiga y la cara anterior del recto reciben una dosis
aproximada a la del cuello uterino.

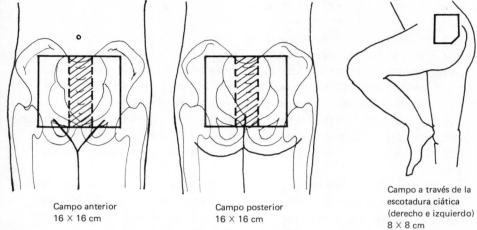

Campo anterior
16 × 16 cm

Campo posterior
16 × 16 cm

Campo a través de la
escotadura ciática
(derecho e izquierdo)
8 × 8 cm

FIG.1.   Técnica de irradiación por radioterapia convencional, 250 kV.
Dosis tumor: 3800 y 4200 rad en el centro de la pelvis
*   4000 y 4600 rad a 5 cm de la línea media*
El campo anterior y posterior pueden ser protegidos durante una parte del tratamiento por
un bloque de plomo (línea de puntos).

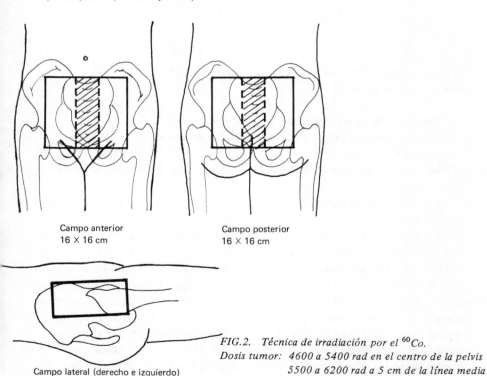

Campo anterior
16 × 16 cm

Campo posterior
16 × 16 cm

Campo lateral (derecho e izquierdo)
8 × 16 cm

FIG.2.   Técnica de irradiación por el ⁶⁰Co.
Dosis tumor: 4600 a 5400 rad en el centro de la pelvis
*   5500 a 6200 rad a 5 cm de la línea media*
La línea de puntos significa protección central de la pelvis.

EFECTOS BIOLOGICOS TARDIOS

Estudiaremos sucesivamente las secuelas producidas por las radiaciones en el tratamiento del cáncer del cuello uterino. Precisamente, y hallándose el cuello uterino y los parametrios con su amplia red linfática en el centro de la pelvis, todo su contenido es sospechoso de estar sembrado, aún en los casos clínicamente en estadio I; es pues necesario irradiar un gran volúmen de tejido sano con una dosis bastante elevada. Tenemos además la piel y el tejido celular subcutáneo, que son ampliamente irradiados cuando hemos empleado los 250 kV. Por ello es a nivel de todos esos órganos que vamos a encontrar las secuelas.

En el conjunto de pacientes estudiadas, un gran número han sido tratadas por cirugía seguida de radioterapia externa; son pacientes operadas fuera de nuestro Instituto y que en su mayoría no han sido sometidas a cirugía radical. La cirugía, después del tratamiento de radioterapia, ha sido indicada en los casos de no esterilización. La radioterapia externa solamente (250 kV o ^{60}Co) ha sido indicada en pacientes en mal estado general y de edad avanzada, a las cuales no ha sido posible aplicar un tratamiento con radio.

Esclerosis severa de la piel y del tejido celular subcutáneo seguida o no de necrosis

Esta secuela ha sido hallada en los siguientes casos:
— Cirugía, más radioterapia externa (250 kV), 40 casos (21%) (15 casos seguidos de necrosis)
— Radioterapia (Ra más 250 kV) exclusiva, 26 casos (14,8%) (3 casos seguidos de necrosis)
— Radioterapia (250 kV) externa solamente, 2 casos (1,2%) (los dos seguidos de necrosis)
En total 68 casos (27,3%) (20 casos seguidos de necrosis (8%)).

Esta secuela ha aparecido entre 3 y 5 años después del tratamiento en pacientes con una sobrevida entre 5 y 14 años. No hemos encontrado influencia de la edad en la aparición de esta complicación. La asociación con la cirugía parece haber influido notoriamente en la aparición de esta secuela, así como la dosis administrada; todos los pacientes de este grupo han recibido entre 4300 y 4600 rad. La obesidad es un factor decisivo en la aparición de esclerosis y necrosis de la piel; del total de 68 pacientes, 55 eran obesas y 13 no lo eran. Pero sobre todo ha sido la calidad de radiación, o sea el uso de la radioterapia convencional, la que ha producido esta complicación.

Edema crónico de las extremidades inferiores y crisis erisipelatosas a repetición

Hemos encontrado verdaderas elefantiasis entre estas pacientes, sobre todo en las pacientes tratadas por la asociación radioquirúrgica.
– Cirugía más radioterapia externa (250 kV), 15 casos (8%)
– Radioterapia (Ra más 250 kV) más cirugía, 3 casos (1,2%)
– Radioterapia externa solamente (250 kV), 2 casos (1%)
– Cirugía más radioterapia externa (^{60}Co), 5 casos (7,6%)
– Radioterapia (Ra más ^{60}Co) más cirugía, 5 casos (7,6%)
– Radioterapia (Ra más ^{60}Co) exclusiva, 5 casos (7,6%)
    En total 35 casos (14%).
Esta secuela ha aparecido entre 1 y 4 años después del tratamiento en pacientes con una sobrevida entre 5 y 18 años. La dosis administrada no ha tenido ninguna influencia, así como tampoco la edad de las pacientes. La asociación con la cirugía ha influido claramente en la aparición de esta complicación, así como los trastornos vasculares ya presentes antes del tratamiento. La aparición de esta secuela también ha sido influenciada por el uso de la radioterapia convencional.

Secuelas óseas

Artrosis coxo-femoral, seguida o no de necrosis de la cabeza del fémur.
– Cirugía más radioterapia externa (250 kV), 7 casos (3,8%) (2 casos de necrosis de la cabeza del fémur, con tres casos bilaterales)
– Radioterapia (Ra más 250 kV) exclusiva, 15 casos (8,1%) (5 casos de necrosis; todos unilaterales)
– Cirugía más radioterapia externa (^{60}Co), 3 casos (4,6%) (ninguna necrosis; todos los casos unilaterales)
– Radioterapia (Ra más ^{60}Co) exclusiva, 2 casos (3%) (ausencia de necrosis; todos los casos unilaterales)
– Radioterapia externa solamente (^{60}Co), 5 casos (7,6%) (4 casos bilaterales; ninguna necrosis)
    En total 32 pacientes (12,8%) (7 casos de necrosis de la cabeza femoral y 7 casos bilaterales).
Las lesiones aparecieron entre 2 y 6 años y la necrosis entre 6 y 8 años después del tratamiento en pacientes con una sobrevida de 7 y 18 años. Evidentemente la necrosis de la cabeza del fémur ha sido más frecuente con la radioterapia convencional; la artrosis lo ha sido con el ^{60}Co. Todas las pacientes de este grupo eran mayores de 45 años. No se ha encontrado ninguna relación con la dosis administrada.

Fractura del cuello del fémur

— Cirugía más radioterapia externa (250 kV), 5 casos (2,7%) (3 casos
   bilaterales)
— Radioterapia (Ra más 250 kV) exclusiva, (3 casos (1,6%) unilaterales)
— Radioterapia externa solamente (250 kV) (2 casos (1%) unilaterales)
— Cirugía más radioterapia externa (^{60}Co), 10 casos (15%) (2 casos bilaterales).

Fractura del pubis

Un caso, en una paciente tratada por radioterapia (Ra más 250 kV)
exclusiva (5%).
En total, 21 casos (8,4%) (5 casos bilaterales).
La fractura ha aparecido entre 2 y 4 años después del tratamiento en
pacientes con una sobrevida entre 6 y 20 años. Esta secuela ha sido también
más frecuente después de los 45 años, y con la radioterapia por ^{60}Co. No se ha
encontrado relación con la dosis administrada.

Cistitis hemorrágica severa, seguida o no de fístula vésico-vaginal

— Cirugía más radioterapia externa (250 kV), 31 casos (16,9%) con 2 fístulas
   vésico-vaginales, que son las únicas del grupo
— Radioterapia (Ra más 250 kV) exclusiva, 7 casos (3,8%)
— Radioterapia (Ra más 250 kV) más cirugía, 1 caso (0,5%)
— Cirugía más radioterapia externa (^{60}Co), 2 casos (3%).
En total 41 pacientes (16,6%), con 2 de fístula vésico-vaginal (0,8%); la
fecha de aparición de esta secuela varía entre 2 y 6 años en pacientes con una
sobrevida entre 5 y 16 años. La edad de las pacientes no parece tener relación
ni tampoco la dosis recibida en el tratamiento con radio. Es la asociación con
la cirugía la que ha influido claramente en la aparición de esta complicación;
se trata en todo caso de una vejiga neurogénica a la que se suman fenómenos
infecciosos agregados por vaciamiento incompleto que hacen que la vejiga sea
más sensible a las radiaciones.

Secuelas rectales

— Radioterapia (Ra más 250 kV) exclusiva, *1 caso de sigmoiditis severa* (0,5%)
   en que fue necesario practicar una colostomia; 31 pacientes con rectitis
   severa, seguida en 4 casos de fístula recto-vaginal (16,9%)
— Radioterapia (Ra más ^{60}Co) exclusiva, 16 casos (24,6%)
— Radio seguido de cirugía, 1 caso (0,4%)
En total 49 pacientes (19,7%) (4 casos de fístula recto-vaginal (1,6%)).

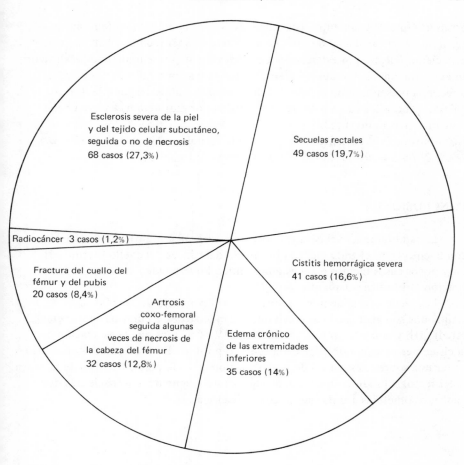

FIG.3. Frecuencia de secuelas en 249 pacientes entre 500 irradiados por cancer del cuello uterino. 251 pacientes han curado sin secuelas.

La fecha de aparición de esta secuela oscila entre 1 y 4 años en pacientes con una sobrevida entre 6 y 10 años. No hemos encontrado influencia por edad, pero la asociación con el radio, aún en dosis baja, es decisiva en la aparición de esta secuela que no tiene ninguna relación con la calidad de la radiación externa empleada.

Radiocáncer

Entre los 249 pacientes que han presentado secuelas graves hemos encontrado tres casos (1,2%) de probable radiocáncer; decimos probable porque es imposible precisarlo histológicamente. Una paciente ha presentado un epitelioma epidermoideo del canal anal después de 10 años de haber recibido tratamiento; la paciente falleció por esta causa. Otra paciente ha presentado una localización en la uretra 7 años después del tratamiento; la paciente falleció también. La tercera ha presentado un epitelioma de la vejiga 12 años después del tratamiento. Todos los casos habían sido tratados por radioterapia externa convencional más radio (fig.3).

En total 249 pacientes han presentado secuelas: 230 una sola, 17 dos a la vez, y 2 tres a la vez. Han curado sin secuelas 251 pacientes.

CONCLUSIONES

La radioterapia exclusiva (radioterapia externa y radio), y en asociación con la cirugía, es el tratamiento obligatorio del cáncer del cuello uterino. Hay muy pocos casos incluso en el estadio clínico I que pueden curarse con intervención quirúrgica solamente.

Las secuelas que hemos encontrado en el conjunto de los 500 casos estudiados son algunas veces inevitables cuando se desea curar pacientes en el estadio III, y aun unos pocos en el estadio IV. Creemos que la asociación con la cirugía es mala, y que debe evitarse en lo posible. En todo caso, es necesario evitar una sobredosis a nivel de la articulación coxo-femoral, y a nivel de la vejiga y del recto. El radioterapeuta debe vigilar estrechamente a las pacientes que han sido sometidas a tratamiento con radiaciones.

BIBLIOGRAFIA

DUBOIS, J.B., POURQUIER, H., Les échecs de la physiothérapie exclusive dans les cancers de l'utérus, J. Radiol., Electrol., Méd. Nucl. 57 5 (1976) 421.

FAYS, J., SIMON, J.M., RICHAUME, B., PARIETTI, R., MACINOT, C., TREHEUX, A., Aspects angiographiques d'une sigmoïdité radique, J. Radiol., Electrol., Méd. Nucl. 52 8–9 (1971) 536.

FLECHTER, G.H., SHUKOVSKY, L.J., The interplay of radiocurability and tolerance in the irradiation of human cancers, J. Radiol., Electrol., Méd. Nucl. 56 (1975) 383.

KOGELNIK, H.D., KÄRCHER, K.H., "Radiobiological considerations of late effects arising from radiotherapy", Radiobiological Research and Radiotherapy (Actas Simp. Viena, 1976) 2, OIEA, Viena (1977) 275.

QUINT, R., ABBATUCCI, J.S., Incidence pratique de la notion N.S.D., J. Radiol., Electrol., Méd. Nucl. 52 11 (1971) 707.

ROUSSEAU, J., FENTON, J., MATHIEU, G., DULAC, G., PICCO, Ch., Les séquelles et complications tardives de la radiothérapie exclusive de haute énergie des carcinomes du col utérin, J. Radiol., Electrol., Méd. Nucl. 57 5 (1976) 409.

SWYNGEDAUW, J., Dose de tolérance tissulaire; dose de stérilisation tumorale en irradiations continues ou discontinues, J. Radiol., Electrol., Méd. Nucl. 56 5 (1975) 369.

TUBIANA, M., DUTREIX, J., DUTREIX, A., JOCKEY, P., Aspects Biologiques, Protection — Les Risques, Ed. Masson, Paris (1946).

DISCUSSION

M. DELPLA: I should first of all like to say, for the benefit of those not familiar with the late complications of radiotherapy — complications well known to doctors — that the stake, i.e. the life of the patient, justifies the risks.

It would be interesting if Mrs Rada could give us an order of magnitude of the doses received at places where a lesion may be caused, for example a radionecrosis or a vesicovaginal fistula.

A. RADA: Radionecroses have resulted from doses of 4300–4600 rads with conventional X-ray radiotherapy at 250 kV. Vesicovaginal fistulas are observed especially after combined surgical and radiation treatment. The tumour doses did not exceed 4100 rads in the case of 250 kV treatment, and 5400 rads in the case of cobalt-60.

R.G. GREGORIO *(Chairman)*: In the Philippine General Hospital we treated about 283 cases of cervix cancer from 1965 to 1969 and found approximately 10% rectal complications. It is well known that the rectum is one of the parts most sensitive to radiation in the pelvic cavity. Are your patients treated with radium under anaesthesia? We have found that rectal complications can be greatly reduced by better packings, which lessen the dose to the rectum considerably.

A. RADA: We use a Delclos applicator (after-loading) which involves placing three tubes of 10 mg each in the uterine canal and a colpostat with two tubes of 10 mg each, and we try to keep the radioactive source away from the rectum and the bladder by packing out the vagina.

IRRADIATION SPINE DEFORMITY
IN CHILDREN TREATED FOR NEUROBLASTOMA

J.K. MAYFIELD
Twin Cities Scoliosis Center,
Department of Orthopaedic Surgery,
University of Minnesota,
Minneapolis,
Minnesota

E.J. RISEBOROUGH
Department of Orthopaedic Surgery,
Children's Hospital Medical Center,
Boston

N. JAFFE
Sidney Farber Cancer Center,
Harvard Medical School,
Boston

M. NEHME
Tufts University School of Medicine,
Boston,
Massachusetts,
United States of America

Abstract

IRRADIATION SPINE DEFORMITY IN CHILDREN TREATED FOR NEUROBLASTOMA.
A retrospective long-term follow-up review of 56 children with neuroblastoma surviving five years and longer following treatment since 1946 revealed that 57% had developed spine deformity (S.D.) following treatment with 250 kilovolt irradiation at the time of review. The average age at diagnosis was 17 months. Irradiation therapy was delivered to most children before 24 months of age. Follow-up averaged 12.9 years with a range of 5−31 years. Eighty-five per cent of the children had developed structural spine deformity at skeletal maturity and 54% of these children had scoliosis greater than 20 degrees. Sixteen per cent of irradiated children developed structural kyphosis. Non-midline opposing anterior and posterior ports were used most frequently. Mean dosage in patients who developed scoliosis of 20 degrees or more was 3588 rads (spine dosage) and 3746 rads in patients who developed kyphosis. Irradiation through opposing anterior and posterior ports was more commonly associated with the development of S.D. Sixty-six per cent of children who had more than 2000 rads developed S.D. The adolescent growth spurt was associated with an increase in the frequency and severity of spine deformity. This study indicated that moderate to severe S.D. was produced by irradiation in excess of 2000 rads administered with a 250-kilovoltage machine. This study would also suggest that children with neuroblastoma treated with orthovoltage irradiation should be followed closely by the orthopaedic surgeon, the oncologist,

the radiotherapist and the paediatrician until the completion of skeletal growth for the development of unsightly structural spine deformity. Early bracing and surgery may be helpful in controlling these deformities in the pre-adolescent to early adolescent years. Continued observation is necessary to determine if current irradiation techniques will minimize or eradicate the incidence and severity of these complications.

INTRODUCTION

Neuroblastoma is the most common extracranial malignant solid tumour in infancy and childhood. It comprises approximately 7—14% of childhood malignancies and 15—50% of neonatal malignancies [1—5]. Treatment usually involves a multi-disciplinary approach with surgery, irradiation and chemotherapy. Most neuroblastomas respond to irradiation treatment [6] and several reports reveal two-year survival rates varying from 32—88% [7—10]. In those children who survive, the frequency and severity of post-irradiation spine deformity are becoming more apparent especially as these children enter and complete their adolescent growth spurts. Thus orthopaedic surgeons are now more frequently facing therapeutic decisions relating to these deformities in this group of children.

Many authors have recognized that the growing skeleton is susceptible to damage by irradiation [11—14]. It has been conclusively demonstrated that the disturbance of growth from irradiation is greater the younger the animal and the larger the irradiation dose [11]. Little attention, however, has been directed towards the methods of irradiation and the spine deformities that are seen in the long-term survivors of this malignancy.

Neuroblastoma is a particularly useful tumour with which to study the late radiation effects on the spine because of the young age of the patients at the time of irradiation and the varied location of the primaries (mediastinal and retroperitoneal) and the frequent asymmetry of the irradiation.

This study is an attempt to analyse the irradiation technique and the spine deformity seen in a large long-term follow-up series of homogeneously treated children with neuroblastoma at the Sidney Farber Cancer Center and the Children's Hospital Medical Center, Boston, Massachusetts, United States of America.

MATERIALS AND METHODS

All patients treated for neuroblastoma at the Sidney Farber Cancer Center and the Children's Hospital Medical Center in Boston, Massachusetts, from November 1946 through November 1976 were reviewed. There were 419 children treated of whom 137 were living at the time of review.

Patients who had no irradiation, patients who had metastatic involvement of the spine by tumour and patients who had a laminectomy or who were rendered paraplegic by their disease, both of which are known to produce spine deformity, were excluded from the study. This sample thus included only those patients whose spine deformity was irradiation-induced. All patients were at least five year survivors at the time of review and their hospital records, roentgenotherapy records and roentgenograms, available from the time of irradiation until their most recent visit, were reviewed.

Twenty-eight were girls and 28 were boys. The staging method proposed by D'Angio and co-workers [15, 16] has been used, and the extent of the disease at the time of treatment was Stage I or II in 32 children and Stage III, IV, or IVs in 24 children. The mean age at diagnosis and treatment was 17 months with a range of one day to 10.4 years. The mean follow-up after irradiation was 12.9 years with a range of 5–31 years.

Forty-six patients had surgical resection of the primary at the time of diagnosis in combination with multi-drug chemotherapy and irradiation. Six patients had irradiation of the primary with chemotherapy but without surgical resection of the primary. Four patients had surgical resection of the primary and irradiation. Fifty-two patients received concomitant multi-drug chemotherapy as a part of their treatment regimen.

The roentgenotherapy record was analysed in all patients and calculations were made of the depth dose in rads delivered to the spine during the irradiation. Fifty-five patients received orthovoltage irradiation in doses of 200 and 250 kilovolts with a mean spine dose of 2657 rads (range 72.5 rads–6250 rads). One patient was treated with a 4 MeV linear accelerator with a spine dose of 2350 rads.

The mean time for administration of the irradiation was 18 days (range 5–49 days). The total dose was delivered in daily doses of 200–250 rads until the total dosage was achieved except in one patient who had a total spine dose of 4988 rads delivered in two separate courses separated by five months between treatments.

The fields of irradiation varied and were single anterior (3 patients), single posterior (8 patients), opposing anterior and posterior (37 patients), multiple ports (4 patients) and the cervical spine (4 patients).

All fields except the lateral fields crossed the midline to include the total width of the spine.

RESULTS

Fifty-seven per cent of the children had developed post-irradiation spine deformity at the time of review. No sex difference was noted; 57% of the boys and 57% of the girls had spine deformity. The stage of the disease at the

TABLE I. PERCENTAGE OF CHILDREN WHO DEVELOPED SPINE
DEFORMITY (S.D.) WITH VARIOUS TREATMENT REGIMES

Treatment	N.D.	S.D.	Percentage deformity
A. Irradiation and surgical resection	2	2	50
B. Irradiation and chemotherapy (Without resection)	2	4	67
C. Irradiation and chemotherapy and surgical resection of the primary	20	26	56

TABLE II. THE EFFECT OF PORTAL OF IRRADIATION ON FREQUENCY
OF SPINE DEFORMITY (S.D.), NO DEFORMITY (N.D.), ANTERIOR
ALONE (A), POSTERIOR ALONE (P) AND OPPOSING ANTERIOR AND
POSTERIOR PORTALS (A & P)

Irradiation portal	N.D.	S.D.	%S.D.
A	4	0	0
P	4	4	50
A & P	12	25	68

TABLE III. MEAN SPINE DOSE
($\bar{X}$ rads) AS DELIVERED THROUGH
THE VARIOUS PORTALS

Irradiation portal	N.D.	S.D.
A	1485	
P	1992	2343
A & P	2106	2634

TABLE IV. IRRADIATION SYMMETRY AND FREQUENCY OF
SPINE DEFORMITY

M = midline; NM = non-midline; A = anterior; P = posterior; A & P = opposing anterior and posterior

	Port Centre					
	M			NM		
Port location	N.D.	S.D.	%S.D.	N.D.	S.D.	%S.D.
A	1	0	0	2	0	0
P	2	3	60	2	1	33
A & P	7	9	56	5	16	76
Total	10	12	55	9	17	65

time of the irradiation did not seem significantly to affect the outcome. Fifty-three per cent in Stage I or II and 63% of patients in Stage III, IV or IVs had developed deformity at the time of review. In addition, surgical resection of the primary did not seem to be a factor in the development of ultimate spine deformity at review (Table I).

Irradiation portals

Irradiation was delivered through various portals as described in Table II. Most of the spine deformities appeared to be associated with delivery of irradiation through opposing anterior and posterior portals, but this increased frequency of spine deformity may have been a reflection of the higher dosage delivered through the opposed ports (Table III). Since the sample size was so small no conclusions can be drawn, but there does not appear to be any difference in the frequency of spine deformity between patients treated with single posterior ports and those treated with opposed anterior and posterior ports. The actual difference can be explained by dose alone.

Irradiation symmetry

An attempt was made to evaluate the relationship between port symmetry (non-midline versus midline) and spine deformity (Table IV). Non-midline irradiation in general was more frequently associated with spine deformity. There was a 65% incidence of deformity associated with non-midline irradiation

TABLE V. IRRADIATION DOSAGE AND SPINE DEFORMITY

Dosage	N.D.	S.D.	No. of patients	%S.D.
< 2000 rads	14	13	27	48
> 2000 rads	10	19	29	66

Scoliosis	$\overset{.}{X}$ dosage (rads)	No. of patients
< 20°	2281	20
≥ 20°	3588	8

TABLE VI. SEVERITY OF SCOLIOSIS IN RELATIONSHIP TO IRRADIATION DOSAGE AND AGE AT FOLLOW-UP

	Spine deformity — scoliosis			
Curve range (degrees)	No. of patients	Average degree	$\overset{.}{X}$ Spine dose	Mean age at follow-up (years)
5−10	10	7	2094	11.6
11−19	10	14	2469	13.1
20−30	4	22	4106	17.7
31−40	2	36	2859	24.0
41−50	0	−	−	−
51−60	1	56	3875	25.0
61−80	1	79	2688	18.0

TABLE VII. THE EFFECT OF GROWTH ON THE FREQUENCY OF SPINE DEFORMITY

	N.D.	S.D.	%S.D.
Prepubertal	17	17	50
Skeletal maturity	2	11	85

compared with 55% in children treated with midline irradiation. This increased
frequency of deformity with non-midline opposing anterior and posterior ports
where 76% developed deformity compared with 56% who had midline irradiation.

Axial skeletal deformity

Thirty-two of 56 patients had structural spine deformity $> 5°$ at review,
most of the deformities being scoliosis or kyphosis. Forty-eight per cent of
children who had < 2000 rads developed deformity and 66% who had > 2000 rads
developed deformity. In those patients who developed scoliosis alone, the
magnitude of the curvature at review was $< 20°$ in 20 patients and $\geqslant 20°$ in
8 patients (Table V). Those patients who developed larger deformities generally
received larger amounts of irradiation (Table VI). The mean dosage received in
those patients who developed scoliosis $\geqslant 20°$ was 3588 rads and 2281 rads in
those patients whose scoliotic curve was $< 20°$.

Nine patients or 16% developed kyphotic spine deformity and the mean
dosage delivered to these patients was 3746 rads. Four patients had scoliosis and
kyphosis, 4 patients had pure kyphosis and 1 patient had scoliosis, kyphosis
and lordosis.

Spine deformity at skeletal maturity

Eighty-five per cent of children followed beyond skeletal maturity had
developed spine deformity and 54% of these patients as adults had deformities
$> 20°$; 50% of children who had not yet entered the adolescent growth spurt
had developed deformity (< 11 years in girls and < 12 years in boys). This
difference in frequency of spine deformity between the prepubertal period
and maturity was statistically significant ($p = 0.05$) and was not dose related,
representing the effect of skeletal growth on the irradiated spine (Table VII).

DISCUSSION

This study is an attempt to analyse the various techniques of irradiation
therapy on the spine in neuroblastoma. A long-term survival study of children
treated for neuroblastoma is an especially useful population to study in order
to determine the late effects of irradiation on the spine. Because of the varied
location of the primary site from midline to non-midline locations in the thoracic,
thoracolumbar and lumbar areas the effects of symmetrical and asymmetrical
irradiation could be analysed. Previous reports [14, 17–21] have documented
scoliosis and kyphoscoliosis as resulting from irradiation treatment in various
childhood malignancies. In 1962 Rubin and co-workers [19] included six
patients with Wilms' tumour, two patients with neuroblastoma and two patients

with medulloblastoma in their review, and noted scoliosis greater than 5° in
nine patients who survived two years or longer after treatment. No correlation
was made with port location and types of ports with the ultimate spine deformity.

In addition, no correlation between port asymmetry and ultimate deformity
was made because of lack of sufficient numbers of long-term survivors for
evaluation. Tachdjian and co-workers [20] in their review of intraspinal tumours
in infants and children of whom 18 had neuroblastoma mention scoliosis as due
to irradiation. No further inquiry was made concerning irradiation technique.
The reports of the effects of growth on the severity of radiation-induced spine
deformity have been inconclusive. Katzman and co-workers [21] felt that
some cases of scoliosis do progress with growth, but usually it was not significant.
This report included cases of paraplegia and laminectomy-induced spine deformity
so that no firm conclusions could be made. Neuhauser and co-workers [18] in
their study concluded that scoliosis caused by irradiation deteriorated little
with growth.

The present study of 56 long-term survivors of neuroblastoma indicates that
57% of these children who were treated with irradiation developed structural
spine deformity at the time of review. Fifty per cent of the children who had
not entered the adolescent growth spurt had deformity compared with 85% of
children who were followed beyond the adolescent growth spurt, reflecting the
effect of rapid growth on the frequency of deformity. Of further interest is the
fact that all the larger degrees of scoliosis ($> 20°$) were seen in children who
had reached skeletal maturity reflecting also the effect of rapid growth on the
severity of deformity.

This increased frequency and severity of spine deformity at maturity differs
distinctly from the reported findings of Neuhauser and co-workers [18]. In their
study the maximum curves were only approximately 12°, and these deteriorated
minimally during subsequent growth. This difference may reflect the small
series of patients (13 patients) and relatively short follow-up (7.6 years) in
Neuhauser's study. This information suggests that these children should
especially be followed by an orthopaedic surgeon until maturity for the detection
and possible treatment of the more severe deformities that may develop during
the adolescent period.

Neuhauser found that more severe deformities were associated with
irradiation in children aged two years or less and when the dosage exceeded
2000 rads using orthovoltage technique [18]. The average age of treatment in
this study was 17 months and the average dosage delivered in patients with
scoliosis less than 20° was 2281 rads and $\geqslant 20°$ 3588 rads, suggesting that
dosages > 2000 rads were associated with mild curves and > 3000 rads were
associated with more severe deformities.

Many authors have recommended caution in using asymmetric irradiation,
and if this has to be used that the fields should cross the midline so that more

uniform exposure of the spine takes place [3, 18, 19]. Rubin and co-workers [19] in their studies felt that the degree of scoliosis which developed was not related to the fields of irradiation, whether they were unilateral or bilateral. In this homogeneously treated population asymmetric irradiation of the spine was more frequently associated with spine deformity than midline irradiation, but no firm conclusions could be made because of the small sample size and the variation in dosage. It is of interest to note, however, that of the four patients who developed scoliosis > 30° three had non-midline irradiation and both patients who had curvatures > 50° had non-midline irradiation.

This study serves to call attention to the fact that irradiation treatment to infants and children with malignancies that includes the spine in the fields of irradiation can produce spinal deformity and can be associated with moderate to severe deformity if these children survive and are followed to skeletal maturity. With the growing number of long-term survivors following pre-operative and post-operative irradiation the incidence and severity of this complication will become more apparent. This study would especially suggest that these children should be followed closely by the orthopaedic surgeon, the oncologist, the radiotherapist and the paediatrician until the completion of skeletal growth for the development of unsightly structural spine deformity. Early bracing and surgical correction and fusion may be helpful in controlling these curves in the pre-adolescent to early adolescent years.

REFERENCES

[1] BODIAN, M., Neuroblastoma, Pediat. Clin. North Am. 6 (1959) 449.

[2] DARGEON, H.W., Neuroblastoma, J. Pediatr. 61 (1962) 456.

[3] ENGEL, D., Experiments on the production of spinal deformities by radium: I, Am. J. Roentgenol., Radium Ther. Nucl. Med. 42 (1939) 217.

[4] EVANS, A.R., Congenital neuroblastoma, J. Clin. Pathol. 18 (1965) 154.

[5] WELLS, H.G., Occurrence and significance of congenital malignant neoplasms, Arch. Pathol. Lab. Med. 30 (1940) 535.

[6] D'ANGIO, G.I., Effects of radiation on the neuroblastoma, J. Pediatr. Surg. 3 (1968) 179.

[7] GROSS, R.E., FARBER, S., MARTIN, L.W., Neuroblastoma sympatheticium; A study and report of 217 cases, Pediatrics 23 (1959) 179.

[8] KOOP, C.E., HERNANDEZ, J.R., Neuroblastoma: experience with 100 cases in children, Surgery 56 (1964) 726.

[9] LINGLEY, J.F., SAGERMAN, R.H., SANTULLI, T.V., WOLFF, J.A., Neuroblastoma: management and survival, New Engl. J. Med. 277 (1967) 1227.

[10] PEREZ, J.F., VIETTI, T.J., ACKERMAN, L.V., JULAPONGS, P., POWERS, W.E., Treatment of malignant sympathetic tumors in children: clinicopathological correlation, Pediatrics 41 (1968) 452.

[11] BARR, J.S., LINGLEY, J.R., GALL, E.A., The effect of roentgen irradiation on epiphyseal growth: I. Experimental studies upon the albino rat, Am. J. Roentgenol., Radium Ther. Nucl. Med. 49 (1943) 104.

[12]   FRANTZ, C.H., Extreme retardation of epiphyseal growth from roentgen irradiation, Radiology **55** (1950) 720.

[13]   RUBIN, P., ANDREWS, J.R., SWARM, R., GUMP, H., Radiation induced dysplasias of bone, Am. J. Roentgenol., Radium. Ther. Nucl. Med. **82** (1959) 206.

[14]   WHITEHOUSE, W.M., LAMPE, I., Osseous damage in irradiation of renal tumors in infancy and childhood, Am. J. Roentgenol., Radium Ther. Nucl. Med. **70** (1953) 721.

[15]   EVANS, A., D'ANGIO, G.J., RANDOLPH, J., A proposed staging for children with neuroblastoma, Cancer **27** (1971) 374.

[16]   POCHEDLY, C., Neuroblastoma, Publishing Sciences Group, Acton, Massachusetts (1976).

[17]   ARKIN, A.M., PACK, G.T., RANSOHOFF, N.S., SIMON, N., Irradiation-induced scoliosis — a case report, J. Bone Joint Surg. **32A** (1950) 401.

[18]   NEUHAUSER, E.B.D., WITTENBERG, M.H., BERMAN, C.Z., COHEN, J., Irradiation effects of roentgen therapy on the growing spine, Radiology **59** (1952) 637.

[19]   RUBIN, P., DUTHIE, R.B., YOUNG, L.W., The significance of scoliosis in post-irradiated Wilm's tumor and neuroblastoma, Radiology **79** (1962) 539.

[20]   TACHDJIAN, M.O., MATSON, D.D., Orthopaedic aspects of intraspinal tumors in infants and children, J. Bone Joint Surg. **47A** (1965) 223.

[21]   KATZMAN, H., WAUGH, T., BERDON, W., Skeletal changes following irradiation of childhood tumors, J. Bone Joint Surg. **51A** (1969) 825.

DISCUSSION

K. NEUMEISTER: Did you find neurological complications after radio-therapy in any of your cases?

J.K. MAYFIELD: No neurological complications from irradiation were noted in this study. All the neurological complications were due to the tumour itself (extradural and spinal cord involvement) and these patients were excluded from the study.

M. DELPLA: From the extreme values of the doses one might think that one group of patients had been subjected to functional radiotherapy and the other to anti-tumoral radiotherapy, which is rather odd.

Was the spine deformity caused by the disease itself or by irradiation? Or did irradiation simply play a supporting role?

J.K. MAYFIELD: All patients were treated for a cure and the fact that all of them survived at least five years reflects this. Certainly many of these patients had chemotherapy and surgery in addition to the irradiation. I do not know why some patients received a much lower dosage than others in the course of treatment.

The spinal deformities were most likely due to the irradiation rather than the disease itself. All patients who developed paraplegia or had a laminectomy or suffered tumour invasion of the bone were excluded from this study, since all the above conditions can produce spine deformity irrespective of irradiation. In addition, five patients who were five-year survivors but who had no irradiation (not included in this study) did not develop scoliosis or kyphosis at follow-up. These five cases can therefore be taken to represent the effect of the disease itself upon the spine, and the spine deformities considered in this study may be regarded as a consequence of radiation alone rather than of the disease itself.

K.R. TROTT: These children are also a valuable source of information on late consequences other than spine deformity, since very large volumes (often approaching half-body irradiation) were treated with moderate doses at an age when follow-up is not complicated by the spontaneous increase in cancer risk above the age of 40. How many of the long-term survivors in your study group developed other malignancies during the follow-up period?

J.K. MAYFIELD: I cannot answer this question, as I did not specifically look at the problem of radiation-induced malignancies in this group of patients.

M. COLMAN *(Chairman):* Most of the patients were treated in the pre-megavoltage era. Was the radiation dose to bone corrected for the type of radiation used (250 kV)?

J.K. MAYFIELD: All doses were corrected for orthovoltage (200–250 kV) irradiation. All doses stated are spine (bone) dosage and not tumour dose.

M. COLMAN *(Chairman):* Presumably the study has been continued to include patients treated with megavoltage therapy. Has any significant finding been noted regarding patients treated with megavoltage therapy compared with those treated with 250 kV X-rays?

J.K. MAYFIELD: I am currently analysing patients who have been treated with megavoltage techniques but no results are available yet. It is suspected that the frequency and severity of spine deformity will be less with megavoltage treatment, but this has yet to be proved.

TUMOURS ASSOCIATED WITH MEDICAL X-RAY THERAPY EXPOSURE IN CHILDHOOD*

M. COLMAN, M. KIRSCH, M. CREDITOR
University of California,
Irvine,
California
and
Michael Reese Hospital,
Chicago,
Illinois,
United States of America

Abstract

TUMOURS ASSOCIATED WITH MEDICAL X-RAY THERAPY EXPOSURE IN CHILDHOOD.
   A total of 5166 persons who were exposed to limited field (80–100 cm^2) X-ray irradiation
to the head, neck and upper chest region during childhood and adolescence have provided an
outstanding opportunity for the study of tumour incidence following medical X-ray therapy.
Initial observations on thyroid cancer were reported at the 1975 IAEA Symposium in Chicago.
An extensive follow-up effort has continued. More than 3254 subjects have been traced, 3108
have completed questionnaires eliciting information on tumour incidence, and 1539 of these
were subjected to a thorough clinical screening procedure that included a thyroid scintigram.
Careful comparison of the screened subgroup with the total population at risk demonstrated
that they were essentially similar in respect of sex distribution, age at the time of irradiation,
radiation dose and year of treatment. The prevalence of thyroid tumours in the 1539 clinically
screened subjects and the prevalence of all other tumours in the 3254 subjects traced can therefore be assumed to reflect the risks in the group of irradiated subjects as a whole. Median age
at irradiation was 3.5 years, and median radiation dose 790 rads (7.9 Gy). Thyroid tumour was
diagnosed in 413 subjects. Of those undergoing surgery (273) 30.3% were found to have thyroid
cancer. A total of 366 surgical pathology specimens of the thyroid, including 93 from subjects
who were diagnosed at other hospitals, were examined revealing 73 papillary carcinomas,
12 follicular carcinomas and 26 microscopic papillary carcinomas. One hundred and eighty-seven
other (non-thyroid) neoplasmas identified included 27 benign and 10 malignant salivary gland
tumours, 16 benign and seven malignant tumours of neural origin (brain, spinal cord, cranial and
peripheral nerves), 37 skin tumours, 9 lymphomas, 8 gonadal tumours, 45 breast tumours and
28 tumours of miscellaneous sites. The incidence of thyroid tumours, salivary gland tumours
and primary brain tumours was considerably in excess of the expected incidence (p values
< 0.0001), and a radiation dose-effect correlation was observed for thyroid and brain tumours.
Comparable incidence rates for many of the benign tumours that were observed are not
available, but gonadal tumours and lymphomas did not occur in excess of the expected incidence.

---

   * This work was supported by grants from the Illinois Division of the American Cancer
Society and the National Cancer Institute (CA22037).

The carcinogenic effects of ionizing radiation have been extensively studied and documented by many authors. Natural radioactivity, occupational exposures, military and medical uses have all been shown to result in an increased prevalence of certain neoplasms [1—4].

The subjects of our study were exposed to therapeutic irradiation using 200 kV X-rays at 50 cm source-to-skin distance (half value layer of 1 mm copper) for various benign conditions, principally in the head and neck area [5]. Approximately 80% of the 5166 persons had received treatment to the tonsils and nasopharynx. Meticulous records had been maintained at the time with exposures recorded as roentgen in air. The treatments were given between 1938 and 1960. The equipment was no longer in use, and dosimetry calculations were carried out assuming a backscatter factor of 1.33 and a roentgen-to-rad conversion factor of 0.945. All treatments to the neck were done using parallel opposed fields of between 80 and 100 cm². Absorbed doses were calculated in the midplane of the neck assuming a cross-sectional diameter of 8 cm (based on the median age of the children). Throughout this report any reference to radiation dose refers to the midplane dose in the neck and not necessarily the tumour site.

Although the treatment of tonsillitis and other benign conditions was discontinued in the late 1950s and early 1960s, our attention was focused on these people through reports that thyroid cancer remained a risk 20 and more years following radiation exposure [6]. A follow-up programme was organized beginning in January 1974 with the object of tracing persons at risk, counselling them, screening them by physical examination and thyroid scintigram, and advising them regarding treatment if thyroid tumour was found [7].

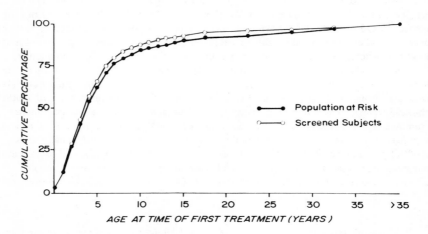

FIG.1. Radiation-induced neoplasia: cumulative percentage against age at treatment.

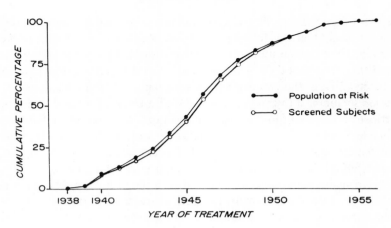

FIG.2. *Radiation-induced neoplasia: cumulative percentage against treatment year.*

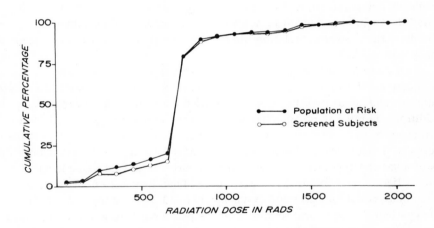

FIG.3. *Radiation-induced neoplasia: cumulative percentage against radiation dose.*

At the International Atomic Energy Agency Symposium in Chicago in 1975, we reported our findings concerning thyroid tumours among the first 1200 screened subjects [5]. The programme has continued and the purpose of this report is to relate our findings concerning other neoplasms in the population at risk, to attempt to determine whether any of these may have occurred in excess attributable to the radiation exposure, and to update the information on the incidence of thyroid tumours in this population.

An exact figure cannot be given for the number of patients located to date but suffice it to say that it is in excess of the 3254 subjects who have completed and returned the initial questionnaire. They comprise the screened group for this report and they represent 63% of the population at risk. A subgroup comprising 1539 subjects (30% of the group at risk) had actually come in for a physical examination including a thyroid scan with $^{99}Tc^m$. Detailed surgical-pathology data pertinent to thyroid tumours was obtained for 366 subjects, and all information available, in some cases only the radiation record, in other cases including the questionnaire and in yet others the full physical examination and thyroid scintigram findings, has been entered on a computerized data file.

The screened group has been compared with the overall population at risk in regard to age at the time of treatment, year of treatment (or number of years lapsed since treatment) and radiation dose. No significant differences have been observed (Figs 1—3).

Although the absolute number of thyroid tumours has increased as more subjects have been located and examined, the proportion of patients with clinically detectable thyroid tumours has remained fairly constant as has the ratio of benign to malignant tumours noted on histological examination. Similarly the dose-effect relationship that we reported previously has remained essentially unchanged [5].

Of those patients subjected to the complete screening procedures, numbering 1539 subjects, 26.9% were found to have clinically detectable thyroid tumours and about two-thirds of that group underwent surgical exploration. In addition a number of patients had been screened and examined elsewhere and arranged for us to receive tissue blocks or microscopy slides and copies of their records. The surgical pathology was reviewed independently by a collaborating pathologist. Altogether we have detailed reports on thyroid tissue from 366 patients. Two hundred and fifty (68.3%) had benign tumours such as adenomas, colloid nodules and cysts, and 111 (33.3%) had thyroid cancers. One patient had equivocal findings that the pathologists were not prepared to categorize as either normal or tumour, one had a hyperplastic lymph node embedded in the thyroid and two had thyrogloccal cysts. Using the pathology classification of Woolner [8], 73 of the malignant tumours were classified as macroscopic papillary carcinoma (including mixed papillary-follicular carcinoma) and 12 were pure follicular carcinomas. Twenty-six patients had microscopic papillary carcinomas less than 5 mm in diameter. These tumours fall within the definition of 'occult' carcinoma of Sampson and co-workers [10] who have reported incidences of 'occult' thyroid cancer of 0.9% in Cleveland, Ohio [9], 5.7% in Ohmsted County, Minnesota [10], 13.7% in Iwate and Shinshu [11], 17.9% and 28.4% in Hiroshima and Nagasaki [12] and 24% in Honolulu [13]. Sampson and his co-workers have reported that these tumours were found incidentally at autopsy (some of these studies involved using a meticulous

TABLE I.　TUMOUR SITES

Site	No. of cases	Mean age at irradiation (years)	Mean latent interval (years)	Mean dose (rads)
Salivary gland	37	6.3	21.8	807
Neural	23	3.8	23.0	954
Skin	37	5.8	24.6	786
Lymphomas	9	4.9	22.7	845
Breast	45	10.6	20.6	801
Gonads	8	3.8	22.5	759
Miscellaneous	28	6.9	20.8	718
Total	187	6.6	22.1	805

TABLE II.　SALIVARY GLAND TUMOURS

Site	Pathology		Total
	Benign	Malignant	
Parotid	24	7	31
Submandibular	1	3	4
Unknown	2	0	2
Total	27	10	37

screening technique of serial sectioning of the tissue specimens [10]), were not clinically apparent before death and had no apparent influence on the cause of death. Sampson maintains that many, if not all, of the thyroid cancers which we have diagnosed may be in this category [14]. Elucidation of this point will require similar screening of a matched non-irradiated population comprising siblings of irradiated subjects (population control) and tonsillectomized patients (disease control) to determine the incidence of clinically detectable thyroid

TABLE III.   SALIVARY GLAND TUMOURS
Type and dose

Type	No. of cases	Mean age at irradiation (years)	Mean latent interval (years)	Mean dose (rads)
Benign	27	5.7	21.4	833
Malignant	10	7.8	22.8	740
Total	37	6.3	21.8	807

TABLE IV.   SALIVARY GLAND TUMOURS
Correlation with radiation dose

Radiation dose (rads)	Number screened	No. of tumours	Incidence (per 1000 subjects)
1– 500	331	2	6
501–1000	2490	31	12
1000–1500	206	4	19
Above 1500	81	0	—
Total	3108	37	12

TABLE V.   NEURAL ORIGIN TUMOURS
Site and pathology

Site	Pathology		Total
	Benign	Malignant	
Brain	3	6	9
Pituitary	2	0	2
Cranial nerve	3	0	3
Peripheral	8	1	9
Total	16	7	23

TABLE VI. NEURAL ORIGIN TUMOURS
Type and dose

Type	No. of cases	Mean age at irradiation (years)	Mean latent interval (years)	Mean dose (rads)
Brain	9	4.0	24 ·	872
Pituitary	2	3.5	21	1200
Cranial nerve	3	3.0	25	1000
Peripheral nerve	9	4.0	21	967
Total	23	3.8	23	954

TABLE VII. NEURAL ORIGIN TUMOURS
Correlation with radiation dose

Radiation dose (rads)	Number screened	No. of tumours	Incidence (per 1000 subjects)
1– 500	331	1	3
501–1000	2490	16	6
1001–1500	206	4	19
Above 1500	81	2	25
Total	3108	23	7

TABLE VIII. LYMPHOMA AND HODKIN'S DISEASE
Pathology and dose

Pathology	Number of cases	Mean age at irradiation (years)	Mean latent interval (years)	Mean dose (rads)
Hodkin's	6	2.3	20.5	942
Lymphoma	2	2.0	24.5	550
Total	8	2.3	21.5	844
Myeloma	1	26	32	850

tumours in the non-irradiated (or zero dose) group. A longitudinal follow-up of patients in the irradiated group who have thyroid tumours but who have elected not to undergo any specific therapy will determine whether these tumours may have clinical significance. This latter group now exceeds 100 subjects and a long-term follow-up has been planned. Similarly efforts have been initiated to identify a control group of about 400 people and to subject them to the same screening procedures.

The questionnaires used in the programme included a question regarding other (non-thyroid) tumours which may have been diagnosed and/or treated. One hundred and eighty-seven other tumours have been recorded to date (Table I). Mean age at the time of irradiation, mean latent interval to tumour diagnosis and mean radiation dose are noted.

Thirty-seven salivary gland tumours have been recorded among 3108 screened subjects for an incidence of 12 per 1000 subjects. Ten of these were malignant and 27 were benign. Most arose from the parotid gland (Table II). The mean age at irradiation, latent interval to diagnosis and radiation dose are recorded (Table III). An apparent dose-effect correlation (Table IV) was not statistically significant. The difference in proportions between various dose groups yielded p values between 0.1 and 0.4. The expected incidence of salivary gland tumours in a non-irradiated population is difficult to establish. Modan and co-workers reported no cases in their control groups numbering 16 400 subject [15]. Takeichi and co-workers reported from 0 to 2 cases per 100 000 yearly from 1953 to 1971 in non-A-bomb exposed residents of Hiroshima [16]. This corresponds to 1.5 per 1000 subjects for a 21.8 year follow-up period similar to that in our study. Bouquot found the incidence in non-irradiated residents of Ohmsted County, Minnesota, to be 0.16 cases per 1000 [17]. If these figures reflect the expected incidence then our study population has a 10—75 fold increase with a p value less than 0.0001.

Twenty-three tumours of neural origin have been identified of which 16 were benign and seven were malignant (Table V). All three cranial nerve tumours were acoustic neuromas. Mean age at irradiation, latent interval to diagnosis and radiation dose are shown in Table VI. Correlation of radiation dose with tumour incidence (Table VII) reveals differences of proportion with p values in the range 0.03 to 0.05 between certain dose groups. These values are significant and suggest a positive correlation between radiation dose and incidence of neural origin tumours. The incidence of malignant brain tumours has been reported to be about 4—6 per 100 000 in the United States of America [18]. We observed six cases among 3108 screened subjects, which is a 32-fold increase and is significant (p < 0.0001). Accurate figures for the expected incidence of other neural origin tumours are not available.

Six cases of Hodgkin's disease, two lymphomas and one case of myeloma have been noted to date (Table VIII). The patient with myeloma was 26 years

TABLE IX.   LYMPHOMA AND HODGKIN'S DISEASE
Correlation with radiation dose

Radiation dose (rads)	Number screened	No. of cases	Incidence (per 1000 subjects)
1– 500	331	2	6
501–1000	2490	5	2
1001–1500	206	2	10
Above 1500	81	0	–
Total	3108	9	3

TABLE X.   GONADAL TUMOURS
Type and dose

Type	No. of cases	Mean age at irradiation (years)	Mean latent interval (years)	Mean dose (rads)
Ovary	3	3.7	20.7	892
Testis	5	3.8	23.6	680
Total	8	3.8	22.5	759

TABLE XI.   GONADAL TUMOURS
Correlation with radiation dose

Radiation dose (rads)	Number screened	No. of tumours	Incidence (per 1000 subjects)
1– 500	331	1	3
501–1000	2490	6	2
1000–1500	206	1	5
Above 1500	81	0	–
Total	3108	8	3

TABLE XII. SKIN TUMOURS
Pathology and dose

Pathology	No. of cases	Mean age at irradiation (years)	Mean latent interval (years)	Mean dose (rads)
Benign	27	6.6	23.6	761
Malignant	10	3.7	27.2	854
Total	37	5.8	24.6	786

TABLE XIII. SKIN TUMOURS
Correlation with radiation dose

Radiation dose (rads)	Number screened	No. of cases	Incidence (per 1000 subjects)
1– 500	331	2	6.0
501–1000	2490	34	13.7
1001–1500	206	0	—
Above 1500	81	1	12.4
Total	3108	37	11.9

TABLE XIV. BREAST TUMOURS
Type and dose

Type	No. of cases	Mean age at irradiation (years)	Mean latent interval (years)	Mean dose (rads)
Benign	42	9.1	20.5	777
Malignant	3	31.7	27	1150
Total	45	10.6	20.6	801

TABLE XV.   BREAST TUMOURS
Correlation with radiation dose

Radiation dose (rads)	No. of subjects screened	No. of cases	Incidence (per 1000 subjects)
1— 500	331	2	6.0
501—1000	2490	40	16.1
1001—1500	206	2	9.7
Above 1500	81	1	12.4
Total	3108	45	14.5

TABLE XVI.   MISCELLANEOUS TUMOURS

Site	Pathology		Total
	Benign	Malignant	
Larynx	5	—	5
Parathyroid	1	—	1
Bone	4	—	4
Nose/sinuses	3	—	3
Dental	3	—	3
Bladder	—	1	1
Uterus	—	1	1
Soft tissue	5	2	7
Colon	—	2	2
Lung	—	1	1
Total	21	7	28

old at the time of irradiation, manifested the disease at the age of 58 years and has been excluded from statistical consideration. No significant correlation of lymphoma and Hodgkin's disease incidence with radiation dose was evident (Table IX). The incidence of Hodgkin's disease and lymphoma reported in the United States of America is about ten cases per 100 000 yearly [11]. For the period of observation of our study population we would have expected 6.7 cases compared with the observed eight cases — an insignificant difference.

Information on gonadal tumours (Tables X and XI), skin tumours (Tables XII and XIII), breast tumours (Tables XIV and XV) and miscellaneous other tumours (Table XVI) are presented for completeness of information and without comment.

In addition, 116 subjects are known to be dead. Twenty-three of the deaths were due to tumour and 16 of these were included in this report. No information is available on the others at present. No deaths attributable to thyroid cancer have been recorded.

ACKNOWLEDGEMENTS

The authors wish to thank the following persons for essential assistance and advice: G.B. Hutchinson, M.D. (Epidemiology), W.M. Recant, M.D., and W.A. Meissner, M.D. (Pathology), L.R. Simpson, M.S. (Radiation Dosimetry and Computing) and B. Kaplan (Computing).

REFERENCES

[1] NATIONAL ACADEMY OF SCIENCES, The Effects on Populations of Exposure to Low Levels of Ionizing Radiation, Advisory Committee on the Biologic Effects of Ionizing Radiation, National Academy of Sciences, Washington D.C. (1972).

[2] UNITED NATIONS, Ionizing Radiation — Levels and Effects, United Nations Scientific Committee on Effects of Atomic Radiation, UN, New York (1972).

[3] AUB, J.C., et al., The late effects of internally deposited radioactive materials in man, Medicine 31 (1952) 221.

[4] HUTCHISON, G.B., Late neoplastic changes following medical irradiation, Cancer 37 (1976) 1107.

[5] COLMAN, M., SIMPSON, L.R., PATTERSON, L.K., COHEN, L., "Thyroid cancer associated with radiation exposure: Dose-effect relationship", Biological and Environmental Effects of Low-Level Radiation (Proc. Symp. Chicago, 1975) 2, IAEA, Vienna (1976) 285.

[6] De GROOT, L., PALOYAN, E., Thyroid carcinoma and radiation — a Chicago endemic, J. Am. Med. Assoc. 225 (1973) 487.

[7] ARNOLD, J., et al., ^{99m}Tc-pertechnetate thyroid scintigraphy in patients predisposed to thyroid neoplasms by prior radiotherapy to head and neck, Radiology 115 (1975) 653.

[8] WOOLNER, L.B., Thyroid carcinoma: pathologic classification with data on prognosis, Semin. Nucl. Med. 1 (1971) 481.

[9]   HAZARD, J.B., KAUFMAN, N., A survey of thyroid glands obtained at autopsy in so-
        called goiter area, Am. J. Clin. Pathol. 22 (1952) 860.
[10] SAMPSON, R.J., et al., Occult thyroid carcinoma in Ohmsted County, Minnesota:
        Prevalence at autopsy compared with that in Hiroshima and Nagasaki, Japan, Cancer 34
        (1974) 2072.
[11] YAGAWA, K., et al., "Clinicopathological study of latent thyroid carcinoma", Proc.
        Japanese Cancer Association (25th Annual Meeting) (1966) 106.
[12] SAMPSON, R.J., et al., Thyroid carcinoma in Hiroshima and Nagasaki: I. Prevalence
        of thyroid carcinoma at autopsy, J. Am. Med. Assoc. 209 (1969) 65.
[13] FUKANAGA, F.H., LOCKETT, L.J., Thyroid carcinoma in the Japanese in Hawaii,
        Arch. Pathol. Lab. Med. 92 (1971) 6.
[14] SAMPSON, R.J., Thyroid carcinoma (Letters to the Editor), New Engl. J. Med. 295
        (1976) 340.
[15] MODAN, B., et al., Radiation-induced head and neck tumours, Lancet i (1974) 277.
[16] TAKEICHI, N., et al., Salivary gland tumors in atomic bomb survivors, Hiroshima,
        Japan, Cancer 38 (1976) 2462.
[17] BOUQUOT, J.E., Personal communication (1977).
[18] NATIONAL CANCER INSTITUTE, Third National Cancer Survey: Incidence Data,
        National Cancer Institute (DHEW Publication No. (NIH) 75–787), Bethesda, Maryland
        (1975).

DISCUSSION

R.E. LINNEMANN: Did you see a linear relationship between dose and increased thyroid cancer incidence? Also, what was the lowest dose at which you found an increase in thyroid cancer incidence?

M. COLMAN: The precise shape of the dose-response curve cannot be determined on the basis of our data. The lowest dose at which thyroid cancer was observed was 150 rads, and several differently shaped curves could be fitted to the data, including a linear response function or a sigmoid function with an initial slope of less magnitude than the subsequent slope. We have not observed a plateau effect nor a diminished slope at higher doses.

K. NEUMEISTER: How can you be sure that all these tumours are not multiple primary malignant tumours, unrelated to radiation?

M. COLMAN: To verify that radiation exposure is a causative factor, one has to demonstrate that the incidence of tumours in the study population exceeds the expected incidence in a similar age group in the United States of America and exceeds that in a control group of unirradiated siblings and patients treated by non-radiation methods such as surgery. We have demonstrated that the incidence of thyroid cancer, salivary gland tumours and primary brain malignancy is greater than expected. A control group will be examined over the next few years.

I. SCHMITZ-FEUERHAKE: In a previous paper by Arnold and co-workers it was reported that there was a greater sensitivity to thyroid cancer among Jewish people, just as had been observed by Hempelmann and co-workers in children irradiated for thymic enlargement. Was this confirmed in your investigations?

M. COLMAN: We have not actually studied this point, as the religious or cultural background of our patients has not been recorded. In any event most of our patients were Jewish, lived in a predominantly Jewish area of Chicago and were treated in a Jewish hospital. The minority of non-Jews in the study population makes it difficult to draw any firm conclusion, however.

H.H. VOGEL: Would you please comment on the methodology used in your retrospective medical study at the Michael Reese Hospital in Chicago? Within a few years, you have received data back from more than 60% of the irradiated population. This is an extraordinary achievement. How did you manage it?

M. COLMAN: The 'trace and search' programme depended heavily on the meticulous and methodical efforts of dedicated staff assistants and the publicity accorded by the Chicago newspapers and television stations to the programme. Most of the subjects sought us out following this publicity. The remainder were traced by use of the Chicago regional telephone directories — calling telephone subscribers or companies having the same name as the patients being searched for.

LATE EFFECTS OF RADIOTHERAPY ON THE LYMPH SYSTEM EXAMINED BY LYMPHOGRAPHY*

E.F. KUHN, Z. MOLNÁR, K. BÖHM
Radiological Clinic,
Medical University,
Pécs,
Hungary

Abstract

LATE EFFECTS OF RADIOTHERAPY ON THE LYMPH SYSTEM EXAMINED
BY LYMPHOGRAPHY.

Twenty-three patients with Hodgkin's disease and malignant testicular tumours had repeat bipedal lymphography 13–73 months following radiotherapy. Cobalt-60 teletherapy was administered either with prophylactic or therapeutic intent by two opposed fields, which encompassed the whole infra-diaphragmatic (inguinofemoral, pelvic and para-aortic) lymph region. Most patients received also radiotherapy to the whole mediastinal lymph region. The lowest tumour dose was of 3000 rads (30 Gy), the highest of 4500 rads (45 Gy) to the infra-diaphragmatic region, with a total weekly dose of 900–1000 rads (9–10 Gy) given in five fractions. Number, calibre and valves of lymphatic vessels, transport capacity, collateral pathways; the filling and width of the thoracic duct, the number, size, shape and storage character of lymph nodes were compared on the first and repeat lymphography films. The number of lymphatic vessels was hardly influenced by radiotherapy, and calibre narrowing was seen in more than half of the patients. The size of lymph nodes was drastically decreased, especially in those who received a tumour dose over 3000 rads (30 Gy). Since new collateral pathways could not be found, it seems obvious that radiotherapy between these dose ranges does not reduce the transport capacity of lymphatic vessels.

INTRODUCTION

It is now universally accepted that bipedal lymphography with oily contrast material is a useful method in staging procedures of malignant tumours of the genito-urinary organs, of the lower limb as well as of malignant lymphomas. The various roentgen-morphologic signs on lymphangiograms and lymphadenograms give valuable information on metastatic spread, and help the radiotherapist on precise field shaping and arrangement. Surveillance films taken during and following radiotherapy are of great importance in judging the effectiveness of radiotherapy and in early detection of recurrences. Since the oily contrast

* Work supported by the Scientific Research Council, Ministry of Health, Hungary (3-25-1002-01-0/K).

material disappears mostly within 12 months, a repeat lymphography might be indicated to obtain information on the actual condition of the pelvic and para-aortic lymph region. This second-look lymphography also enables a study to be made of those changes that could have been caused by previous radiotherapy.

MATERIALS AND METHOD

Between the years 1971–77 28 patients had repeat lymphography, three of the patients also having a third-look lymphography. Of these 28 patients 23 could be evaluated. There were 14 females and 9 males, 3 had malignant testicular tumours, the others Hodgkin's disease. The youngest patient was 19, the eldest was 66 years old. The shortest interval between the first and repeat lymphography was 13 months, the longest 73 months. The first lymphography was made as part of a radiologic evaluation at the first admission before any treatment had begun. One millilitre of contrast material (Lipiodol Ultra Fluid) per 10 kg body weight was injected into each lower limb with the restriction that the whole quantity of contrast material must not exceed 7.5 ml into each lower limb. The injection was performed by a motor-driven pump with a constant flow rate of 0.8–1.0 ml contrast material during 10 minutes. Films were taken during and one hour after the end of injection to visualize the opacified lymphatic vessels as well as thoracic duct. Other films in antero-posterior and oblique directions were exposed after 24 hours to obtain detailed information on the storage picture of the lymph nodes. The inguinofemoral, common and external iliac as well as para-aortic lymphatic regions were examined bilaterally in each patient.

The second lymphography was performed under the same conditions. The identity of the technical parameters in each examination seems to be a sound basis in comparing results.

Treatment consisted of radiotherapy administered by ^{60}Co teletherapy with a SSD of 70–80 cm. Two opposed anterior and posterior fields were used which encompassed the inguinofemoral, pelvic and para-aortic lymph node areas to the level of the diaphragm. Tumour dose was calculated at the midplane level. Treatment was given five days weekly, and all fields were irradiated every day by a tumour dose of 180–200 rads (1.8–2.0 Gy). The total tumour dose varied between 3000–4500 rads (30–45 Gy) depending on the histology and aiming at prophylactic or therapeutic intent.

The mediastinum was irradiated by two opposed anterior and posterior fields. The tumour dose was calculated at the midplane level without lung correction. Treatment was given five days weekly, every field being treated at each session by a tumour dose of 180–200 rads (1.8–2.0 Gy). The tumour dose varied between 3060–5660 rads (30.6–56.6 Gy), most patients receiving

TABLE I. CHANGES POST IRRADIATION

	Unchanged	Reduced	Increased
Lymph vessels (23[a])			
Number	21	2	–
Calibre	10	13	–
Lymph flow (23[a])	21	–	2
Thoracic duct (18[a])			
Filling	8	3	7
Calibre	12	3	3
Lymph nodes (23[a])			
Number	21	2	–
Size	3	20	–

[a] Number of patients.

4200–4400 rads (42–44 Gy). The mediastinal irradiation always preceded
infra-diaphragmatic irradiation in patients with Hodgkin's disease. Patients with
malignant testicular tumours first received infra-diaphragmatic irradiation,
followed by mediastinal irradiation in those patients in which the para-aortic
lymph nodes were thought to be metastatic.

On the lymphography films the following signs were studied: the number,
calibre and valves of lymphatic vessels, transport capacity, the possible lympho-
venous anastomoses and collaterals; the width and length of filling of the
thoracic duct; the number, size, shape and storage character of lymph nodes.

RESULTS

The summarized results are shown in Table I. It is obvious that the number
of lymphatic vessels was hardly influenced by radiotherapy. The calibre width
of the lymphatic vessels showed more significant changes. The lumen of the
lymphatic vessels was narrower than before radiotherapy in 13 patients, and
one had the impression that these vessels have partly lost their elasticity and
become somewhat stretched and rigid. In spite of these findings the transport
capacity of the lymphatic vessels, judging by the length of that period in which

TABLE II. CHANGES IN CONNECTION WITH DOSE ABSORBED
(3000–4500 rads)

Alteration dose	Lymph vessels (23[a])		Thoracic duct (18[a])		Lymph nodes (23[a])	
	Number	Calibre	Filling	Calibre	Number	Size
rad = 3000 Unaltered	6	4	2	4	6	1
rad ≈ 4000	15	6	6	8	15	2
rad = 3000 Decreased	–	2	–	–	–	5
rad ≈ 4000	2	11	3	3	2	15
rad = 3000 Increased	–	–	2	–	–	–
rad ≈ 4000	–	–	5	3	–	–

[a] Number of patients.

the contrast material disappeared from the vessels as well as by the length of the opacified vessels, was not disturbed. In no case could we detect any sign of dermal backflow, new collateral vessels or lympho-venous shunts. It is obvious that blocking of the lymph flow never occurred. Acceleration of lymph flow was seen in two patients.

Filling of the thoracic duct was partly the same as before irradiation, three patients showing decreased and seven increased filling. The calibre of the thoracic duct remained unaltered in 12 patients, it became narrower in three, and in three its dilatation could be observed.

The number of lymph nodes decreased in two cases only. In contrast to this the size of the lymph nodes decreased in 20 patients with a factor of about 50%. The shape of the lymph nodes was not influenced by radiotherapy. The storage picture of the lymph nodes, which decreased in size, was mostly altered, the density of contrasting being markedly increased.

Table II shows the changes in connection with the absorbed dose. It seems clear — as one expected — that the changes mentioned above became more frequent with increasing absorbed dose. Doses over 3000 rads (30 Gy) drastically decreased the size of the lymph nodes. Calibre narrowing and rigidity of the lymphatic vessels also became striking above this dose level.

We investigated the influence of the time elapsed following radiotherapy on the frequency of the observed changes. It was found that calibre narrowing of the lymphatic vessels and decrease in size of the lymph nodes did not significantly progress with time elapsed, and all changes that could be detected following radiotherapy at these dose levels were already present within two years.

DISCUSSION

It has been for long well known that cellular elements of lymphatic tissue belong to the most radiosensitive structures of organisms, and there is much literature discussing the processes of cellular damage and repair. A good deal has been stated, mostly by surgeons, on the fibrosing effect on the lymphatic vessels caused by radiotherapy, claiming that lymphoedema observed in patients who had undergone combined surgery and radiotherapy was caused by radio-therapy. Macroscopic changes of the irradiated lymphatic system could only be examined in vivo after introduction of repeat lymphography. The literature discussing the late effects of radiotherapy on morphologic and functional changes of the lymphatic system is rather scanty. It has been uniformly pointed out that a total blocking of lymph flow never develops, not even as a result of doses of the range of 6100–8000 rads (61–80 Gy), although these doses do obliterate a few lymphatic vessels [1–8]. Our experiences are in good agreement with these findings, though the doses administered in our tests fell below these dose levels. Gregl and co-workers [1] emphasize that lymphatic blockade develops in those patients only who underwent surgery that mechanically dissected lymphatic vessels.

The frequency of calibre narrowing of the lymph vessels found by us is of about the same range as mentioned in the literature [4, 6, 8]. In contrast to data in the literature we could not observe the destruction of the valves of the lymphatic vessels [6, 8], and some acceleration of the lymph flow, also mentioned in the literature [6, 8] was seen, especially in the thoracic duct. This seems to be closely connected with the decreased storage capacity of the lymph nodes, which were decreased in volume, since we gave the same quantity of contrast material as previously. The on-flow rate was constant, yet the capacity of the storage pool diminished, so that the out-flow rate must be speeded up to be able to transport the increased quantity of contrast material. In this sense the acceleration of lymph flow seems to us to be artificial, and it is therefore questionable whether it occurs under normal conditions. The increased in-flow rate of the contrast material into the subclavian vein is well demonstrated on chest X-ray pictures, which show diffuse disseminated micro-embolization of the contrast material.

The significant decrease in the size of the lymph nodes is emphasized also by other authors [1, 3, 5, 6, 8], and it is pointed out that after doses over 6000 rads (60 Gy) this occurs in 100% of cases.

Segenidze and Zyb [6] believe that radiotherapy-induced changes increase with the time elapsed following radiotherapy. Our experiences show that changes can already be seen after two years, and seem not to increase later.

CONCLUSIONS

The results of repeat lymphographies following radiotherapy permit us to draw the following conclusions:

(1) Radiotherapy administered within therapeutic dose levels does not influence lymph circulation significantly enough to cause lymphoedema.

(2) Favourable results of pre-operative irradiation do not depend on 'lymphatic vessel's obliteration' as often quoted in the literature, since obliteration of all lymphatic vessels actually does not occur.

REFERENCES

[1]   GREGL, A., KIENLE, J., KRACK, U., YU, D., Röfo 112 (1970) 26.
[2]   LÜNING, M., WILJASALO, M., WEISSLEDER, H. (Eds), Lymphographie bei malignen
       Tumoren, G. Thieme, Leipzig (1976).
[3]   MACDONALD, J.S., Clin. Radiol. 20 (1969) 447.
[4]   MALINA, J., BRÜCKNER, F., BESKA, F., CERNY, J., KLEGA, J., Radiol. Clin. Biol.
       34 (1965) 357.
[5]   MARKOVITS, P., BLACHE, R., GASQUET, C., CHARBIT, A., Ann. Radiol. 12
       (1969) 835.
[6]   SEGENIDZE, G.A., ZYB, A.F., Lymphographie bei malignen Tumoren (LÜNING, M.,
       WILJASALO, M., WEISSLEDER, H., Eds), G. Thieme, Leipzig (1976) 292.
[7]   WILJASALO, M., PERTTALA, Y., Ann. Med. Intern. Fenn. 55 (1966) 57.
[8]   ZYB, A.F., NESTJAKO, O.W., Radiol. Diagn. 14 (1973) 332.

DISCUSSION

R.G. GREGORIO *(Chairman):* I wonder if the lymphatics of the breast would be of the same nature.

E.F. KUHN: We carried out breast lymphographies before any treatment was started, but repeat lymphographies were not performed. It seems to me, however, that the same changes may occur in the lymphatics of the breast after radiotherapy.

RADIOGENIC LATE EFFECTS IN THE EYE AFTER THERAPEUTIC APPLICATION OF BETA RADIATION

P. LOMMATZSCH
Ophthalmic Clinic,
Berlin-Buch

H.J. CORRENS
Nuclear Medicine Clinic of the
    Humboldt University,
Berlin

K. NEUMEISTER
Nuclear Safety and Radiation Protection
    Board of the German Democratic Republic,
Berlin,
German Democratic Republic

Abstract

RADIOGENIC LATE EFFECTS IN THE EYE AFTER THERAPEUTIC APPLICATION OF BETA RADIATION.

Although beta irradiation of the eye produces less risk of radiation-induced damage than other methods of irradiation, such side effects have to be expected after a long period. Beta irradiation with $^{90}Sr/^{90}Y$ is used to treat epibulbar tumours (carcinoma, melanoma) and irradiation with $^{106}Ru/^{106}Rh$ is used to treat intra-ocular tumours (melanoma, retinoblastoma). Two studies have been carried out. In the first, radiation-induced late damage after epibulbar beta irradiation was studied. Since 1960, 185 patients with epibulbar pigment tumours and 15 patients with conjunctiva carcinomas have been treated with $^{90}Sr/^{90}Y$-applicators and observed for several years. The dose applied was 10 000 to 20 000 rads at the focus depending on the type and extent of the tumour. Apart from teleangiectasias of the conjunctiva, there were only a few cases of severe radio-induced complications such as keratopathies and secondary glaucoma, which were regarded as the lesser evil in comparison with the main disease. The radiation cataract after beta irradiation remains peripheral and does not impair vision. The second study was of radiation-induced late damage after transscleral beta irradiation with $^{106}Ru/^{106}Rh$ of intra-ocular tumours. So far 39 patients with choroid melanomas and 22 children with retinoblastomas have been observed for more than 5 years after beta irradiation with $^{106}Ru/^{106}Rh$. The dose applied at the sclera surface was 40 000 to 100 000 rads for 4 to 8 days. In 39 patients with successfully irradiated choroid melanomas, radio-induced late complications developed such as macula degeneration, opticus atrophy and retinal-vessel ablations, which may impair vision. In the 22 children irradiated, only 7 cases of late complications with impaired functions could be observed. Whereas radiation-induced late damage after beta irradiation of the front section of the eye is of small clinical importance, especially in older patients, intra-ocular tumours with radio-induced late damage in the retinal vessel and capillary system have to be expected after high-dose beta irradiation.

187

Because of the high radiosensitivity of certain parts of the organ of vision, an effective radiotherapy of eye diseases faces more difficulties than in the case of other organs. By good co-operation among ophthalmologists, radiologists and radiophysicists, however, it is possible, particularly in treating primary malignant eye tumours, to apply a high dose to the diseased part without destroying the healthy parts by means of beta radiation. In the treatment of epibulbar processes the decay pair $^{90}Sr/^{90}Y$ in particular, and because of its somewhat greater penetration depth of radiation in the treatment of intra-ocular tumours, the decay pair $^{106}Ru/^{106}Rh$ have proved successful as sources of beta radiation. The maximum beta energy of ^{90}Y is 2.27 meV corresponding to a half-life layer in water of 15 mm. Rhodium-106 has a maximum beta energy of 3.53 meV and a half-life layer in water of 2.4 mm [1–8].

A report is here given on the radiogenic late effects in the eye after beta radiation. These observations were made on patients treated in the eye and tumour clinics of the Berlin Humboldt University (Charité) between 1960 and 1974.

1.   STRONTIUM-90/YTTRIUM-90 IRRADIATION OF PIGMENTED EPIBULBAR TUMOURS

From 1960 to 1974, 185 patients suffering from pigmented conjunctival tumours (69 melanomas, 107 pigmental naevi, 9 precancerous melanoses) were irradiated with $^{90}Sr/^{90}Y$-devices. Depending on the extent of the finding, the applied dose was 15 000 to 20 000 rads at the surface (daily dose: 1000 rads). The therapeutic results obtained will be reported elsewhere. During check-ups over many years the following radiogenic late effects could be observed:

1.1. In 65 patients teleangiectasias of conjunctival vessels developed in the irradiated region which, apart from cosmetic disadvantages, did not cause any functional disturbances.

1.2. In 15 cases a typical beta-radiation cataract developed after several years' latency (Fig. 1). In this type of cataract, the opacity of the lens was limited to the irradiated sector of the lens and always had a wedge-like shape with one base oriented towards the periphery. This did not cause any impairment of the patient's vision.

1.3. After inevitable co-irradiation of the cornea, in six patients keratopathies developed shortly after irradiation, which, however, quickly waned after medication.

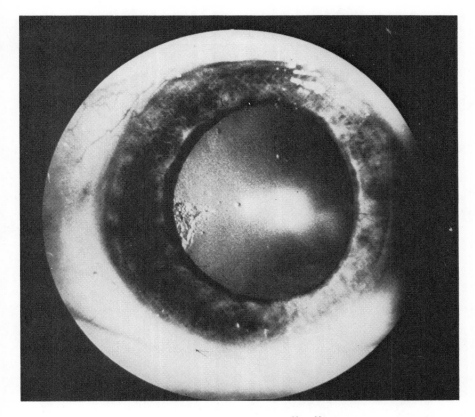

FIG.1.   Beta-radiation cataract 11 years after successful ^{90}Sr/^{90}Y-irradiation for conjunctival melanoma with 18 000 rads. Vision = 6/6.

1.4. In two patients there was a secondary glaucoma after irradiation, perhaps due-to the obliteration of the vessels offering aqueous humour (Schlemm's channel).

2.   CLINICAL EXPERIENCES WITH RUTHENIUM-106/RHODIUM-106 DEVICES

So far, 162 patients (124 choroid melanomas, 38 retinal blastomas) have been treated for intra-ocular tumours with ^{106}Ru/^{106}Rh-devices. For the time being, 61 patients suffering from choroid melanomas have been followed up for less then five years, 39 for more than five years. In 24 of them, enucleation could not be avoided because of continuing tumour growth. Out of a total of

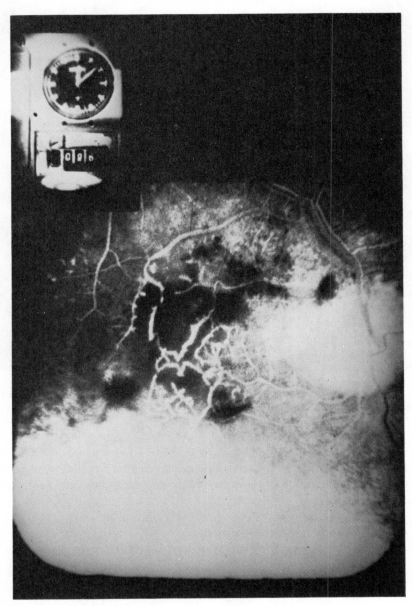

FIG.2.   Expanded and enlarged capillaries in macular region with capillary-free zones;
arteriovenous connections, three years after $^{106}Ru/^{106}Rh$-beta irradiation of choroid melanoma
above macula of left eye with 126 000 rads.   Vision = 6/36.

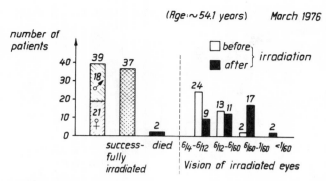

FIG.3.   Radiogenic late effects in 39 patients suffering from choroid melanoma more than five years after $^{106}Ru/^{106}Rh$-beta irradiation.

38 children suffering from bilateral retinal blastoma, 16 have so far been checked up for less and 22 for more than five years after irradiation. For assessing radiogenic damages, however, only those patients are reported on here who could be followed up for more than five years after treatment. These are 39 patients suffering from choroid melanomas and 22 children suffering from retinal blastomas.

2.1. Choroid melanoma (39 patients)

On an average, the applied dose was 80 000 to 100 000 rads at the scleral surface, for four to eight days. In spite of successful tumour irradiation, vision in 33 patients was worse after treatment than before, as radiogenic late effects destroyed the capillary vessel system (Fig. 2). The nearer the tumour to macula or opticus, the worse were the functional results at the end of the treatment. The following radiogenic late effects could be observed in the fundus (Fig. 3):

Macula degeneration	27
Partial opticus atrophy	7
Atrophy of larger vessels	3
Hard exsudates	2
Reversible corpus haemorrhage	1
Papillitis	1
Central venous occlusion	1

As fluorescence-angiographic investigations have shown, radiogenic vessel damage plays a great role in vision-decreasing side-effects. In the immediate neighbourhood of the irradiated tumour high-degree vascular constrictions and

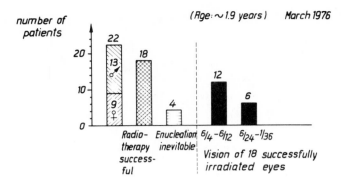

FIG.4.   *Radiogenic late effects in 22 patients suffering from retinal blastoma more than five years after* $^{106}Ru/^{106}Rh$-*beta irradiation.*

obliterations occur, so that a filling is hardly visible in the angiogram. Arterial walls are considerably thickened, the lumen closed. At the fringe of the irradiated region capillary micro-aneurysms with prolonged filling time, arteriovenous anastomoses and tele-angiectasias in the venous side develop under dye extravasation as a symptom of pathologically changed vessel walls. The region of irradiation effects is characterized by an extreme atrophy expressed in fluorescence angiography by the atrophy of retinal vessels, pigmental epithelium and choroid vessels. The papillar fading frequently observed is caused by the ascending atrophy of the retinal nerve fibres of the irradiated region. If the irradiation device was in the immediate neighbourhood of the opticus, direct damage to opticus capillaries occurs. Although obliterations of the arterial branch occur also after $^{106}Ru/^{106}Rh$-irradiations, the ischaemic regions seem to be not so extensive as after ^{60}Co-application. The radiation scars have more clear-cut borderlines. Fluorescence angiography, however, shows an effect by far exceeding the tumour region also in the case of irradiation devices.

2.2. Retinal blastoma

Out of 22 children suffering from retinal blastomas, 18 could be successfully irradiated with $^{106}Ru/^{106}Rh$-devices. The dose applied was 80 000 rads at the scleral surface, for four to eight days. In seven children radiogenic late effects developed, the destruction of the macula being always explained by an unfavourable tumour position near the posterior ocular pole (Fig. 4).

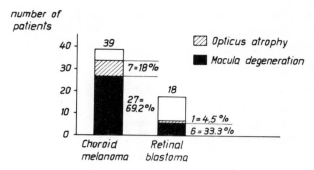

FIG.5.   Comparison of radiogenic late effects after beta irradiation of 57 patients suffering from choroid melanoma and retinal blastoma.

A comparison of the frequency of radiogenic vascular late effects of patients suffering from choroid melanomas (average age: 54.1 years) with those suffering from retinal blastomas (average age: 1.9 years) clearly shows that the complication rate is much higher in older patients than in children (Fig. 5). Of course this is partly due to the higher dose in melanoma irradiation; it cannot be excluded, however, that after radiation exposure of the infantile eye the threshold of damage to intra-ocular vessels is higher. The impression arises that ionizing radiation accelerates the sclerosing aging processes in the vascular system during biomorphosis. This agrees with the clinical observation that, particularly in older patients, radiogenic vascular late effects and the respective functional impairments have to be expected after irradiation treatment, the ophthalmoscopic picture of the posterior pole corresponding to late states of other vascular diseases.

3.   SUMMARY

3.1. Following beta irradiation (^{90}Sr/^{90}Y) of the anterior bulbar section in epibulbar tumours, the following late effects can develop after surface doses of more than 10 000 rads:

>   Teleangiectasias of the conjunctiva
>   Beta-radiation cataract
>   Keratopathies
>   Secondary glaucoma

3.2. In 39 patients (average age: 54.1 years) suffering from choroid melanomas who could be followed up for at least five years after ^{106}Ru/^{106}Rh-irradiation, the following radiogenic late effects were found to induce impairment of vision:

> 27 cases of macula degeneration
> 7 cases of opticus atrophy
> 3 cases of atrophy of large vessels
> 2 cases of hard exudates
> 1 case of central nervous thrombosis
> 2 cases of reversible corpus haemorrhages

The dose applied was 60 000 to 100 000 rads at the scleral surface (Fig. 5).

3.3. In 22 children irradiated with ^{106}Ru/^{106}Rh-devices for retinal blastomas and who could be followed up for at least five years, the following radiogenic late effects were found:

> 5 cases of macula destruction
> 1 case of macula degeneration
> 1 case of opticus atrophy

The dose applied was 40 000 to 80 000 rads at the scleral surface (Fig. 5).

3.4. Radiogenic late effects of choroid and retina develop several months only after irradiation:

> Construction and obliteration of retinal arteries, veins
> and capillaries
> enlarging of retinal capillary system with formation of
> aneurysms
> atrophy of the opticus
> atrophy of the choroid

3.5. Radiogenic vessel changes do not show a typical picture. They recall well-known changes of the vascular fundus due to other causes. In older patients there are more distinct vascular complications than in children. Under ionizing radiation, the processes of biomorphosis seem to be increased and accelerated.

3.6. The possibility of potential radiogenic late effects has to be particularly allowed for in making indications for radiotherapy of intra-ocular tumours near macula and papilla.

REFERENCES

[1]   BEDFORD, M.A., Trans. Ophthalmol. Soc. U.K. **XCIII** 1973 (1974).
[2]   HAYREH, S.S., Br. J. Ophthalmol. **54** (1970) 705.
[3]   LOMMATZSCH, P., Surv. Ophthalmol. **19** (1974) 85.
[4]   LOMMATZSCH, P., Albrecht v. Graefes Arch. Opthalmol. **176** (1968) 100.
[5]   LOMMATZSCH, P., Die therapeutische Anwendung von ionisierenden Strahlen in der Augenheilkunde, Georg Thieme, Leipzig (1977).
[6]   McFAUL, P.A., BEDFORD, M.A., Br. J. Ophthalmol. **54** (1970) 237.
[7]   MERRIAM, G.R., SZECHTER, A., FOCHT, M.F., Front. Radiat. Ther. Oncol. **6** (1972) 346.
[8]   VELHAGEN, K.H., LOMMATZSCH, P., GODER, G., Wiss. Z. Humboldt-Univ. Berl., Math.-Naturwiss. Reihe **XXII** (1973) 494.

DISCUSSION

W.A. MÜLLER: Do you think that beta irradiation is always to be preferred to other types of radiation, both from the point of view of the therapeutic results and the possible radiogenic late effects?

K. NEUMEISTER: Beta radiotherapy is the best type of radiation therapy for small tumours in the eye, in particular because it gives a very good dose distribution between the various parts of the organ. Late effects from beta radiotherapy may appear in very small parts of the eye. This is better than enucleation of the eye.

R.E. LINNEMANN: In the cataract complication, what was the dose to the lens and when did the cataract develop?

K. NEUMEISTER: The dose to the lens was more than 10 000 rads and the cataract developed after more than one year. We don't have any experience with lower beta-radiation doses.

RADIATION-ASSOCIATED CHRONIC MYELOGENOUS LEUKAEMIA IN YOUNGER PEOPLE

K. SHIMAOKA, J.E. SOKAL
Roswell Park Memorial Institute,
Buffalo,
New York,
United States of America

Abstract

RADIATION-ASSOCIATED CHRONIC MYELOGENOUS LEUKAEMIA IN
YOUNGER PEOPLE.
Chronic myelogenous leukaemia (CML) is known to be induced by exposure to
ionizing radiation, as is acute leukaemia. However, CML has been recorded only rarely as
a complication of radiation exposure early in life. This is partly because of the rarity of
this disease in childhood and young adulthood. During the period from 1973 to 1976,
75 patients with CML were admitted to Roswell Park Memorial Institute (RPMI). In addition,
64 patients admitted to RPMI previously were also available for study in 1973. Among
79 patients who were born after 1925, information regarding radiation exposure was
obtained in 89%; 49 were interviewed and 21 responded to a mailed questionnaire.
Consultation with parents was achieved in 52 of the 70 responding cases (74%). Replies
were obtained from 15 of the 18 patients below the age of 25, and were confirmed by
parents or siblings in all instances. Replies to the mailed questionnaire were obtained from
45 age- and sex-matched controls. In addition to two patients already known to have
radiation exposure for treatment of malignant neoplasms, these inquiries yielded a total of
nine patients with histories of radiation exposure for benign conditions. Three had therapeutic
irradiation, two for thymic enlargement and one for eczema. Three had exposure in utero
by pelvimetry. Two had diagnostic exposure during the perinatal period and one had
occupational exposure as a nurse. Four of these patients were below the age of 25. All nine
patients had the Ph' chromosome. The course of CML in these patients was not different
from that of other patients with Ph' chromosome-positive CML without a history of radiation
exposure. A history of radiation exposure was elicited in one-fourth of the younger patients
($<$ 25) in this study, compared with one of 45 age- and sex-matched controls without leukaemia
($p < 0.02$). Unless a specific inquiry had been made, and consultation with parents achieved,
this information would not have been uncovered.

It is known that exposure of human populations to ionizing radiation is
followed by an increase in the incidence of leukaemia [1−7]. Various forms of
leukaemia appear to be induced, except chronic lymphocytic leukaemia. There
are many reports of chronic myelogenous leukaemia (CML) following radiation
exposure among adult populations [3−23]. However, CML has been recorded

TABLE I. NUMBER OF CML PATIENTS IN THIS STUDY

	Total pts with CML	No. pts born after 1925	No. pts below age 25 at diagnosis	No. pts above age 25 at diagnosis
New RPMI patients, 1973–76	75	48	8	40
Old RPMI patients, available for study in 1973	64	31	10	21
Total	139	79	18	61
Replies to special inquiry obtained		65	15	50
History of radiation exposure	11	10	4	7
Percentage of patients			22%	11%
Percentage of responding patients			27%	14%

only rarely as a complication of radiation exposure early in life, and most follow-up studies of irradiated pediatric populations report no cases [24—30]. The development of CML in children and young adults following radiation exposure early in life appears to be a rare event. Recently, we studied a young adult with CML who had developed a thyroid nodule during the course of his disease [31]. During investigation of his thyroid disease, a history of thymic irradiation in infancy was elicited. We then initiated the present, detailed inquiry regarding radiation exposure among our patients with CML.

MATERIALS AND METHODS

Seventy-five patients with CML were admitted to Roswell Park Memorial Institute in a four-year period from 1 January 1973 to 31 December 1976. All the patients who were born after 1925 were either interviewed by the authors or sent detailed questionnaires regarding radiation exposure. In addition, 64 of 272 patients with CML admitted to Roswell Park between 1914 and 1972 were available in 1973 and were studied in a similar manner. Patients were requested to consult their mother, father or an older sibling before completing these interviews or questionnaires.

This inquiry supported our routine practice, in which radiation exposure was identified in the course of admission interviews by clerical staff of the Epidemiology Department or medical history-taking by junior professional staff. These procedures had uncovered cases with previous therapeutic irradiation for neuplastic disease, ankylosing spondylitis or uterine fibroid, but no exposure during infancy.

A total of 79 patients were born after 1925 and were available for detailed questioning regarding radiation exposure (Table I). Of these, 44 were interviewed and 21 responded to a mailed questionnaire, for a total response rate of 82%. Consultation with parents was achieved in 46 of the 65 responding cases (71%). There were 18 patients below the age of 25 at diagnosis of CML; replies were obtained from 15 and were confirmed by parents in all instances.

Patients attending the clinic of the School of Dentistry of the State University of New York at Buffalo[1], and students of the State University of New York at Buffalo, were asked to complete the same questionnaire. Among those whose replies indicated consultation with parents or older siblings, 45 were matched for age and sex with our younger CML patients and used as controls for this study.

---

[1]   The authors gratefully acknowledge the assistance of M. Sciascia and M. LaMastar, dental students at the State University of New York at Buffalo, School of Dentistry.

RESULTS

Eleven of these 139 patients with CML were found to have histories of radiation exposure. There were three females and eight males. The mean age at diagnosis of CML in these patients was 29.7 ± 3.3, with a range of 15 to 49 years. This is much younger than that of our population of patients with CML whose mean age was 51.6 ± 1.0 years ($p < 0.02$). The mean interval between radiation exposure and diagnosis of CML was 18.6 ± 2.8 years, with a range of 2 to 31 years. The average survival after diagnosis of these patients was 61 ± 12.5 months. This is somewhat longer than the average survival of all our patients with CML, but the difference is not statistically significant. Two patients received radiation therapy for malignant tumours: one for hypernephroma and the other for carcinoma of the breast. Three patients were treated for benign conditions, two for thymic enlargement and one for eczema. Three had exposure in utero via pelvimetry. Two had diagnostic exposures during the perinatal period and one had occupational exposure as an X-ray technician-nurse.

Four of these patients were below the age of 25 at the time of diagnosis of CML; two had received thymic irradiation and two pelvimetry. Among 45 age- and sex-matched controls, none had received thymic irradiation and only one gave a history of intra-uterine exposure; the mother had an abdominal X-ray examination (KUB film) in the second trimester of pregnancy for an obscure abdominal ailment. Comparison of the CML patients with these controls indicates that there is a statistically significant difference in radiation exposure ($p < 0.02$).

Chromosomal analyses were carried out on all 11 patients, and revealed the Philadelphia chromosome in 10 of them. The eleventh patient had a normal karyotype, but otherwise typical CML.

DISCUSSION

There is no doubt that exposure of human populations to ionizing radiation may induce CML as well as various forms of acute leukaemia. Occurrence of CML has been associated with radiation therapy for benign and malignant gynaecological disease [3, 4, 8, 9], exposure to the atomic bomb [7, 10, 11, 32], exposure to thorium [6, 12], radioiodine therapy [13–16], radiation therapy for polycythaemia [17] and various other types of radiation exposure [5, 18–22]. Our results appear to indicate that CML may develop many years after radiation exposure as well as after the usual leukaemia latency period, and that there is a greater spread of latency period than in acute leukaemia. An association with radiation is more likely to be recorded in younger populations, since radiation histories are more readily available. However, there is no way at present to identify an individual case of CML as radiation induced, since CML following radiation exposure does not differ from the 'spontaneous' disease [33].

CML is extremely rare in childhood, for reasons not yet understood. We have previously reported a paucity of childhood CML in the literature [31]. This is also recorded in a large-scale study of leukaemias [34]. The pediatric population appears to be much more susceptible to acute leukaemia, and the ratio of CML to acute leukaemia is very small, averaging 0.03 [35]. Although there is a decline in incidence of acute leukaemia in the late teens and early 20s, acute leukaemia is still much more common than CML, which is encountered much more frequently after the age of 30. Various cohort analyses of populations irradiated in utero or during infancy have indicated an increased incidence of acute leukaemia [24, 30]. However, they failed to identify any case of CML in these populations. This is probably because the number of subjects in these series was not large enough [31]. In addition, insufficient follow-up may have contributed to the failure to record CML among these cohorts; most such studies are terminated well before the subjects reach the age of 20. Our data indicate that a longer period of observation is necessary to detect all cases of radiation-associated CML. This conclusion is supported by studies of the Hiroshima bomb survivors, among whom an increased incidence of CML was still being recorded 25 years later.

When cases of CML are studied for previous radiation exposure, the yield for the association becomes much higher, as in our experience and that of others [5]. There are two other reports of CML following thymic irradiation [36,37]; these were associated with more typical incubation periods of nine and less than five years respectively, whereas our two cases had incubation periods of 18 and 22 years [31]. Our series includes three patients who had prenatal radiation exposure via pelvimetry; leukaemia was discovered at 15, 20 and 26 years of age. Such in-utero exposure to radiation has also been implicated as a possible cause of CML in one pediatric case reported in the literature [38]. It is of interest to note that pelvimetry has been performed twice in two of our three cases, and in the case reported by Barrett and co-workers [38].

It is noteworthy that although routine epidemiologic interview and medical history-taking successfully identified significant radiation exposure in adult life among our patients, these procedures completely failed to record exposure in infancy or in the prenatal period. Before undertaking the special inquiry reported herein, we would have underestimated the frequency of radiation-associated cases in our series of patients with CML. We suspect that this is also true in most other series, especially in so far as radiation in the perinatal period and early childhood is concerned.

We conclude that our patients probably represent examples of radiation-associated CML, and that the paucity of reports of CML following radiation exposure early in life is probably due to the following reasons: (1) the much

greater likelihood that acute leukaemia will be induced rather than CML;
(2) incomplete or too short follow-up periods in studies of radiation-exposed
populations; and (3) failure to obtain an accurate history of radiation exposure
in many cases of CML.

REFERENCES

[1] LEWIS, E.B., Leukemia, multiple myeloma and aplastic anemia in American radiologists,
     Science 142 (1963) 1494.
[2] COURT BROWN, W.M., ABBATT, J.D., Incidence of leukaemia in ankylosing spondylitis
     treated with X-rays: Preliminary report, Lancet i (1955) 1283.
[3] DOLL, R., SMITH, P.G., The long-term effects of irradiation in patients treated for
     metropathia haemorrhagica, Br. J. Radiol. 41 (1968) 363.
[4] SIMON, N., BRUCER, M., HAYES, R., Radiation and leukemia in carcinoma of the
     cervix, Radiology 74 (1960) 905.
[5] GUNZ, F.W., ATKINSON, H.R., Medical radiations and leukaemia: Retrospective survey,
     Br. Med. J. i (1964) 389.
[6] DaSILVA, J.H., DaMOTTA, L.C., Follow-up study of thorium dioxide patients in
     Portugal, Ann. N.Y. Acad. Sci. 145 (1967) 830.
[7] BRILL, A.B., TOMONAGA, M., HEYSSEL, R.M., Leukemia in man following exposure
     to ionizing radiation: Summary of findings in Hiroshima, Nagasaki and comparison
     with other human experience, Ann. Intern. Med. 56 (1962) 590.
[8] SØRENSEN, B., Late results of radium therapy in cervical carcinoma, Acta Radiol. Suppl.
     169 (1958) 1.
[9] LOUITIT, J.F., Malignancy from radium, Br. J. Cancer 24 (1970) 195.
[10] WATANABE, S., SHIMOSATO, Y., OHKITA, T., EZAKI, H., SHIGEMATSU, T.,
     KAMATA, N., "Leukemia and thyroid carcinoma found among A-bomb survivors in
     Hiroshima", Recent Results in Cancer Research 39 (GRUNDMANN, E., TULINIUS, H.,
     Eds), Springer-Verlag, Berlin (1972) 57.
[11] LIU, P.I., ISHIMARU, T., McGREGOR, D.H., Autopsy study of blast crisis in patients
     with chronic granulocytic leukemia, Hiroshima & Nagasaki 1949–1969, Cancer 33
     (1974) 1062.
[12] VAN KAICK, G., DRINGS, P., LOHOLTER, H., Chronische myelogische Leukaemie
     27 Jahre nach Thorotrastinkorporation, Strahlentherapie 43 (1973) 341.
[13] OZARDA, A., ERGIN, U., BENDER, M.A., Chronic myelogenous leukemia following
     I^{131} therapy for metastatic thyroid carcinoma, Am. J. Roentgenol., Radium Ther. Nucl.
     Med. 85 (1961) 914.
[14] WERNER, A.C., GITTELSOHM, A.M., BRILL, A.B., Leukemia following radioiodine
     therapy of hyperthyroidism, J. Am. Med. Assoc. 177 (1961) 649.
[15] BRINCKER, H., HANSEN, H.S., ANDERSEN, A.P., Induction of leukaemia by ^{131}I
     treatment of thyroid carcinoma, Br. J. Cancer 28 (1973) 232.
[16] BUNDI, R.S., SCOTT, J.S., HALNAN, K.E., Chronic myeloid leukaemia following radio-
     iodine therapy for carcinoma, Br. J. Radiol. 50 (1977) 61.
[17] MODAN, B., LILIENFELD, A.M., Polycythemia vera and leukemia: The role of radiation
     treatment; A study of 1222 patients, Medicine 44 (1965) 305.
[18] ENGEL, E., FLEXNER, J.M., ENGEL-DE MONTMOLLIN, M.L., FRANK, H.E., Blood
     and skin chromosomal alterations of a clonal type in a leukemic man previously
     irradiated for lung cancer, Cytogenetics 3 (1964) 228.

[19] ALBERT, R.E., OMRAN, A.R., Follow-up study of patients treated by X-ray epilation for tinea capitis: I. Population characteristics, post-treatment illnesses and mortality experience, Arch. Environ. Health **17** (1968) 899.

[20] SHIFFMAN, N.J., STECKER, E., CONEN, P.E., GARDNER, H.A., Males with chronic myeloid leukemia and the 45, XO, Ph' chromosome pattern, Can. Med. Assoc. J. **110** (1974) 1151.

[21] WHANG-PENG, J., GRALNICK, H.R., JOHNSON, R.E., LEE, E.C., LEAR, A., Chronic granulocytic leukemia during the course of chronic lymphocytic leukemia: Correlation of blood, marrow and spleen morphology and cytogenetics, Blood **43** (1974) 333.

[22] CANELLOS, G.P., Second malignancies complicating Hodgkin's disease in remission, Lancet i (1975) 1294.

[23] WAKISAKA, G., YONEDA, M., UCHINO, H., MIYATA, H., ENOMOTO, H., "Leukemia in radiological workers and in patients treated with irradiation", IX Congress International Society of Hematologists (1962) 511.

[24] STEWART, A., WEBB, J., HEWITT, D., Survey of childhood malignancies, Br. Med. J. i (1958) 1495.

[25] STEWART, A.M., KNEALE, G.W., Age distribution of cancer caused by obstetric X-rays and their relevance to cancer latent periods, Lancet ii (1970) 4.

[26] CONTI, E.A., PATTON, G.D., CONTI, J.E., HEMPELMANN, L.H., Present health of children given X-ray treatment to the anterior mediastinum in infancy, Radiology **74** (1960) 386.

[27] SAENGER, E.L., SILVERMAN, F.N., STERLING, T.D., TURNER, M.E., Neoplasia following therapeutic irradiation for benign conditions in childhood, Radiology **74** (1960) 889.

[28] PIFER, J.W., HEMPELMANN, L.H., DODGE, J.H., HODGES, F.J., Neoplasms in the Ann Arbor series of thymus-irradiated children, Am. J. Roengenol., Radium Ther. Nucl. Med. **103** (1968) 13.

[29] HEMPELMANN, L.H., HALL, W.J., PHILLIPS, M., COOPER, R.A., AMES, W.R., Neoplasms in persons treated with X-rays in infancy: Fourth survey in 20 years, J. Natl. Cancer Inst. **55** (1975) 519.

[30] JANOWER, M.L., MIETTINEN, O.S., Neoplasms after childhood irradiation of the thymus gland, J. Am. Med. Assoc. **215** (1971) 753.

[31] SHIMAOKA, K., SOKAL, J.E., Thymic irradiation and chronic myelogenous leukemia, New York State J. Med. **77** (1977) 2226.

[32] ICHIMARU, M., ISHIMARU, T., Leukemia and related disorders, J. Radiat. Res. Suppl. **16** (1975) 89.

[33] SHIMAOKA, K., EZDINLI, E.Z., HAN, T., FRIDMAN, M., Chronic myelocytic leukemia (CML) following irradiation, Proc. Am. Ass. Cancer Res. **12** (1971) 48.

[34] CUTLER, S.J., AXTELL, L., HEISE, H., Ten thousand cases of leukemia: 1940—1962, J. Natl. Cancer Inst. **39** (1967) 993.

[35] SHIMAOKA, K., SOKAL, J.E., "Chronic myelogenous leukemia developing after thymic irradiation", Proc. Third Int. Symposium on Detection and Prevention of Cancer, Part I: Prevention I: Etiology (NIEBURGS, H.E., Ed.), Marcel Dekker, New York (1977) 819.

[36] REISMAN, L.E., TRUJILLO, J.M., Chronic granulocytic leukemia of childhood, J. Pediatr. **62** (1963) 710.

[37] BURGERT, E.O., Jr., NIERI, R.L., MILLS, S.D., LINMAN, J.W., Non-lymphocytic leukemia in childhood, Mayo Clin., Proc. **48** (1973) 255.

[38] BARRETT, O., Jr., CONRAD, M., CROSBY, W.H., Chronic granulocytic leukemia in childhood, Am. J. Med. Sci. **240** (1960) 587.

DISCUSSION

G.W. DOLPHIN: It is an assumption that the existence of radiation exposure at some previous time in the history of CML patients has induced the leukaemia. Have you investigated the existence of any exposures to other carcinogenic agents such as chemicals?

K. SHIMAOKA: We have also been looking into other agents such as chemicals, pharmaceuticals and immunizations in our questionnaires. The 139 patients concerned in this survey failed to report any significant such exposures. However, among the CML cases previously reported from our institute (33), there were two patients (one with Hodgkin's disease and the other with ovarian cancer) who had received both radiation therapy and chemotherapy. We are also carrying out a study at present on patients with plasmacytoma; we have found some acute leukaemias but have yet to find a CML.

M. DELPLA: This paper prompts me to mention that, according to observations on Hiroshima survivors, the frequency of chronic granulocytic leukaemia appears to be higher even in the categories that were only slightly irradiated. I would add, however, that this is but one of the possible clinical forms of leukaemia and that the frequency of all the clinical forms together appears to be lower in the categories where the dose was not very high.

AGE- AND TIME-DEPENDENT CHANGES IN THE RATES OF RADIATION-INDUCED CANCERS IN PATIENTS WITH ANKYLOSING SPONDYLITIS FOLLOWING A SINGLE COURSE OF X-RAY TREATMENT

P.G. SMITH, R. DOLL
DHSS Cancer Epidemiology and
  Clinical Trials Unit,
Department of the Regius Professor
  of Medicine,
University of Oxford,
Oxford,
United Kingdom

Abstract

AGE- AND TIME-DEPENDENT CHANGES IN THE RATES OF RADIATION-INDUCED CANCERS IN PATIENTS WITH ANKYLOSING SPONDYLITIS FOLLOWING A SINGLE COURSE OF X-RAY TREATMENT.

The causes of death have been analysed in 14 111 patients with ankylosing spondylitis following a single course of X-ray treatment. Patients who were re-treated with X-rays were followed until the end of the year following their second course of treatment and deaths subsequent to this time were ignored. An attempt was made to follow the remaining patients to 1 January 1970, or their date of death or emigration, whichever was the earlier. A total of 7455 (52.8%) patients were re-treated before 1 January 1970, 1759 (12.5%) patients had died and 269 (1.9%) had emigrated. A total of 208 (1.5%) patients were lost to follow-up and the remaining 4420 (31.3%), who had all received one course of treatment, were alive. The number of deaths from all causes was 66% greater than the expected number computed from national age and sex specific mortality rates. There were 31 deaths from leukaemia (6.5 expected), 259 from cancers of 'heavily irradiated' sites (167.5 expected) and 79 from cancers of 'lightly irradiated' sites, which was not significantly higher than the 65.6 expected. The ratio of observed to expected deaths and the excess death rate from leukaemia was greatest in the period three to five years after first treatment and subsequently declined. The ratio of observed to expected deaths from cancers of heavily irradiated sites was high in the two years following treatment, fell to a minimum six to eight years after treatment and then rose. At longer intervals after treatment there was no significant trend with time in either the ratio of the observed to the expected number of deaths or in the excess death rate. Data for individual heavily irradiated sites showed little variation in the ratio of observed to expected numbers of deaths, apart from those due to tumours of the spinal cord. The ratio of observed to expected deaths for both leukaemia and cancers of the heavily irradiated sites showed no apparent change according to the age of the patients at their first treatment but the excess death rate showed a highly significant increase with increasing age at first treatment. This suggests that radiation is interacting with other factors that are inducing cancer.

205

INTRODUCTION

In the mid 1950s Court Brown and Doll identified over 14 000 patients who had been treated with X-rays for ankylosing spondylitis between 1935 and 1954 at any of 87 radiotherapy clinics in Great Britain and Northern Ireland. An attempt was made to follow up all these patients from the time of their original treatment until a fixed date to ascertain their mortality rates from various causes to determine if these could be related to the radiation treatment which the patients had received. Two major reports have been published on their mortality experience. The first dealt primarily with deaths from leukaemia [1] and the second compared death rates from other causes, particularly those due to cancer, with the corresponding rates in the general population of England and Wales [2]. Both of these earlier reports included deaths among patients who had been treated with X-rays for their spondylitis on more than one occasion. This complicated the interpretation of the late effects of the treatment on mortality as it was not clear to what extent the second or subsequent treatments contributed to the excess of deaths from leukaemia and cancers of heavily irradiated sites that persisted for many years after the first radiation treatment. We have avoided this problem in the present analysis by examining the death rates from leukaemia and radiation-induced cancers at different times after a single course of treatment. Patients who were re-treated have been included in the analysis up to 18 months following their second treatment course but any deaths occurring after this time have been ignored.[1]

By restricting the analysis to patients receiving only one treatment course we can examine the variation in the late effects of radiation according to both the age of the patient at the time of treatment and the time since the radiation exposure without any subsequent treatment being a complicating factor. The ways in which the risk of developing a radiation-induced cancer is dependent upon both these factors is clearly of relevance when considering both the biological mechanism by which radiation induces cancer and also in setting standards for radiological protection.

---

[1] Re-treated patients have been included for this period following their second course as, in some instances, the early symptoms of a cancer may have been mis-diagnosed as a recurrence of spondylitis and treated accordingly. Thus to exclude re-treated patients from the date of their second course might have biased the estimate of the carcinogenic effects of the initial course. It is unlikely that any carcinogenic effects of the second treatment course would have resulted in a patient dying within the 18 months following the treatment.

THE DATA

The study group consists of 14 111 patients who were first treated with X-rays for ankylosing spondylitis between 1935 and 1954 [1, 3]. An attempt has been made to trace all these patients up to the earliest of the following dates: (1) their date of death, (2) the end of the year following their second course of radiation treatment, (3) their date of emigration from the United Kingdom, or (4) 1 January 1970. Only 208 (1.5%) patients could not be fully traced in this way; 1759 (12.5%) patients had died; 7455 (52.8%) patients were found to have been re-treated before 1 January 1970, 269 (1.9%) had emigrated, and the remaining 4420 (31.3%) were alive at 1 January 1970. Of the initial group of 14 111 patients, 2335 (17%) were women. Similar proportions of men and women were traced and just over 50% of patients of each sex had been re-treated. As the results of all our analyses are similar for men and women we present here only the results for the two sexes combined. Most patients who were re-treated received their second course soon after the first, and these patients were followed, on average, for 3.5 years after their first course. The average follow-up period for patients receiving only one course was 16.2 years.

Causes of death were obtained from death certificates and coded according to the seventh revision of the International Classification of Diseases. Person years at risk were computed for each patient in the study in five-year age groupings and quinquennial time periods. Expected numbers of deaths were computed by multiplying the appropriate number of person years at risk by the corresponding age and sex specific mortality rates for England and Wales.

RESULTS

Mortality rates of spondylitic patients compared with national rates

In Table I the numbers of deaths from various causes are compared with the numbers expected if the patients in this study suffered the same age, sex and time specific death rates as the population of England and Wales. The total number of deaths, 1759, is 66% greater than the expected number, and this excess is statistically highly significant. Both the number of deaths from neoplasms and from non-malignant conditions are significantly in excess of the expected numbers. Of greatest interest for our present purpose are the deaths from cancer, and these have been divided into four groups. Deaths from leukaemia are shown separately as radiation exposure has a proportionately greater effect on deaths from this cause than on deaths from other cancers. This is apparent from Table I in which the ratio of observed to expected deaths from leukaemia

TABLE I. NUMBER OF DEATHS AMONG PATIENTS WITH ANKYLOSING
SPONDYLITIS COMPARED WITH THE NUMBERS EXPECTED BASED ON
NATIONAL MORTALITY RATES

	Observed	Expected	Observed/ expected	P (one-sided)
All causes	1759	1061.7	1.66	< 0.001
All neoplasms	397	256.9	1.55	< 0.001
Leukaemia	31	6.5	4.79	< 0.001
Cancer of colon	28	17.3	1.62	< 0.05
Cancers of H.I.S. [a]	259	167.5	1.55	< 0.001
Cancers of L.I.S. [b]	79	65.6	1.20	= 0.06
All other causes	1362	804.8	1.69	< 0.001

[a]   H.I.S. = heavily irradiated sites.
[b]   L.I.S. = lightly irradiated sites.

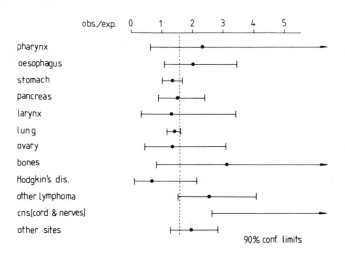

FIG.1.   Ratio of observed to expected number of deaths from cancers of heavily irradiated
sites three or more years after first treatment.   Upper confidence limits not shown in the
figure and for cancer of the pharynx, 6.0, and for cancer of the bones, 8.1.   For tumours of
the spinal cord and nerves the ratio of observed to expected deaths was 7.8 with upper
confidence limit of 18.0.   The dotted vertical line corresponds with the ratio of observed to
expected deaths for cancers of all heavily irradiated sites combined.

(4.8 to 1) is considerably greater than that for all other neoplasms combined (1.5 to 1). Cancer of the colon may be associated with spondylitis independently of any radiation effects through the increased risk of ulcerative colitis suffered by patients with spondylitis. Deaths from other cancers have been divided between those involving 'lightly irradiated' and 'heavily irradiated' sites. The former group consists of cancers of those sites not likely to have been included directly in the radiation field[2], and, though there is an excess of deaths from cancers of these sites, the difference of the observed from the expected number is not quite statistically significant (P = 0.06). In contrast, the excess over expectation of the number of deaths from cancers of those sites that were directly in the radiation field is statistically highly significant.

Some of the cancer deaths that occurred in the period immediately following the entry of patients into the study were due to tumours which were present at the time of first treatment and, indeed, may have been the cause of symptoms that were incorrectly ascribed to spondylitis and thus prompted the radiation treatment. Such deaths must be excluded from any analysis designed to estimate the carcinogenic effect of the treatment. Careful review of the case notes of the patients dying of leukaemia indicated that the three patients who died in the same year as they were first treated for spondylitis had developed their leukaemia before entry into the study, and these deaths have been excluded from subsequent analyses. The period of start of risk for leukaemia for all patients in the study has been taken from the beginning of the second year following first treatment. Examination of the data for cancers of other individual sites for a similar bias led us to exclude from further analysis all observations made up to three years immediately following first treatment for spondylitis [3].

In the period three or more years after first treatment, 68 deaths were ascribed to cancers of lightly irradiated sites and 56.2 were expected. This difference is not statistically significant and, furthermore, none of the individual sites included in this category showed significantly raised numbers of cancer deaths. The ratio of the observed to the expected numbers of deaths from cancers of those individual sites classed as heavily irradiated are shown in Fig.1 together with the 90% confidence intervals on the ratios. If tumours of the spinal cord and nerves are excluded the variation in the ratios between the remaining sites is not statistically significant. Two of the four deaths from tumours of the spinal cord and nerves which were recorded three or more years after first treatment occurred four years after first treatment, but we have no evidence that the tumours were present when these patients were first treated.

---

[2] These sites were: brain (excluding tumours of the spinal cord and nerves), mouth, tongue, liver, rectum, breast, uterus, prostate, testes, kidney, bladder, lip, vulva, vagina, penis, scrotum, jaw and nose.

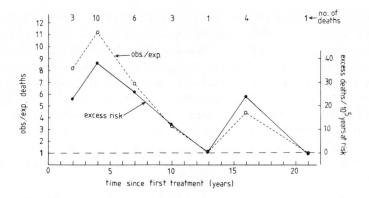

FIG.2.   Observed and expected numbers of deaths from leukaemia according to the time since first treatment.

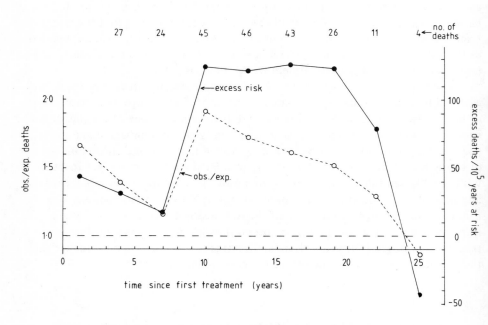

FIG.3.   Observed and expected deaths from cancers of 'heavily irradiated' sites, according to the time since first treatment.

Time since first treatment

Figure 2 shows the change in the ratio of the number of deaths from leukaemia to the number expected according to the time since first treatment. This ratio is highest in the period three to five years after first treatment, and the decline subsequent to this period is statistically significant ($P < 0.01$). In the period 15 to 17 years after entry four deaths from leukaemia occurred whereas only 0.9 were expected. Subsequent to this period one death occurred and about one was expected. Also shown in Fig.2 is the change in the excess death rate from leukaemia with time since first treatment.[3] This rate also is highest in the period three to five years after first treatment, and subsequently shows a statistically significant decline.

Figure 3 shows similar data for deaths from cancers of the heavily irradiated sites. The ratio of the number of observed to expected deaths was low in the period six to eight years after first treatment and then rose. At longer intervals the ratio declined steadily but the trend downwards is not statistically significant (χ^2(1 d.f.) = 3.35; $P < 0.10$). The excess death rate also fell to a minimum at six to eight years following treatment, and then rose to maintain a level that was approximately constant up to 20 years after first treatment. The decline 20 or more years after treatment is not statistically significant — in this period there were 15 deaths whereas 13.18 were expected.

Age at first treatment

The ratio of the observed number of deaths from leukaemia two or more years after first treatment to the number expected is shown in Table II according to the age of the patients at their first treatment for spondylitis. The differences in the ratios in the five age groups are not statistically significant. However, in the general population the leukaemia death rate increases markedly with age and thus the excess death rate from leukaemia shows a considerable increase with age at first treatment, which is statistically significant ($P < 0.01$). Deaths from cancers of heavily irradiated sites showed a similar trend (Fig.4). The ratio of observed to expected deaths from cancers of heavily irradiated sites does not change significantly with age at first treatment but when the excess death rate is calculated a steep rise with age at first treatment is seen which is highly statistically significant ($P < 0.001$).

---

[3] The excess risk is computed, for each of the periods following first treatment, as (no. of deaths − expected no.) $\times 10^5$/(no. of person years at risk).

TABLE II. NUMBERS OF DEATHS FROM LEUKAEMIA TWO OR MORE
YEARS AFTER FIRST TREATMENT ACCORDING TO THE AGE AT
FIRST TREATMENT

Age at first treatment (years)	Observed	Expected	Observed/ expected	Excess deaths/10^5 person years at risk
< 25	1	0.40	2.5	4
25–34	7	1.35	5.2	13
35–44	8	1.71	4.7	19
45–54	8	1.39	5.8	43
⩾ 55	4	1.00	4.0	52
Total	28	5.85	4.8	19.6

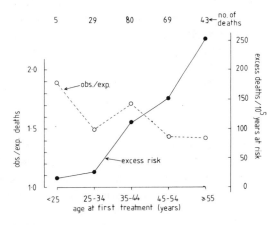

FIG.4. *Observed and expected deaths from cancers of the 'heavily irradiated sites' three or more years after first treatment according to age at first treatment.*

DISCUSSION

The present analysis, confined to patients with ankylosing spondylitis who had received only one course of X-ray treatment, indicates that the risk of developing a radiation-induced cancer is raised for many years following the X-ray exposure. The rate of induced leukaemia deaths is greatest in the period three to five years following first treatment and subsequently declines such that after 20 years little or no excess risk may remain. In contrast, the excess of

deaths from cancers of 'heavily irradiated' sites reaches a maximum nine to
eleven years following treatment, and the excess death rate remains approximately
constant from this time up until 20 years after the radiation exposure. The fall
in the rate after this time (Fig.3) is not statistically significant, and clearly it will
be necessary to extend our present observations to obtain a firmer estimate of
the effects in this late period. Part of the fall in the excess death rate in the period
long after the radiation exposure may be attributable to the lower rates of
radiation-induced cancers seen among patients first irradiated at a young age
(Fig.4). In the 20-year period following first treatment many of the patients who
were first treated for their spondylitis at an older age will have died from causes
unrelated to the treatment. Death rates for younger patients are lower and thus
as the time since treatment increases, the patients who were younger at first
treatment form an increasing proportion of the surviving population. Furthermore,
as the rate of radiation-induced cancers appears to be lower in younger patients
there will be an apparent decline in the overall excess death rate with time
since first treatment. We have attempted to adjust for this bias by standardizing
for the effect of age at first treatment when examining the change in the excess
cancer death rate with time since first treatment [3]. The effect of doing this
is to make the decline 20 or more years after first treatment (Fig.4) less marked,
but the procedure does not remove the fall completely though, of course, it is
still not statistically significant. Application of the same technique to the data
on leukaemia deaths, shown in Fig.2, slightly raises the estimate of the number
of radiation-induced leukaemias at long periods after treatment but this effect
is small.

Our findings are largely in agreement with those obtained from study of
the survivors of the atomic bomb explosions of Hiroshima and Nagasaki. Jablon
and Kato [4] found that both the ratio of observed to expected deaths and the
excess death rate for leukaemia declined with time, though there was evidence
of some excess risk remaining more than 20 years after the radiation exposure.
The excess death rate from cancers other than leukaemia among the atomic
bomb survivors is elevated for many years after the explosions, and shows some
signs of increasing in the period 20 or more years after exposure [5]. Thus,
whereas it is likely that most of the radiation-induced leukaemia deaths will
have occurred within 20 years of exposure in both patients with spondylitis and
in the atomic bomb survivors, deaths from other cancers induced by radiation
are still occurring, and it will be necessary to follow carefully the survivors in
both populations for a number of years yet before a final estimate can be made
of the total carcinogenic effects of the original radiation exposures.

Our data strongly suggest that susceptibility to radiation-induced cancer
and leukaemia is dependent upon a person's age at the time of exposure, those
exposed at older ages being at greatest risk. Such effects have also been reported
for the survivors of the atomic bomb explosions, with the exception that those

aged 0 to nine years at the time of the explosion seem to have suffered a greater
risk of radiation-induced cancers and leukaemia than those in the nearby older
age groups [4, 5]. We can offer no data in support of this observation as none
of the patients in our series were irradiated in this young age group. It may be
that the very young are particularly susceptible to radiation-induced cancers.
It is clear, however, that the age at exposure to radiation is important when
assessing an individual's risk of developing a radiation-induced cancer, and
also this factor should be taken into account when comparing the rates of
radiation-induced cancers in different populations.

For most sites our data are compatible with the risk of cancer developing
in particular sites included among those 'heavily irradiated' being directly
proportional to the risk of a tumour in the absence of radiation. Similarly, the
risk of radiation-induced death from leukaemia and from cancers of heavily
irradiated sites combined appears to vary with the patient's age at first treatment
in direct proportion to the number of tumours expected in the absence of
radiation. This multiplicative relationship suggests that radiation is interacting
with other factors which are inducing cancer. Thus we would speculate that
in situations where persons are exposed to radiation and another carcinogenic
hazard the effects of the two exposures on cancer induction are likely to
be greater than simply additive.

REFERENCES

[1]   COURT BROWN, W.M., DOLL, R., Leukaemia and aplastic anaemia in patients
       irradiated for ankylosing spondylitis, Spec. Rep. Ser. Med. Res. Coun. (Lond.),
       No. 295 (1957).
[2]   COURT BROWN, W.M., DOLL, R., Mortality from cancer and other causes after radio-
       therapy for ankylosing spondylitis, Br. Med. J. ii (1965) 1327.
[3]   DOLL, R., SMITH, P.G., Causes of death among patients with ankylosing spondylitis
       following a single treatment course with X-rays (in preparation).
[4]   JABLON, S., KATO, H., Studies of the mortality of A-bomb survivors: 5. Radiation
       dose and mortality, 1950–1970, Radiat. Res. **50** (1972) 649.
[5]   BEEBE, G.W., KATO, H., LAND, C.E., Studies of the mortality of A-bomb survivors:
       8. Mortality experience of A-bomb survivors, 1950–74, Radiation Effects Research
       Foundation, RERF Technical Report 1–77 (1977).

DISCUSSION

A.M. STEWART: Have you observed the effect of grouping cancers following
the ICRP classification of tissues according to their sensitivity to the cancer-
induction effects of radiation? Since this is a 4-point classification, it automatically avoids the difficulty of choosing suitable groups from the ICD classificati

(which is too detailed for most epidemiological studies) and it might show you that some of your residual cancers (e.g. pharynx) properly belong to radio-sensitive categories.

P.G. SMITH: At present the only specific grouping of cancers we have made has been into those involving 'heavily irradiated' or 'lightly irradiated' sites. This grouping was made solely on the basis of the parts of the body which were likely to have been located directly in the radiation beams as treatment was usually given. We have examined deaths from cancers by individual site and, as I mentioned in my presentation, none of the 'lightly irradiated' sites showed a statistically significant excess of cancer deaths. Among the heavily irradiated sites the excess of deaths seems to involve different sites roughly in proportion to the numbers of deaths that would be expected if the spondylitic patients had suffered the same death rates as the general population. An exception to this was the number of deaths from tumours of the spinal cord and nerves (Fig.1), and the larger excess for this site suggests perhaps increased sensitivity compared with other sites. The ratio of observed to expected deaths from lymphomas other than Hodgkin's disease was also high (2.6 to 1; Fig.1). Multiple myeloma has been included in this category in the figure but is not responsible for the high ratio; there were three deaths from this cause, whereas about two were expected. With respect to the specific example you cite, in the period three or more years after first treatment there were three deaths from cancer of the pharynx and 1.3 were expected. We shall be presenting our data on observed and expected deaths by individual sites in such a way that it will be possible for others to make groupings other than the specific ones we choose.

A.M. STEWART: Have you taken into account that, if cancers lower resistance to other causes of death before they are clinically recognizable, any exposed group of persons that has a high non-cancer mortality rate (e.g. patients with ankylosing spondylitis and A-bomb survivors) would be unsuitable for studying how age affects tissue radiosensitivity?

P.G. SMITH: The hypothesis that cancers lower resistance to other causes of death before their clinical recognition is an interesting one but, if it were true, I should have expected to see evidence of a radiation-related excess risk of death from non-malignant conditions. Mr. Beebe indicated earlier in this meeting that he could find no such evidence among the data on A-bomb survivors and, though our data is limited, we have not seen an excess of deaths from non-malignant causes which can be related to the radiation exposure (SMITH, P.G., DOLL, R., RADFORD, E.P., Cancer mortality among patients with ankylosing spondylitis not given X-ray therapy, Br. J. Radiol. 50 (1977) 728).

D. BENINSON: Mrs. Stewart mentioned an ICRP classification of sensitivity and from the context I believe she was referring to ICRP publication 14. The only ranking present in the new ICRP recommendations (ICRP 26) is implicit and given indirectly by the factors W_T.

A.M. STEWART: Yes, I was referring to the ICRP 14 classification (which is one of tissue radiosensitivity, however imperfect), because any independent classification that is focused on radiosensitivity and only recognizes a small number of diagnostic groups is better than the ICD classification (which leaves the choice of suitably large groups to the investigator — with the obvious risk of introducing unnecessary bias).

C. STREFFER: Mr. Smith, at the end of your presentation you stated that the interaction of ionizing radiation with other cancerogenic agents has a multiplicative (or, rather, higher-than-additive) effect for tumour induction. Do you believe this to be a general situation, and of which substances are you thinking in this connection? I would add that experimental experience is not in agreement with such a general statement. The combination of substances with irradiation can lead to effects higher-than-additive, additive or even less-than additive in comparison with the effects of single treatments.

P.G. SMITH: The statement I made was based on our finding that the risk of a radiation-induced cancer seems to increase with age at exposure in direct proportion to the expected number of deaths from cancer that would be suffered by persons first treated at a particular age. This suggests to us that radiation is interacting with whatever other factors are inducing cancer. I had no specific substance in mind and the effect may be fairly general though, of course, there may be exceptions. Direct epidemiological observations on this issue are very limited and more are needed, but there is, for example, some evidence that the combined effect of radiation and tobacco smoking may be greater than an additive model would suggest.

G.W. DOLPHIN: I have two points. First, as the age-specific incidence of the various types of leukaemia differs, the relative risk must be applied separately to each type of leukaemia. The other point concerns the use of 'years at risk' from first treatment to 18 months after the second treatment for those who were treated more than once. As the risk of leukaemia changes with time after irradiation, the limitation of the 'years at risk' in this arbitrary way may lead to overestimation of the excess leukaemia rate.

P.G. SMITH: Our analysis of the leukaemia deaths by type is not completed yet and we will be presenting this data at a later date.

With respect to your second comment, we have discussed why we considered it necessary to include the first 18 months following the second course of treatmen in the period of risk for patients in the study. We have calculated the risk of leukaemia in different time intervals following first treatment and, in this way, we are able to derive risk estimates that take account of patients who were removed from further study because of subsequent treatment. The method we have used does not lead to an overestimate of the excess leukaemia death rate. In our analysis, second treatment is treated in essentially the same way as competing causes of death.

D. GRAHN: Since your observations on irradiated human subjects demonstrate a close similarity of response to that seen in irradiated mouse populations, it is likely that excess risk from all cancers other than leukaemia will remain elevated for the balance of lifetime after the initial latent period. Do you expect that it will be possible in your study to evaluate this issue for man? This remains an important matter, since most risk analyses use a 20–30 year limit as the duration of excess cancer risk.

Second, did you determine that the elevated risk for causes of death other than cancer was not radiation-induced by relating this mortality ratio to that seen among the unirradiated spondylitic patients?

P.G. SMITH: It is our intention to follow the patients in our series until they have all died, and we will be able to determine if the excess death rate from cancers of heavily irradiated sites persists. We have recently studied a smaller group of some 1000 patients with ankylosing spondylitis, who were diagnosed during the same period as patients in the main series, but who were not treated with X-rays for their disease (RADFORD, E.P., DOLL, R., SMITH, P.G., Mortality among patients with ankylosing spondylitis not given X-ray therapy, New. Eng. J. Med. 297 (1977) 572; SMITH, P.G., DOLL, R., RADFORD, E.P., Cancer mortality among patients with ankylosing spondylitis not given X-ray therapy, Br. J. Radiol. 50 (1977) 728.) We found that these patients also had mortality rates from non-malignant conditions which were similar to those of patients in the irradiated series, and this strongly suggests that the X-ray treatment is not responsible for the marked increase in deaths from non-malignant conditions which we see in the irradiated spondylitics. There is no evidence in our data that radiation has produced a general life-shortening effect other than through the induction of certain cancers.

G.W. BEEBE: What is the status of the dosimetry programme? Will the next report contain any dosimetric data?

P.G. SMITH: Mr. Ellis at the University of Leeds has developed a computer program for estimating the mean bone marrow dose received by patients in our study, and we will shortly be reporting our results with respect to leukaemia. He is also working on dose estimates to other organs, specifically the lungs, stomach and pancreas. These are unlikely to be available in time for our next report, but we will, of course, be analysing this information as soon as it becomes available.

R. WICK: You stated that there appears to be a higher incidence of leukaemia in ankylosing spondylitis patients after X-ray treatment. As you know, there is another quite effective form of therapy, namely treatment with ^{224}Ra. After this treatment most patients are free of pain or, at least, greatly relieved. I have been continuing the work of F. Schales on the follow-up of ankylosing spondylitis patients treated with ^{224}Ra, and have traced and analysed nearly 2000 patients. Up to now in the low-dose group (up to about 12 MBq in total) no cases of osteosarcoma have been found, but there is one fibrosarcoma in the left ileosacral joint and one reticulosarcoma of the bone marrow. A connection with the ^{224}Ra treatment cannot be ruled out. However, the incidence of bone tumours in the lower dose group does not seem to have increased and certainly not in the manner of leukaemia incidence after X-ray treatment. Are there still indications for X-ray treatment today, or would you decline to give any irradiation, even with alpha emitters like ^{224}Ra?

P.G. SMITH: I am interested to learn of your series of patients treated with ^{224}Ra, and I hope that it will be possible for the mortality experience of these patients to be compared with that of ours. I am not a radiotherapist and therefore can only report views that have been put to me regarding possible therapeutic benefits of treating ankylosing spondylitis with X-rays. I know that some radiotherapists in Britain have been concerned about the movement away from this method of treatment since the original publications of Court Brown and Doll on the carcinogenic effects of radiation treatment. They consider that X-ray treatment may be more effective in alleviating the symptoms of the disease than other therapies. Furthermore, advances in radiation treatment since 1954 (when the last patient in our series was treated) have been considerable, and it is likely that the use of smaller fields and smaller radiation doses in modern treatments would reduce the carcinogenic effect. As far as I am aware, clinical trials comparing the effects of radiation therapy with other methods of treating spondylitis have not been conducted, and we have suggested that these might be considered (SMITH, P.G., DOLL, R., RADFORD, E.P., Cancer mortality among patients with ankylosing spondylitis not given X-ray therapy, Br. J. Radiol. 50 (1977) 728). However, any benefits in the relief of symptoms brought about by radiation therapy would have to be balanced against the increased risk of cancer when deciding the method of treatment for individual patie

M. DELPLA: From the point of view of numbers involved, it is interesting to compare the group that has just been presented to us with the groups of survivors of Nagasaki and Hiroshima. We find that these are respectively 14 000, 20 000 and 60 000 people.

It is a pity that you did not divide your group into categories according to the dose. Court Brown and Doll (1957) did not find any leukaemia in the category that had received less than 250 R. What is the situation now? It is also a pity that you have not distinguished between different types of leukaemia; according at least to the Hiroshima observations, they appear to react independentl to the aggression constituted by irradiation.

The study being performed by your group could supply us with more information — precisely in those areas where it is particularly lacking.

P.G. SMITH: We will be presenting data on the different types of leukaemia and the dose response relationship in a paper we are now preparing. With respect to your question about leukaemia deaths in spondylitics receiving doses in the lower range, we have an excess of leukaemia deaths among patients with a mean bone marrow dose of less than 100 rads.

RISK ESTIMATION OF RADIATION-INDUCED THYROID CANCER IN ADULTS

I. SCHMITZ-FEUERHAKE, E. MUSCHOL,
K. BÄTJER, R. SCHÄFER
University of Bremen,
Bremen,
Federal Republic of Germany

Abstract

RISK ESTIMATION OF RADIATION-INDUCED THYROID CANCER IN ADULTS.
Studies on radiation-induced thyroid cancer by several investigators show that the mean latency period is very high when the follow-up time is long. Estimations of the life time risk will therefore strongly depend on assumptions about the development of the induction rate with time. Risk estimations are given related to person years and person years 'at risk' assuming a negligible rate up to eight years after irradiation and a following plateau. This latter assumption will lead to a value of 170 cases per million per rem in 30 years after irradiation (range 50–440). The data do not show that children are more sensitive to cancer induction than adults. No dose rate effect in the low dose region can be derived, but further studies are required on patients examined by an ^{131}I-uptake test.

Carcinoma of the thyroid is an effect of radiation that has been most frequently investigated in man up to now. A large range of dose is covered by the data of several investigators (Fig.1). The incidence figures are given as excess rates against the control group. Data from the same source are linked by filled lines. In the high dose region reliable information is taken only from persons who were adults at the time of the therapy. The study of 34 600 cases by Dobyns and co-workers ('X-ray, I-131-therapy') clearly shows the effect of cell sterilization which suppresses the development of carcinoma at high doses [9]. The exact dose in every case is unknown. There were only 30 persons < 10 years of age at time of irradiation in the ^{131}I-therapy group of Dobyns and co-workers. In Fig.1, a summarized value for them and 19 other irradiated children [10–13] is plotted ('I-131-therapy'), related to only one case of carcinoma.

Several studies have been undertaken on the atomic bomb survivors, the most recent follow-up being by Parker and co-workers [2, 3] ('A-Bombs 74'). This study deals with only a small group < 10 years ATB, so that data of Jablon and co-workers [1] are reported also ('A-Bombs 71'). Autopsy data [16] of the atomic bomb survivors show a higher incidence, but they are not quite comparable with the other findings because they include small and occult carcinoma which would not be discovered in living beings or as a cause of death. For dose estimation of the A-bomb survivors an RBE = 10 for neutrons is taken and the T-65 D was

SCHMITZ-FEUERHAKE et al.

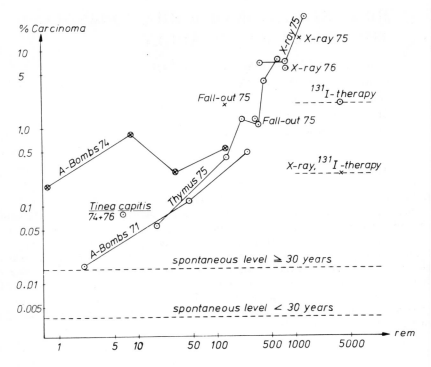

FIG.1. Radiation-induced thyroid carcinoma reported by several authors.

Signs and symbols: ⊙ *Age at irradiation < 10 years*
                 × *Age at irradiation ⩾ 10 years*
                 ⊗ *All ages*

A-Bombs *Incidence in Hiroshima and Nagasaki* [1–3]
Tinea capitis *Children irradiated at the head for tinea capitis* [4, 5]
Thymus *Irradiation for thymic enlargement* [6]
X-ray *Irradiation for benign diseases in the region of head, neck and upper thorax* [7, 8]
X-ray, Iodine-131-therapy *Radiation therapy for hyperthyroidism* [9–13]
Fall-out *Marshall islanders exposed through Bikini atomic bomb test* [14]
Spontaneous level *Tumour registry of the Saarland, W. Germany* [15]

corrected [17]. The data 'A-Bombs 74' show a poor correlation with dose. This may be explained by the effect of fall-out which is not regarded in the T-65 D. It is reported by Watanabe [18] that there were significant effects in the 'early entrants' to Hiroshima. Twenty-three cases of thyroid cancer were found in persons who entered the city one to eight days after the explosion (out of a total of about 45 000). As about 1 MCi of ^{131}I may have been disseminated by the bomb at Hiroshima and 1 μCi produces about 1 rad to the adult thyroid, the error of conventional dose estimations in the survivors may be extreme in the low dose classes.

'Fall-out' data in Fig.1 are obtained from the studies on the Marshallese affected by the Bikini atomic bomb test in 1954 [14]. The development of thyroid nodules in 80% of those who were ⩾ 10 years old at the time of the accident was a striking fact as well as the incidence of three carcinoma in the rather small group of adults. The data from these and from others in the low dose region are given in Table I.

The results of the two recent studies on *tinea capitis* children are summarized in Fig.1. Whereas Modan and co-workers [4] found an incidence of 0.09% for 6.5 rads, no case of carcinoma was reported by Shore and co-workers [5]. This is not significant, however, because the latter investigation concerned no more than 2124 persons so that only 1.9 cases of carcinoma would have been expected based on the values of Modan and co-workers.

The spontaneous incidence in Fig.1 is taken from the cancer registry of the Saarland [15], a region in W. Germany with 1.1 million inhabitants. Two age groups were chosen for comparison: those radiated in childhood with a latency period and those radiated later. The incidence in 1972–74 was 3.7 cases per 100 000 persons of <30 years of age and 15.2 cases per 100 000 persons of ⩾30 years of age.

LATENCY PERIOD

Block and co-workers [20] who investigated 296 thyroid carcinoma after irradiation at ages of 1–50 years found no age dependency in the latency periods, i.e. the time between radiation and occurrence of cancer. Latency periods in 132 cases were previously reported by Beach and Dolphin [19]. They found no dependency of thyroid dose, age at irradiation and sex, but looked at irradiated children only. The maximum in their frequency distribution was at eight years. This maximum has shifted in our summary (Fig.2) of 120 cases more recently reported. This may be a consequence of the longer observation time of patients in these studies [1, 4, 6, 14, 21–26]. The later decrease with time in Fig.2 appears to be only an effect of insufficient follow-up periods, because there is no evidence in the studies for a real decrease with time [6, 18, 23].

AGE SENSITIVITY

The values in Fig.1 give no evidence for a greater sensitivity in children to radiation. Parker and co-workers [2, 3] report that there were nearly three times more carcinoma in the group <10 years ATB than in the older group. This may be an effect of incorrect dose estimation because ^{131}I-fall-out would affect the thyroid of children to a higher degree. Sampson and co-workers [16] found no age differences in sensitivity in their autopsy studies of the atomic bomb survivors.

TABLE I. DATA DERIVED FROM REPORTS ON RADIATION-INDUCED THYROID CANCER IN THE LOW DOSE RANGE

Source	Age at irrad.	Dose (rem)	Irradiated group					Control			Remarks
			No. of persons	No. of carcinomas	PYR	Excess incid. (‰)	Mean obs. time (years)	No. of persons	No. of carcinomas	PYR	
Jablon et al. [1] 'A-Bombs 71'	<10	2.1[a]	10 729	4		0.17	15	5 025 (NIC)	1		Not used
		45.5[a]	3 669	5		1.2	15				10 rem added
Modan et al. [4], Shore et al. [5] 'Tinea capitis 74+76'	<10	6.5	13 026	12		0.76	15	12 233	2		Data of authors combined
Hempelmann et al. [6] 'Thymus 75'	<10	17.2	1 637	1	35 028	0.61	21	5 055	0	115 921	
		137	211	1	5 310	4.7	25				
Conard [14] 'Fall-out 75'	≥10	135	156	3		19.2	15	133	0		
Parker et al. [3] 'A-Bombs 74'	≥10	0.73[a]		13	46 364	~1.6	13		7	44 472 (NIC)	Not used
		8.5[a]		6	9 592	~6.2	13				Not used
		31[a]		9	27 052	~2.3	13				
		103[a]		14	} 29 574	~6.0	13				Data combined
		153[a]		4							

[a] According to T-65 D.

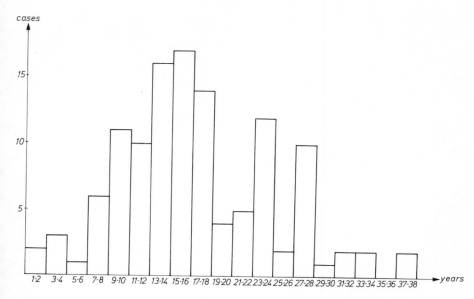

FIG.2. Distribution of latency periods for 120 cases of radiation-induced thyroid carcinoma.

The data of Refetoff and co-workers ('X-ray 75'; [7]) showed twice as high a risk for the younger group, but there was only one case in seven people ⩾ 10 years. Much of the evidence for a nearly as high risk for adults may be drawn from the findings on the Marshall islanders [14], where three carcinoma were detected among 156 persons in the older group.

RISK ESTIMATION IN THE LOW DOSE REGION

Risk estimations have been carried out using a linear non-threshold model. Only values below 150 rem have been used following the recommendations of Gray [27]. The absolute risk is expressed in a conventional manner related to person years (PYR). All values that were used for calculation are presented in Fig.3. They are derived from the data given by the authors in Table I. The low dose values of the A-bomb victims were not used for calculation because of the suspected distortions from fall-out. For the higher dose values 5 rem were added for adults and 10 rem for children in Fig.3. This was a rough estimate based on the incidence in the 'early entrants'. The risk for children, using only the values <10 years at irradiation is calculated to be 1.40×10^{-6} rem^{-1} PYR^{-1}. The best fit for all values results in a risk of 4.44×10^{-6} rem^{-1} PYR^{-1} for all ages.

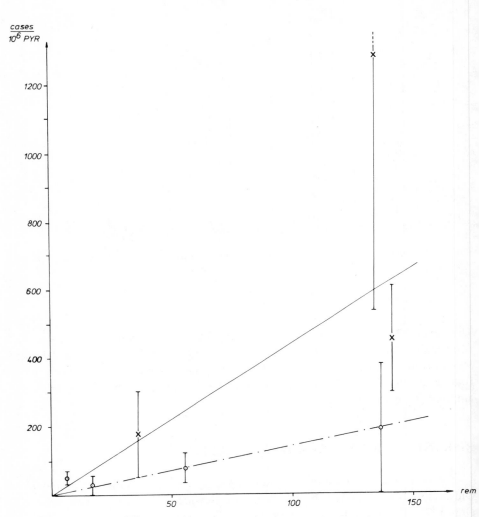

FIG.3.   Values in the low dose region used for risk estimation of thyroid cancer.
⊙ *< 10 years at time of irradiation*
✕ *≥ 10 years at time of irradiation*

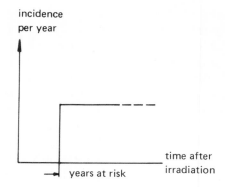

FIG.4. Theoretically derived course of cancer rate with time.

The above risk values will be an underestimation for the case of a high expectation of lifetime because of the long latency periods and the insufficient length of observation in the studies. Therefore, a calculation was made related to person years 'at risk' (PYR*). According to the distribution of latency periods in Fig.2, an eight-year period without occurrence of carcinoma was assumed and a following plateau (Fig.4). This would mean that in a period of 30 years following the irradiation the risk is calculated to be 0 for 8 years and as below for 22 years 'at risk'. According to these assumptions the results are:

2.25×10^{-6} rem^{-1} PYR*$^{-1}$ for persons < 10 years at irradiation
7.94×10^{-6} rem^{-1} PYR*$^{-1}$ for all ages

With regard to the risk for adults we take the above value of 2.25×10^{-6} rem^{-1} PYR^{-1} as a lower limit. As a higher limit we obtain 20.35×10^{-6} rem^{-1} PYR^{-1} using only the higher values PYR* according to 6.5 rem and 135 rem. The risk in 30 years after irradiation will then be

170×10^{-6} rem^{-1}, range $50-440(\times 10^{-6}$ rem$^{-1})$

for persons $\geqslant 10$ years at irradiation.

DISCUSSION

In relation to its cellular mass the thyroid seems to be most sensitive for cancer induction by radiation. In contradiction to our risk estimations and apart from the investigation of Shore and co-workers [5] on *tinea capitis,* there are two studies in which no malignant effects were found after irradiation. Rallison and co-workers [28] investigated 1378 young persons of Utah and Nevada where areas had been affected by fall-out of the atom bomb tests in 1952—55. The thyroid dose for children has been estimated up to 120 rads by Tamplin and Fisher [29]. Rallison and co-workers found 1.3% of nodules in the irradiated group against 0.9% in people of Arizona used as control, the difference being considered not significant. No carcinoma was found in the irradiated group. Several carcinoma should have been expected after our risk estimations, but there was no control of dose by measurements, and the mean time of observations was probably much less than 19 years. No increase of thyroid nodules was found in Kerala [30] where the dose is estimated to reach 1.5—3.5 rem yearly. But as the mean organ dose is unknown and two-thirds of the people were younger than 30 years, which means that only about 4000 persons above 30 were living there, no positive conclusions may be drawn from this study.

The lack of effects in both investigations may also be a consequence of low dose rates. But the data used for our risk estimations (Fig.3) tend to show a dose rate effect in the adverse direction. The findings of Modan and co-workers [4] at a dose of 6.5 rads were originated by fractions of scattered X-rays of probably less than 2 rads/min [31]. Moreover, the extremely high incidence in the Marshalles group [14] was caused by a radiation of very low dose rate. Although many animal studies have been carried out on radiation-induced thyroid tumours, there is no reliable information about a dose rate effect in the low dose range. In a review by Lindsay [32] the optimum dose for tumour induction in rats is reported to be 500—1000 rads for X-rays and after application of 25—40 mCi of ^{131}I (about 12 000—20 000 rads). But this may only mean that the declining part of the dose-effect curve is taken into account where a different behaviour because of cell sterilization has to be expected. If there is no dose-rate effect the spontaneous incidence of thyroid carcinoma can be regarded as an upper limit because of the natural background radiation. Our risk estimation for children < 10 years would lead to 5.0×10^{-5} in those < 30 years old assuming 80 mrad yearly, which is somewhat higher than 3.5×10^{-5} as indicated in the Saarland but not in contradiction. Further analysis of natural occurrences in certain regions of the world, which has not yet been done by us, could be helpful in obtaining a definite upper limit for risk values.

Differences of sensitivity between the sexes were not studied in our estimation. Refetoff and co-workers [7] found no difference in incidence in females and males but investigated only seven persons who were adults at the time of irradiation in contrast with 96 children. The three carcinoma in the Marshallese occurred only in females [14]. Other differences are suspected to be of genetic origin. Hempelmann and co-workers [6] found a 3.4 times higher rate in the Jewish subgroup of their collective than in the others, all irradiated for thymic enlargement in their first year of life. These findings are confirmed by investigations of Arnold and co-workers [33].

The uncertainties discussed as well as those of dose estimations and the various methods of investigation chosen in the studies will lead to the conclusion that the risk for a certain collective cannot be guaranteed to lie in the range of values estimated in this paper. They should lead, however, to a critical view of our so-called laws of radiation 'protection'. The 'Strahlenschutzverordnung' of 1976 in the Federal Republic of Germany is based on a maximum permissible thyroid dose of 30 rem for people occupationally exposed. More restrictions should also be recommended for the use of ^{131}I in nuclear medicine. In Germany, some 100 000 people have been diagnosed by an ^{131}I-uptake test which will deliver 30—100 rads to the thyroid. Studies on these persons could answer some questions about the extent of the dose-effect relationship and the influence of dose rate.

REFERENCES

[1] JABLON, S., TACHIKAWA, K., BELSKY, J.L., STEER, A., Cancer in Japanese exposed as children to atomic bombs, Lancet 1 (1971) 7706.

[2] PARKER, L.N., BELSKY, J.L., YAMAMOTO, T., KAWAMOTO, S., KEEHN, R.J., Thyroid carcinoma after exposure to atomic radiation, Ann. Intern. Med. 80 (1974) 600.

[3] PARKER, L.N., BELSKY, J.L., YAMAMOTO, M.D., KAWAMOTO, S., KEEHN, R.J., Thyroid carcinoma diagnosed between 13 and 26 years after exposure to atomic radiation, ABCC Technical Rep. 5-73 (1973).

[4] MODAN, B., BAIDATZ, D., MART, H., STEINITZ, R., SHELDON, G.L., Radiation-induced head and neck tumours, Lancet 1 (1974) 7852.

[5] SHORE, R.E., ALBERT, R.E., PASTERNACK, B.S., Follow-up study of patients treated by X-ray epilation for tinea capitis, Arch. Environ. Health 31 (1976) 21.

[6] HEMPELMANN, L.H., HALL, W.J., PHILIPS, M., COOPER, R.A., AMES, W.R., Neoplasms in persons treated with X-rays in infancy: fourth survey in 20 years, J. Natl. Cancer Inst. 55 (1975) 519.

[7] REFETOFF, S., HARRISON, J., KARANFILSKI, B.T., KAPLAN, E.L., De GROOT, L.J., BEKERMANN, C., Continuing occurrence of thyroid carcinoma after irradiation to the neck in infancy and childhood, N. Engl. J. Med. 292 (1975) 172.

[8] FAVUS, M.J., SCHNEIDER, A.B., STACHURA, M.E., ARNOLD, J.E., RYO, U.Y., PINSKY, S.M., COLMAN, M., ARNOLD, M.J., FROHMAN, L.A., Thyroid cancer occurring as a late consequence of head and neck irradiation, N. Engl. J. Med. 294 (1976) 1019.

[9] DOBYNS, B.M., SHELINE, G.E., WORKMAN, J.B., TOMPKINS, E.A., McCONAHEY, W.M., BECKER, D.V., Malignant and benign neoplasms of the thyroid in patients treated for hyperthyroidism: a report of the cooperative thyrotoxicosis therapy, J. Clin. Endocrinol. Metab. 38 (1974) 976.

[10] CRILE, G., SCHUMACHER, O.P., Radioactive iodine treatment of Graves disease: results of 32 children under 16 years of age, Am. J. Dis. Child. 110 (1965) 501.

[11] HAYEK, A., CHAPMAN, E.M., CRAWFORD, J.D., Long-term results of treatment of thyrotoxicosis in children and adolescents with radioactive iodine, N. Engl. J. Med. 283 (1970) 949.

[12] SAFA, A.M., SCHUMACHER, O.P., RODRIGUEZ-ANTUNEZ, A., Long-term follow-up results in children and adolescents treated with radioactive iodine (131-I) for hyperthyroidism, N. Engl. J. Med. 292 (1975) 167.

[13] SAFA, A.M., SCHUMACHER, O.P., Follow-up of children treated with 131-I, N. Engl.
      J. Med. **294** (1976) 54.

[14] CONARD, R.A., et al., A 20-year Review of the Findings in a Marshallese Population
      accidentally exposed to Radioactive Fallout, National Technical Information Service,
      U.S. Dep. of Commerce, 5285 Port Royal Road, Springfield, Virginia 22161 (Sep. 1975).

[15] STATISTISCHES AMT DES SAARLANDES, Saarländische Krebsdokumentation
      1972–1974: Einzelschriften zur Statistik des Saarlandes Nr. 51, Saarbrücken (1976).

[16] SAMPSON, R.J., KEY, C.R., BUNCHER, C.R., IIJIMA, S., Thyroid carcinoma in
      Hiroshima and Nagasaki: I. Prevalence of thyroid carcinoma at autopsy, J. Am. Med.
      Assoc. **209** (1969) 65.

[17] JONES, T.D., AUXIER, J.A., CHEKA, J.S., KERR, G.D., In vivo dose estimates for
      A-bomb survivors shielded by typical Japanese houses, Health Phys. **28** (1975) 367.

[18] WATANABE, S., "Cancer and leukemia developing among atom-bomb survivors",
      Handbuch der allg. Pathologie **VI** (5), Springer, Berlin, Göttingen, Heidelberg (1974) 461.

[19] BEACH, S.A., DOLPHIN, G.W., A study of the relationship between X-ray dose delivered
      to the thyroids of children and the subsequent development of malignant tumours,
      Phys. Med. Biol. **6** (1962) 583.

[20] BLOCK, M.A., MILLER, M.J., HORN, R.C., Carcinoma of the thyroid after external
      radiation to the neck in adults, Am. J. Surg. **118** (1969) 764.

[21] SOCOLOW, E.L., HASHIZUME, A., NERIISHI, S., NIITANI, R., Thyroid carcinoma
      in man after exposure to ionizing radiation, N. Engl. J. Med. **268** (1963) 406.

[22] McDOUGALL, I.R., KENNEDY, J.S., THOMSON, J.A., Thyroid carcinoma following
      iodine-131 therapy, J. Clin. Endocrinol. Metab. **33** (1971) 287.

[23] De GROOT, L., PALOYAN, E., Thyroid carcinoma and radiation, J. Am. Med. Assoc.
      225 (1973) 487.

[24] SMITH, D.G., LEVITT, S.H., Radiation carcinogenesis: an unusual familial occurrence
      of neoplasia following irradiation in childhood for benign disease, Cancer **34** (1974) 2069.

[25] BECKER, F.C., ECONOMOU, S.G., SOUTHWICK, H.W., EISENSTEIN, R., Adult
      thyroid cancer after head and neck irradiation in infancy and childhood, Ann. Intern.
      Med. **83** (1975) 347.

[26] CHANG-CHIEN, Y., LIAW, K., WANG, D., CHEN, F., Thyroid cancer after radiation,
      Int. Surg. **62** (1977) 112.

[27] GRAY, L.H., "Radiation biology and cancer", Cellular Radiation Biology (ANDERSON,
      M.D., Ed.), 18th Ann. Symp. on Fundamental Cancer Research, 1964, Williams and
      Wilkins, Baltimore (1965).

[28] RALLISON, M.L., DOBYNS, B.M., KEATING, F.R., RALL, J.E., TYLER, F.H., Thyroid
      nodularity in children, J. Am. Med. Assoc. **233** (1975) 1069.

[29] TAMPLIN, A.R., FISHER, H.L., Estimation of Dosage to Thyroids of Children in the
      U.S. from Nuclear Tests conducted in Nevada during 1952 through 1955, Lawrence
      Radiation Lab., University of Calif., Livermore, Rep. UCRL-14707 (1966).

[30] KOCHU PILLAI, N., THANGAVELU, M., RAMALINGASWAMI, V., "Nodular lesions
      of the thyroid in an area of high background radiation in coastal Kerala, India", Proc.
      1st World Congress Nucl. Med. Tokyo, Oct. 1974, Indian J. Med. Res. **64** (1976) 537.

[31] MODAN, B., RON, E., WERNER, A., Thyroid cancer following scalp irradiation,
      Radiology **123** (1977) 741.

[32] LINDSAY, S., "Ionizing radiation and experimental thyroid neoplasms: a review",
      Thyroid Cancer (HEDINGER, C.E., Ed.), Springer UICC Monograph Series **12** (1969).

[33] ARNOLD, J., PINSKY, S., RYO, U.Y., FROHMAN, L., SCHNEIDER, A., FAVUS, M.,
      STACHURA, M., ARNOLD, M., COLMAN, M., 99m-Tc-Pertechnetate thyroid scintigraphy
      in patients predisposed to thyroid neoplasms by prior radiotherapy to the head and neck,
      Radiology **115** (1975) 653.

DISCUSSION

V. VOLF: You criticize the present maximum permissible thyroid dose. What change would you suggest?

I. SCHMITZ-FEUERHAKE: I think the maximum permissible doses should be lowered by a factor of 10 at least.

D. BENINSON: A comment on the remark about dose limits. They are not levels to be reached, or to be used for design or planning. They are in fact boundaries for cost-effectiveness analyses (optimization requirement). In this sense, doses above the limit are automatically prohibited, but doses under the limit are not automatically acceptable.

I. SCHMITZ-FEUERHAKE: If the maximum permissible doses are not reached, there is no reason not to lower them. The individual risk from 30 rem thyroid dose is much too high.

K.J. OLSEN: I agree with you that the use of ^{131}I for diagnostic uptake studies should be restricted. A high proportion of thyroid glands are nodular, which means that the dose distribution is inhomogeneous. How would that affect your risk estimates?

I. SCHMITZ-FEUERHAKE: This is a problem I cannot solve. For our risk estimations we of course need something like the mean thyroid dose.

J.L. WEEKS: I entirely accept the validity of Mr. Beninson's comment, and I am sure that we here all recognize that ICRP recommendations relate to a lower level of an impermissible level of exposure. However, this concept is difficult to get across to those who are not concerned with radiological protection, and it must be repeatedly emphasized that these recommendations are not speed limits.

I. SCHMITZ-FEUERHAKE: Everybody who is concerned with radiological protection knows that these limits will be reached by a lot of people, especially in the nuclear industry.

R.A. CONARD: I should like to comment on the use of a guideline of 30 rads for the thyroid with regard to iodine-131. It is generally conceded that iodine-131 is one tenth to one fortieth as effective as X-radiation in producing tumours. Therefore such a dose to the thyroid from use of iodine-131 would be rather conservative.

INTERACTION BETWEEN RADIATION
AND OTHER BREAST CANCER
RISK FACTORS

J.D. BOICE, Jr.
Harvard University,
Boston, Massachusetts;
Bureau of Radiological Health,
Rockville, Maryland;
National Cancer Institute,
Bethesda, Maryland

B.J. STONE
National Cancer Institute,
Bethesda,
Maryland,
United States of America

Abstract

INTERACTION BETWEEN RADIATION AND OTHER BREAST CANCER RISK
FACTORS.

A follow-up study was conducted of 1764 women institutionalized for pulmonary
tuberculosis between 1930 and 1954. Among 1047 women exposed to fluoroscopic chest
X-rays during air collapse therapy of the lung, an excess of breast cancer was observed and
previously reported (41 cases observed versus 23.3 expected). Among 717 comparison
patients who received other treatments, no excess breast cancer risk was apparent (15 cases
observed versus 14.1 expected). To determine whether breast cancer risk factors modify
the carcinogenic effect of radiation, analyses were performed evaluating the interaction of
radiation with indicators of breast cancer risk. The greatest radiation risk was found when
radiation exposure occurred just before and during menarche. This suggests that during
the time of breast budding and early breast development, proliferating breast tissue is
particularly sensitive to ionizing radiation. Similarly, exposures during first pregnancy
appeared substantially more hazardous than exposures occurring before or after first
pregnancy, suggesting that the condition of the breast at the time of pregnancy modifies
the effect of radiation in such a way as to enhance the risk. Nulliparous women were found
to be at a three to four-fold greater excess radiogenic breast cancer risk than women who
had given birth; this difference, however, was not statistically significant (p = 0.14). A
family history of breast cancer was associated with a two-fold excess radiogenic breast
cancer risk, but the numbers were too small to be reliable. Age at menopause did not appear
to influence the risk of radiation exposure. Other than radiation, benign breast disease was
the most significant breast cancer risk indicator. Benign breast disease was not seen to modify
the effect of radiation exposure; however, excessive radiation exposure might have increased
the incidence of benign breast disease, complicating the interaction analysis. Women possessing

231

one or more breast cancer risk factors were found to be at greater risk of developing radiogenic breast cancer than women possessing no known risk factors. This difference in radiogenic breast cancer risk was not, however, statistically significant (p = 0.19). Because of the uncertainty due to small-number sampling variation, these study results will require confirmation by a larger series. They do, however, suggest that stages when breast tissue undergoes high mitotic activity, e.g. menarche and pregnancy, are times of special vulnerability to the harmful effects of ionizing radiation.

INTRODUCTION

It is fairly well accepted that excessive radiation exposure increases the risk of breast cancer development [1]. Excessive breast cancer cases have been observed in Japanese women exposed to the atomic bomb [2], in women treated therapeutically with x-rays for acute [3] and chronic [4] breast conditions and in women with pulmonary tuberculosis whose artificial pneumothorax treatments were repeatedly monitored with fluoroscopic chest x-rays [5, 6]. Because of the presumptive radiation risk associated with low-dose mammographic x-ray exposures, the screening of asymptomatic women for the early detection and treatment of breast cancer has been criticized [7, 8], and it has been suggested that mammographic examinations be conducted only on women at high risk of developing breast cancer. It is not determined however, whether women at high risk of breast cancer are particularly sensitive to the carcinogenic effects of ionizing radiation. The purpose of this report is to examine the interaction of radiation with known breast cancer risk factors in a population of women exposed repeatedly to fluoroscopic chest examinations, and also to examine the effects of radiation exposure during times of breast stimulation, e.g. menarche and pregnancy. The analyses are directed toward generating hypotheses on whether underlying risk factors or breast conditions interact with radiation in such a manner as to ennance the carcinogenic potential of irradiation.

SUBJECTS AND METHODS

To investigate the long-term effects of repeated x-ray exposure to the chests of adolescent girls and adult women, a follow-up study was conducted of 1 764 female patients who were discharged alive from 2 tuberculosis sanatoria in Massachusetts between 1930 and 1954. One of the sanatoria treated children and adolescents exclusively, while the other treated adults. The study population included 1 047 women who had been exposed to an average of 102 fluoroscopic examinations of the chest in the course of air-collapse therapy (artificial pneumothorax) and a comparison group of 717 women who were treated by other procedures, such as surgery or drugs. A 1975 mailing address or a death certificate was obtained for 93.6% of the subjects, and a questionnaire sent to 1 146 living patients resulted in a response rate of 78%. The initial study objectives were to determine whether there is a relationship between breast cancer risk and radiation dose received and whether susceptibility to late radiation effects is related to age at exposure [6].

The estimation of radiation dose to the breasts of those patients undergoing repeated fluoroscopic chest examinations was a major endeavor and the results have recently been published [9]. The reported methodology attempted to improve the estimation of fluoroscopic breast doses by interviewing physicians who conducted the examinations, questioning patients fluoroscopically examined and coupling measurements of fluoroscopic exposure rates with an absorbed-dose Monte Carlo computation.

Summarizing the overall findings, 41 breast cancer cases were observed versus 23.3 expected among those patients fluoroscopically examined. Among the comparison patients, no excess breast cancers were apparent--15 breast cancers observed versus 14.1 expected. Expected breast cancer cases were computed using Connecticut Tumor Registry age-calendar year incidence rates. The average cumulative breast dose was determined to be 150 rad, delivered in small fractions of approximately 1.5 rad per examination. (The fluoro-scopic examinations were performed every few weeks in order to monitor the collapse of the lung and to determine the quantity of air to inject to maintain the lung collapse.) The pneumothorax treatments and exposures lasted an average of 3.3 years. The best estimate of excess breast cancer absolute risk was 6.2 cases per million women per year per rad, computed excluding the first 10 years of follow-up. The radiation dose required to double the 'spontaneous' incidence of breast cancer was estimated as 170 rad, the percent relative risk increase was estimated as 0.51% per rad, and the estimated lifetime radiation risk was 1 to 2 breast cancer cases per 10 000 women irradiated per rad based on an average follow-up period of 25.4 years. Because of the difficulty in determining retrospectively the fluoroscopic procedures and their associated doses, the computed risk estimates must be interpreted with some caution.

The relative risk for breast cancer among women fluoroscopically examined was estimated to be 1.8; i.e. women frequently exposed to fluoroscopic chest x-rays were 80% more likely to develop breast cancer than a comparable unexposed population. These results could not be accounted for by any differences between exposed and comparison patients with respect to several known risk factors for breast cancer: age, family history of breast cancer, age at menarche, nulliparity, age at first pregnancy, history of benign breast disease, age at menopause. The greatest absolute excess breast cancer risk occurred among exposed women who were first treated between the ages of 15 and 19 (13 breast cancers observed versus 3.4 expected), and no elevated breast cancer risk was detected among women 30 years of age or older at the time of first exposure (8 breast cancers observed and 8.1 expected); a 50% increased risk, however, could not be excluded among the older women due to the small numbers involved. These data were inter-preted to suggest that exposures occurring before the age of 30 were par-ticularly hazardous and that young women may be especially susceptible to environmental insult [6].

When radiation dose was considered, a linear dose-response relationship was found to be consistent with the data, although other relationships could not be excluded [9]. The excess breast cancer risk was not detected until 15 years after the initial exposure and was still present after 40 years of observation. These findings reaffirmed that repeated, relatively low radiation doses pose some future risk of breast cancer, that the risk may be cumulative, and that multiple radiation doses may convey the same breast cancer risk as a single exposure of the same total dose.

Current analysis

For the present analysis, breast cancer risk factors were identified from several sources: sanatorium medical records, patient responses to a mailed questionnaire and information obtained during the tracing of the study population. Because the presence or absence of particular breast cancer risk factors was not always obtained, analyses were conducted only on women for whom risk factor information was known.

To evaluate whether radiation interacts with various conditions associated with breast cancer risk, radiogenic risk estimates among women possessing and not possessing known risk factors were compared. Relative risk was computed as the ratio of breast cancer incidence rates between

TABLE I. BREAST CANCER RISK FACTORS POSSESSED BY TUBERCULOSIS
PATIENTS WHO DID AND DID NOT DEVELOP BREAST CANCER

Relative risks controlling for radiation exposure[a]

Risk factors	Women who developed breast cancer	Women who did not develop breast cancer	Relative risk
Multiple fluoroscopic exposures	73.2% (41/56)	41.1% (702/1708)	1.8[b]
Benign breast disease	32.1% (9/28)	14.7% (123/837)	2.6[b]
Family history of breast cancer	7.1% (2/28)	6.2% (51/828)	1.2
Nulliparous	45.2% (19/42)	42.1% (625/1485)	1.4
Age at first pregnancy 25 years or greater	31.0% (13/42)	28.6% (424/1481)	1.2
Menarche 14 years or under	78.1% (25/32)	78.5% (662/843)	0.7
Menopause 45 years or greater	62.5% (15/24)	73.7% (521/707)	0.6

[a] Only patients with known presence or absence of risk factors are included.
[b] $p < 0.05$.

exposed and non-exposed (comparison) women. Rate differences specific for dose were computed as the difference of breast cancer incidence rates between exposed and comparison women divided by radiation dose. Interaction, for the purposes of this paper, was defined as a departure from the absolute risk model, i.e. a statistically significant difference between the dose specific rate differences among women possessing and not possessing the factor under evaluation. In other words, if a particular breast cancer risk factor influences the effect of radiation exposure, it would be expected that the 'excess breast cancer cases per million women per year per rad' would be statistically significantly different between women possessing and not possessing the risk factor. A maximum likelihood chi-square test for heterogeneity was used to determine whether a statistically significant difference existed between two risk estimates [10].

Tests of significance were also made using the Mantel-Haenszel procedure [11]. Age and calendar-year adjusted relative risks were estimated following a method described by Jablon and Kato that utilized population expected values [12], and adjusted rate differences were similarly computed as discussed by Shore [3]. Confidence limits about rate differences were determined by the method of Miettinen [13].

In some instances the age-calendar year breast cancer incidence rates from the Connecticut Tumor Registry were applied to compute expected numbers of breast cancer cases. Ratios of observed to expected cases and absolute excess risks (observed minus expected cases divided by women-years at risk) were calculated, and 90% confidence limits determined, assuming the observed number of breast cancer cases to be distributed as a Poisson variable.

The period of risk for breast cancer development began at the date of first fluoroscopic examination among exposed patients and at the date of first sanatorium admission among comparison patients. The end of the period of risk was taken as July 1, 1975, for those located alive, the date of death for those who had died, the last date at which the patient is known to have been alive for those lost to follow-up and the date of breast cancer diagnosis for those found to have had a breast malignancy.

RESULTS

Table I presents the distribution and percentage of breast cancer risk factors that were present among women who did and did not develop breast cancer. The relative risks associated with these factors, adjusted for radiation exposure, are also presented. Benign breast disease (BBD), family history of breast cancer (FHBCA), nulliparity, and increased age at first birth (AAFB) were found to be independent indicators of breast cancer risk, although only the risk for BBD was statistically significant. Early age at menarche and late age at menopause were not seen to be associated with an increased risk of breast cancer.

Menarche

Radiogenic breast cancer risk was computed as a function of age at initial fluoroscopic exposure and age at menarche (Table II). Although the number of women who were exposed before or during the time of first menses is small, only 30, a statistically significant (p = 0.003) excess of breast cancer was detected (3 observed and 0.28 expected). It should be noted that all of these women were over 10 years of age at initial exposure. The excess absolute risk associated with exposure before menarche was computed to be 18.6 breast cancers per million women per year per rad, with 90% confidence limits of 3.7 to 51.2 cases/10^6WY-rad. Exposures occurring after menarche but before the age of 20 also resulted in a statistically significant (p = 0.001) breast cancer excess risk, but

TABLE II. RADIOGENIC BREAST CANCER RISK AS A FUNCTION
OF AGE AT EXPOSURE AND AGE AT MENARCHE

	Exposure before and during menarche	Exposure after menarche but before age 20	Exposure after age 20
No. fluoroscopically examined	30[a]	302	689
Breast cancer cases			
Observed (O)	3	12	26
Expected (E)	0.28	3.92	18.51
O/E	10.9	3.1	1.4
Woman-years at risk (WY)	785	7967	18 557
Average breast dose (rad)	186	185	130
$(O-E)/10^6$ WY-rad	18.6	5.5	3.1
90% C.I.	(3.7, 51.2)	(2.0, 10.5)	(−0.1, 7.3)

[a] No exposures occurred before age 10.

apparently of lower magnitude, 5.5 cases/10^6WY-rad. The risk estimate for
exposures among women over 20 was even less, 3.1/10^6WY-rad (p = 0.06).
It is unlikely that these results simply reflect an age effect, since the
previously reported analysis suggested that adolescence (ages 15 to 19)
was the particularly sensitive time for increased breast cancer risk [6].
An analysis performed using the comparison population gave similar risk
estimates to those above, and the difference among the three risk estimates
was statistically significant (p = 0.04). It seems, then, that exposures
before and during menarche are more harmful than exposures after menarche.
Possibly, the exposures that occur before menarche, during the period of
breast budding [14, 15], are particularly damaging. This conclusion is in
accord with the recent study of atomic bomb survivors in which the greatest
increased incidence of breast cancer among young females exposed to less
than 100 rad occurred among those exposed at ages 10 through 13. In this
Japanese study, it was also suggested that breast tissue at early stages
of development may be especially sensitive to the carcinogenic effects of
radiation [2].

Pregnancy

Pregnancy is one of the most important risk indicators for breast
cancer, and it is known that nulliparous women are at increased risk for

TABLE III.   RADIOGENIC BREAST CANCER RISK IN PAROUS AND
NULLIPAROUS WOMEN, TESTS FOR INTERACTION, AND RADIATION
RISK ESTIMATES COMPUTED ADJUSTING FOR PREGNANCY

	Parous women		Nulliparous women	
	Exposed	Comparison	Exposed	Comparison
No. women	510	373	409	235
Breast cancer cases				
Observed (O)	16	7	17	2
Expected (E)	12.68	7.97	8.15	4.00
Woman-years at risk (WY)	14 973	11 091	9 635	5038
Average breast dose (D) (rad)	150		145	
Relative risk (crude)[a,b]	1.7		4.4	
Relative risk (adjusted)[c] χ_1^2 (heterogeneity) = 1.4, p = 0.24	1.4		4.2	
Rate difference				
(crude)[d,e]	2.9/10^6WY-rad		9.4/10^6WY-rad	
90% C.I.	(−1.2, 7.0)		(2.3, 16.5)	
Rate difference				
(adjusted)[f] χ_1^2 (heterogeneity) = 2.2, p = 0.14	1.8/10^6WY-rad		8.7/10^6WY-rad	

[a] $(O_1/WY_1)/(O_0/WY_0)$ where 1 and 0 are subscripts for the exposed and comparison women
respectively.

[b] Radiation risk estimate adjusting for pregnancy;
$\widehat{RR}$ (Maximum likelihood) = 2.3, p = 0.01.

[c] $(O_1/E_1)/(O_0/E_0)$ termed the relative risk (RR_a) of exposed women compared with non-
exposed, adjusting for age and calendar year [12].

[d] $(O_1/WY_1 - O_0/WY_0)/D$.

[e] Radiation risk estimate adjusting for pregnancy;
$\widehat{RD}$ (Maximum likelihood) = 4.9/10^6WY-rad, p = 0.01.

[f] $(RR_a - 1)$ $(O_0/WY_0)/D$ [3].

TABLE IV.   RADIOGENIC BREAST CANCER RISK AS A FUNCTION
OF AGE AT EXPOSURE AND AGE AT FIRST BIRTH (AAFB)

	Exposure before AAFB	Exposure equal to AAFB	Exposure after AAFB
No. fluoroscopically examined	263	20	230
Breast cancer cases			
Observed (O)	7	2	7
Expected (E)	5.67	0.34	6.72
O/E	1.2	5.9	1.0
Woman-years at risk (WY)	8617	513	5846
Average breast dose (rad)	177	189	114
$(O-E)/10^6$WY-rad	0.9	17.1	0.4
90% C.I.	(−1.6, 4.9)	(0.2, 61.4)	(−5.2, 9.6)

developing breast cancer [16].   When evaluating radiogenic breast cancer
risk by pregnancy status (Table III), it is seen that nulliparous women
were at a 3- to 4-fold increased radiation risk when contrasted with parous
women: 8.7 breast cancers/10^6WY-rad versus 1.8/10^6WY-rad. Although the
difference between these two groups of women is not statistically significant (p = 0.14), the difference is in the direction of an enhanced radiation
effect among nulliparous women, or more correctly, among exposed women who
had not been pregnant or who did not become pregnant after irradiation.
    The radiogenic relative risk estimate, controlling for pregnancy, is
2.3 and differs from the crude risk estimate of 1.8 (Table III), computed
using the entire study population.   The crude relative risk computed among
women responding only to the questionnaire, however, was 2.4 and is perhaps
the appropriate one for comparison purposes in this table and in subsequent
tables.

Age at exposure and AAFB
    When considering only exposed women who have borne children, it appears
from Table IV that exposures before or after the age at first birth produce
less of a radiation risk than exposures occurring during the time of first
pregnancy.   Although the numbers are small (among 20 women, 2 breast cancers
were observed versus 0.33 expected) the computed absolute excess risk of
17.1 cancers/10^6WY-rad is statistically significant (p = 0.03).   The data
further suggest that exposures occurring at the time of first pregnancy are
especially hazardous and that the condition of the breast may modify the
carcinogenic potential of radiation.   This increased radiogenic risk at
first pregnancy may also hold for subsequent pregnancies, but the data were
not available for analysis.

TABLE V.   RADIOGENIC BREAST CANCER RISK AS A FUNCTION
OF BENIGN BREAST DISEASE (BBD), TESTS FOR INTERACTION
AND RADIATION RISK ESTIMATES COMPUTED ADJUSTING FOR BBD

| | Benign breast disease | | | |
| | Present | | Absent | |
	Exposed	Comparison	Exposed	Comparison
No. women	83	49	440	293
Breast cancer cases				
Observed (O)	6	3	16	3
Expected (E)	2.10	1.0	12.09	7.50
Woman-years at risk (WY)	2698	1588	14 377	9622
Average breast dose (rad)	187	—	154	—
Relative risk (crude)[a,b]	1.2		3.6	
Relative risk (adjusted)[a] χ_1^2 (heterogeneity) = 1.36, $\quad$ p = 0.24	1.0		3.3	
Rate difference (crude)[a,c] 90% C.I.	$1.8/10^6$WY-rad (− 11.0, 14.5)		$5.2/10^6$WY-rad (1.2, 9.2)	
Rate difference (adjusted)[a] χ_1^2 (heterogeneity) = 0.10, $\quad$ p = 0.80	$− 0.5/10^6$WY-rad		$6.7/10^6$WY-rad	

[a] See footnotes, Table III.

[b] Radiation risk estimate adjusting for BBD;
$\widehat{RR}$ (M.L.) = 2.4, p = 0.03.

[c] Radiation risk estimate adjusting for BBD;
$\widehat{RD}$ (M.L.) = $4.9/10^6$WY-rad, p = 0.03.

TABLE VI.   DISTRIBUTION OF BENIGN BREAST DISEASE BY RADIATION BREAST DOSE

	Dose (rad)						
	0	<100	100–199	200–299	300–399	400–499	500 +
Average breast dose	0	32	150	242	336	433	669
No. women	342	208	148	100	36	11	20
Benign breast disease (BBD)	49	28	27	15	3	2	8
Women-years at risk (WY)	11 210	6514	4775	3409	1279	393	704
BBD/10^3WY[a]	4.4	4.3	5.7	4.4	2.3	5.1	11.4

[a] Age-adjusted values are not appreciably different from these crude rates.   The difficulty in interpreting this distribution, however, is the uncertainty whether the BBD was present at time of irradiation or developed subsequent to irradiation.

Benign breast disease

A somewhat imprecise definition for benign breast disease was used on the patient questionnaire. Anyone who reported having cysts, nodules or tumors other than cancer was classified as having benign breast disease. Of the 865 women who responded to this question, 132 (15.2%) had benign breast disease. Although benign breast disease was found to be associated with an increased risk of breast cancer after controlling for radiation exposure (RR = 2.6, Table I), there was no indication that benign breast disease increased the effect of radiation exposure (Table V). In fact, the radiation effect appeared restricted to those women without benign breast disease. Complicating factors, however, include the uncertainty about whether the benign breast disease appeared before or after the radiation exposure as well as the possibility that benign breast disease was caused by the radiation exposure. Another difficulty is the possibility that women with breast cancer were subsequently intensely screened after diagnosis so that benign breast disease was more likely to be detected and reported.

In Table VI, distribution of the incidence of benign breast disease by radiation breast dose is shown. Although no trend is apparent at relatively low doses, there is a suggestion of an increased incidence of benign breast disease among the high-dose categories. It might be, then, that radiation causes both breast cancer and benign breast disease. This conclusion is supported by the recent Rochester study of women who received therapeutic doses of radiation for acute postpartum mastitis, in that an apparent dose-response relationship, compatible with linearity, was reported between radiation dose and benign breast disease [13].

Family history

Among 31 exposed patients with a family history of breast cancer, 2 breast cancers were observed, in contrast to 0 cancers among 22 comparison patients with similar family histories. The numbers are particularly sparse and the radiogenic risk estimates not statistically significant (p = 0.30); the data, however, are in the direction of a 2-fold increase in radiogenic risk among women with a family history of breast cancer: $10.8/10^6$WY-rad versus $4.3/10^6$WY-rad (Table VII).

Age at menopause

The data (Table VIII) on the risk of breast cancer among women who have experienced menopause suggest that women who experienced menopause after age 45 were at decreased breast cancer risk compared to women who experienced menopause before age 45 (RR = 0.6, controlling for radiation exposure). The apparent absence of a protective effect of early menopause is contrary to current understanding [16] and chance is a possible explanation (90% C.I.: 0.3 and 1.2). On the other hand, tuberculosis and the frequently associated condition of malnutrition might have played a role in minimizing the protective effect of early menopause by being correlated with reduced fertility, erratic menstrual cyles and minimally active ovarian estrogen cycles. Menopause was also not found to influence the effect of radiation exposure to any appreciable degree.

Multiple risk factors

Table IX presents breast cancer radiogenic risk estimates by number of risk factors. Women for whom no information was known with regard to specific risk factors were assumed not to possess the risk factor. The excess radiogenic risk, adjusted for age and calendar year, for women possessing 0, 1, 2 and 3 or more breast cancer risk factors was 0.2, 4.8, 5.2 and 14.8 cancers/10^6WY-rad respectively, assuming the unadjusted risk to approximate the adjusted risk for the 3+ category. The heterogeneity

TABLE VII. BREAST CANCER RISK AS A FUNCTION OF FAMILY
HISTORY OF BREAST CANCER (FHBCA), TESTS FOR INTERACTION
AND RADIATION RISK ESTIMATES COMPUTED ADJUSTING
FOR FHBCA

| | Family history of breast cancer | | | |
| | Yes | | No | |
	Exposed	Comparison	Exposed	Comparison
No. women	31	22	479	324
Breast cancer cases				
Observed (O)	2	0	20	6
Expected (E)	0.78	0.49	13.72	8.24
Woman-years at risk (WY)	1022	709	16 402	10 912
Average breast dose (rad)	182	—	157	—
Relative risk (crude) [a,b]	∞		2.2	
Relative risk (adjusted) [a]	∞		2.0	
χ^2_1 (heterogeneity) = 1.04, p = 0.31				
Rate difference (crude) [a,c]	$10.8/10^6$ WY-rad		$4.3/10^6$-rad	
90% C.I.	(− 4.3, 25.8)		(0.3, 8.3)	
Rate difference (adjusted) [a]	∞		$3.5/10^6$ WY-rad	
χ^2_1 (heterogeneity) = 1.1, p = 0.30				

[a] See footnotes, Table III.

[b] Radiation risk estimate adjusting for FHBCA;
$\widehat{RR}$ (M.L.) = 2.4, p = 0.02.

[c] Radiation risk estimate adjusting for FHBCA;
$\widehat{RD}$ (M.L.) = $5.1/10^6$ WY-rad, p = 0.02.

TABLE VIII. RADIOGENIC BREAST CANCER RISK AS A FUNCTION
OF AGE AT MENOPAUSE AMONG WOMEN OVER 45 YEARS OF AGE,
TESTS FOR INTERACTION AND RADIATION RISK ESTIMATES
COMPUTED ADJUSTING FOR AGE AT MENOPAUSE

	Age at menopause			
	45 +		< 45	
	Exposed	Comparison	Exposed	Comparison
No. women	323	213	120	75
Breast cancer cases				
Observed (O)	11	4	7	2
Expected (E)	9.37	5.55	3.07	2.02
Woman-years at risk (WY)	10 795	7113	3888	2592
Average breast dose (rad)	163	—	168	—
Relative risk (crude) [a,b]	1.8		2.3	
Relative risk (adjusted) [a] χ_1^2 (heterogeneity) = 0.07, p = 0.79	1.6		2.3	
Rate difference (crude) [a,c]	$2.8/10^6$ WY-rad		$6.1/10^6$ WY-rad	
90% C.I.	(− 1.7, 7.3)		(− 3.1, 15.4)	
Rate difference (adjusted) [a] χ_1^2 (heterogeneity) = 0.35, p = 0.55	$2.2/10^6$ WY-rad		$6.0/10^6$ WY-rad	

[a] See footnotes, Table III.

[b] Radiation risk estimate adjusting for age at menopause;
$\hat{RR}$ (M.L.) = 2.0, p = 0.07.

[c] Radiation risk estimate adjusting for age at menopause;
$\hat{RD}$ (M.L.) = $3.4/10^6$ WY-rad, p = 0.07.

[d] Risk of late menopause controlling for exposure is $\hat{RR}$ (M.L.) = 0.6,
90% C.I. of (0.3, 1.2).

TABLE IX. RADIOGENIC BREAST CANCER RISK BY NUMBER OF RISK FACTORS

| | Number of risk factors | | | | | | | |
| | 0 | | 1 | | 2 | | 3+ | |
	Yes	No	Yes	No	Yes	No	Yes	No
Fluoroscopically examined	Yes	No	Yes	No	Yes	No	Yes	No
No. women	271	267	445	316	278	126	27	8
Breast cancer cases								
Observed (O)	9	8	17[d]	4	12	3	3	0
Expected (E)	5.89	5.39	9.87	5.70	6.12	2.82	0.82	0.23
Woman-years at risk (WY)	7102	7633	11 827	7816	7448	3279	932	297
Average breast dose (D) (rad)	130		155		149		217	
Relative risk (crude)[a,b]	1.2		2.8		1.8		∞	
Relative risk (adjusted)[a]	1.0		2.5		1.8		∞	
χ^2_3 (heterogeneity) = 2.33, p = 0.51								
Excess risk difference (crude)[a,c]	1.7/10^6 WY-rad		6.0/10^6 WY-rad		4.7/10^6 WY-rad		14.8/10^6 WY-rad	
90% C.I.	(−5.4, 8.8)		(0.9, 11.0)		(−4.0, 13.3)		(−10.1, 39.8)	
Excess risk difference (adjusted)	0.2/10^6 WY-rad		4.8/10^6 WY-rad		5.2/10^6 WY-rad		∞	
χ^2_3 (heterogeneity) = 4.79, p = 0.19								

[a] See footnotes, Table III.

[b] Radiation risk estimate adjusting for breast cancer risk factors; $\widehat{RR}$ (M.L.) = 1.9, p = 0.02.

[c] Radiation risk estimate adjusting for breast cancer risk factors; $\widehat{RD}$ (M.L.) = 6.2/10^6 WY-rad, p = 0.02.

[d] One risk factor only

	No. cancers/No. exposed with one risk factor only
Menarche at 14 years or under	7/179
Nulliparous	7/185
Age at first birth 30 years or greater	2/50

chi-square with 3 degrees of freedom was 4.8 (p = 0.19), indicating that the differences are not statistically significant. Although by no means conclusive, and limited to only 5 breast cancer risk factors (early menarche, personal history of benign breast disease, family history of breast cancer, nulliparity and age at first birth greater than 30 years), the data do not exclude the possibility that underlying host conditions could interact with radiation in such a manner as to increase the carcinogenic potential of irradiation.

DISCUSSION

Because of the small numbers involved when looking at interaction effects between radiation and other breast cancer risk indicators in this study, interpretations cannot be made with any degree of certainty, and the results must be regarded as generating hypotheses that need to be confirmed by larger series. Other uncertainties include the unknown effects of the 22% non-response rate for the questionnaire, the inability to obtain breast cancer risk factor information on most of the women who had died, and the imprecision associated with the retrospective determination of fluoroscopic procedures and associated radiation breast doses. Another general difficulty is that the breast cancer risk factors, with the exception of benign breast disease, do not seem to clearly operate as risk factors in the comparison women. Thus, a portion of the difference in radiogenic risks might be explained by a lower than 'expected' rate in the comparison group. Certainly the small size of the comparison group contributes to this difficulty. Care should also be taken in extrapolating these results to populations of women undergoing periodic x-ray mammography examinations. Breast cancer screening is apparently effective in reducing breast cancer mortality among women over age 50 [17]; few women in this study, however, were over age 50 at initial exposure and not all of the breast cancer risk factors were present at the time of irradiation, e.g., menopause and benign breast disease.

Keeping in mind the above criticisms, several hypotheses regarding radiogenic breast cancer risk do, however, seem plausible: (1) menarche and pregnancy are times of particular breast susceptibility to tumor induction by irradiation and (2) nulliparous women appear more susceptible to radiogenic breast cancer induction than parous women. An alternate interpretation for (2) might be that pregnancy can protect against radiogenic breast cancer development.

Since menarche and pregnancy are times of breast proliferation, and since dividing cells are more sensitive to the cell-killing effects of irradiation, it may be that proliferating tissue is more susceptible to tumor induction by irradiation. Interestingly, among atomic bomb survivors, exposures before age 10 have not been associated with an increased breast cancer risk [2], suggesting either that radiation damage was repaired before breast budding took place or that the exposed women have not been followed to the age when the induced breast cancers will occur.

Since the pregnant and lactating breast undergoes active cell division and proliferation, radiation might have more effect on these dividing cells than on quiescent cells. Radiation to the lactating breast or the newly pregnant breast may be particularly harmful if the opportunity to repair radiation damage is minimized because of the increased rate of cell division. If this hypothesis can be evaluated in other populations, it may have implications with regard to radiation risk estimates that derive from populations of parous women who were treated for acute inflammatory disease of the breast. For example, a high risk of radiogenic breast cancer has been reported for postpartum mastitis patients [3]. Possibly these high

risk estimates are associated with the condition of the breast at the time
of irradiation.

The apparent increased radiogenic breast cancer risk of nulliparous
women compared to parous women might be due to an appreciable protective
effect of pregnancy rather than an increased susceptibility among nulliparous
women. The concentration of excess risk among women under 30 years of age
at exposure supports the theory that reproductive life is a time of particular vulnerability to environmental carcinogens [16], but it may be that
pregnancy protects against the development of radiogenic breast cancer unless
perhaps,   the exposure occurs at the time of pregnancy.

When considering radiation risks among women possessing multiple breast
cancer risk factors, an enhancement of the radiogenic risk cannot be
excluded. Although the chi-square for heterogeneity indicated that there
was no statistically significant difference (p = 0.19) among the 4 risk
factor categories, women possessing no breast cancer risk factors appeared
to be at much less radiogenic risk. Farewell [18] has reported the
apparent interaction of breast cancer risk factors to enhance the risk of
breast cancer development, i.e. the factors were found to interact in
a multiplicative rather than additive manner. Also, Japanese A-bomb
survivors, at low 'natural' risk of breast cancer, have lower absolute
radiation risk estimates than irradiated Western women who are at higher
'natural' risk, although variations in the ages at exposure and the durations
of follow-up may partially explain this difference [9]. It may be, then,
that the carcinogenic potential of irradiation is somewhat enhanced among
women with multiple breast cancer risk factors, but the sample size of
this study is too small to be convincing.

In conclusion, the interaction of radiation with underlying breast
cancer risk factors or breast conditions has been evaluated in a population
of women who received repeated fluoroscopic chest examinations during
treatment for pulmonary tuberculosis. The smallness of the sample size,
however, makes interpretations uncertain, and chance must always be included
as a possible explanation. The current evaluations should be considered
as hypothesis-generating and not hypothesis-testing. The data do suggest,
however, that menarche and pregnancy are times of particular sensitivity
to the carcinogenic effects of ionizing radiation.

REFERENCES

[1] United Nations Scientific Committee on the Effects of Atomic Radiation, Sources
     and Effects of Ionizing Radiation, Rep. E77IX1, UN, New York (1977).

[2] MCGREGOR, D.H., LAND, C.E., CHOI, K., et al., Breast cancer incidence among
     atomic bomb survivors, Hiroshima and Nagasaki, 1950—69, J. Natl. Cancer Inst. 59 3
     (1977) 799.

[3] SHORE, R.E., HEMPELMANN, L.H., KOWALUK, E., et al., Breast neoplasms in
     women treated with X-rays for acute postpartum mastitis, J. Natl. Cancer Inst. 59 3
     (1977) 813.

[4] BARAL, E., LARSSON, L., MATTSSON, B., Breast cancer following irradiation
     of the breast, Cancer 40 6 (1977) 2905.

[5] MACKENZIE, I., Breast cancer following multiple fluoroscopies, Br. J. Cancer 19 1
     (1965) 1.

[6] BOICE, J.D., Jr., MONSON, R.R., Breast cancer in women after repeated fluoroscopic
     examinations of the chest, J. Natl. Cancer Inst. 59 3 (1977) 823.

[7] BAILAR, J.C., III, Mammography: a contrary view, Ann. Intern. Med. **84** 1 (1976) 77.

[8] UPTON, A.C., BEEBE, G.W., BROWN, J.M., et al., Report of NCI ad hoc working group on the risks associated with mammography in mass screening for the detection of breast cancer, J. Natl. Cancer Inst. **59** 2 (1977) 481.

[9] BOICE, J.D., Jr., ROSENSTEIN, M., TROUT, E.D., Estimation of breast doses and breast cancer risk associated with repeated fluoroscopic chest examinations of women with tuberculosis, Radiat. Res. **73** (1978).

[10] ROTHMAN, K.J., BOICE, J.D., Jr., Epidemiologic Analysis with a Programmable Calculator, in press.

[11] MANTEL, N., HAENSZEL, W., Statistical aspects of data from retrospective studies of disease, J. Natl. Cancer Inst. **22** 4 (1959) 719.

[12] JABLON, S., KATO, H., Mortality among A-bomb Survivors, 1950–70, Report 6, Atomic Bomb Casualty Commission Technical Report 10–71 (1971) 319.

[13] MIETTINEN, O.S., Estimability and estimation in case-referent studies, Am. J. Epidemiol. **103** 2 (1976) 226.

[14] TANNER, J.M., Growth at Adolescence, Blackwell Scientific Publ., Oxford (1962).

[15] MARSHALL, W.A., TANNER, J.M., Variations in pattern of pubertal changes in girls, Arch. Dis. Child. **44** (1969) 291.

[16] MACMAHON, B., COLE, P., BROWN, J., Etiology of human breast cancer: a review, J. Natl. Cancer Inst. **50** 1 (1973) 21.

[17] SHAPIRO, S., STRAX, P., VENET, L., et al., "Changes in five-year breast cancer mortality in a breast cancer screening program", Proc. Seventh National Cancer Conference, J.B. Lippincott Co., Philadelphia (1973) 633.

[18] FAREWELL, V.T., The combined effect of breast cancer risk factors, Cancer **40** 2 (1977) 931.

DISCUSSION

Y. NISHIWAKI: What would be the effects of other factors such as smoking or taking contraceptive pills?

J.D. BOICE: Smoking was not found to be associated with an increased breast cancer risk in our study. None of the women were taking birth control pills at the time the fluoroscopic exposures occurred.

Y. NISHIWAKI: Are the various risk factors you studied to be considered just additive or synergistic?

J.D. BOICE: There is little information on whether breast cancer risk factors interact in an additive or multiplicative fashion. One recent small-scale study by Farewell, however, suggests that the risk factors for breast cancers interact in a multiplicative fashion, and thus synergistically with respect to an additive model. The National Cancer Institute is currently conducting a very large case-control study to obtain more definitive information on this important question. In our study, the numbers were too small to evaluate the interaction of the breast cancer risk factors themselves.

W.A. MÜLLER: You mentioned that the same effect was observed when the dose was delivered in one exposure as when the identical total dose was delivered in several fractions. Do you think this is a general law, or is it restricted to low doses, or is there perhaps a threshold?

J.D. BOICE: The conclusion made regarding the effects of a single exposure versus multiple exposures of the same total dose was based upon the similarity of the radiation risk estimates of women who received multiple fluoroscopic chest examinations and women who were exposed to the atomic bomb. For breast cancer I feel there is good evidence to believe that the radiogenic risk is approximately proportional to the total dose received from numerous low-dose fractionated exposures. However, this might not be the case if the dose fraction is large enough to produce cell-killing effects. The postpartum mastitis study indicated a turn-down of the dose-response relationship at very high total breast doses, of the order of 400+ rads, whereas no turn-down was apparent in the Canadian fluoroscopy study at cumulative doses of several thousand rads. I'm not sure what effect might be expected if the dose fractionations were substantially less than one rad or if the dose rate were lower than those during fluoroscopy.

I am also uncertain as to whether or not a threshold exists for cumulative breast doses. We were not able to detect a significant breast cancer risk at cumulative breast doses under 100 rads (10 breast cancers observed versus 9.6 expected), but the number of women was too small to detect an effect at these dose levels (32 rads average) even if it existed. The atomic bomb data do, however, suggest a statistically meaningful risk following doses of the order of 17 rads. Practically all human radiogenic breast cancer studies indicate a linear relationship between dose and cancer incidence, and there is little evidence to support the existence of a threshold.

L.R. KARHAUSEN: Did you take account of age at first pregnancy, which is known to be a significant risk factor, especially since your exposed population is likely to have had a delayed first pregnancy compared with your control population?

J.D. BOICE: Yes, age at first birth was allowed for in the interaction analyses. Late age at first birth in the control group without radiation exposure was found to be associated with an increased breast cancer risk, though the numbers were too small to be statistically meaningful.

H.H. VOGEL: As you know, there have been several animal studies which show that, in rats, radiation and female œstrogenic hormones are synergistic in the induction of mammary neoplasms (Shellabarger, Segaloff, Maxfield, et al.). The times of increased sensitivity you reported in women (parity and menarche) are clearly times of endocrine changes. Did you consider œstrogens as a risk factor in your work?

J.D. BOICE: The average age of the population was 26 years at the time of initial fluoroscopic exposure so it is unlikely that many women were receiving postmenopausal œstrogens then. However, I agree that it would be of value to consider exogenous œstrogens as a risk factor, and I will try to obtain this information during the next follow-up in 1980.

K. SHIMAOKA: If the thyroid was in the fluoroscopy field, I would expect a substantial number of thyroid cancers in this population. Have you looked into the prevalence of thyroid cancer?

J.D. BOICE: Yes, we did attempt to evaluate the possible occurrence of thyroid cancer on the basis of medical records, mailed questionnaires and death certificates. No thyroid cancers were detected, however. We also interviewed many of the physicians who performed the fluoroscopy examinations and learnt that it was unlikely for the thyroid to be in the direct radiation field during fluoroscopy. Thus the absence of an observable effect could be related to our method of ascertainment which did not include physical examination, or it could be due to the thyroid not being in fact directly exposed.

RADIATION HAZARDS OF
X-RAY MAMMOGRAPHY

J.C. BAILAR III
National Cancer Institute,
Bethesda,
Maryland,
United States of America

Abstract

RADIATION HAZARDS OF X-RAY MAMMOGRAPHY.
X-ray mammography delivers significant amounts of ionizing radiation to the breast, and the female breast is more susceptible to radiation carcinogenesis than any other human organ. On the other hand, breast cancer is least likely to cause serious illness and death when it is detected at a very early stage. The risks and benefits of mammography can be estimated. This paper summarizes current risk estimates, then proceeds to a comparison of risks and benefits. As for breast cancer mortality, the addition of mammography to a programme of annual breast examinations of average U.S. women is of questionable value for women under age 50 but it is probably beneficial for older women. However, the break-even point is closely related to the average radiation exposure of breast tissue, and would be earlier in a few centres now using optimum techniques and equipment. For women with below-average risks of breast cancer, the age would be higher, and for a few women with a high probability of developing breast cancer it would be lower. The break-even point should be significantly exceeded before mammographic screening becomes worth the time, trouble and other costs. Breast cancer screening programmes have been improved significantly since criticisms were first publicized in mid-1975. Partial improvements include reduction in radiation exposure (at least in some centres), guidelines from the National Cancer Institute (NCI) and the American Cancer Society (ACS) for restricting the screeening of women under age 50, and changes in the patient consent form signed by participants in the NCI-ACS programme. Professional and public awareness of the need to balance the benefits of screening with its risks and costs has rapidly and markedly increased. Future improvements should further define the optimum design and application of breast cancer screening programmes.

In the United States of America there has been much public debate (and much public misunderstanding) about the benefits and risks of breast cancer screening. This report briefly reviews the history of this debate, assesses the data on which decisions must be based, comments on the many serious questions remaining, and describes current guidelines. Radiation hazards have been important elements in the debate, and their impact on opinions and conclusions will be described. Various aspects of this matter have been discussed in other publications [1—3], with which this paper forms a continuous series.

In this paper, 'screening' refers to the periodic examination of women who have no symptoms that specifically suggest breast cancer. Thus the diagnostic study of suspected cancers is excluded. Most women have minor breast complaints from time to time; such women are not considered symptomatic unless there is real suspicion that the symptoms may indicate cancer.

This paper does not re-examine the basic data on radiation carcinogenesis in the human breast. Upton and co-workers [4] recently considered all available human data suitable for this purpose; no additional data have been reported since then; and I know of no other significant data sources that could add to our knowledge on this matter within the next few years. Upton and co-workers concluded that

> ...... the risk may be assumed to approximate 3.5–7.5 cases of breast
> cancer per million women of ages 35 or older at risk per year per rad
> to both breasts, from the tenth year after irradiation throughout the
> remainder of life.

I accept that estimate as the best that can be derived today. It implies a strictly additive, linear, non-threshold dose-response relationship, and those who believe that other models should be used may come to significantly different risk estimates (For discussion of these points see Refs [5–11].) This estimate also implies that the female breast is one of the most sensitive human organs for radiation carcinogenesis [12]. This fact is important in determining how X-ray examinations of the breast, called mammography, should be used in screening programmes.

The well-known study of the Health Insurance Plan of Greater New York (H.I.P.) [13] showed, beyond serious question, that annual screening by a combination of modalities (medical history, physical examination and mammography) can reduce mortality from breast cancer for women over age 50. The mortality reduction was almost 40% in that age group, a result of great practical importance. In contrast, no mortality reduction whatever occurred in younger women. These results refer to the effect of the three screening modalities together. The H.I.P. study was not designed to provide reliable assessments of the effect of each modality separately, and the problems involved in attempts to obtain such estimates include length bias, lead-time bias, self-selection, and many other factors [1–3]. We do not know, therefore, how much mammography contributed to the good results from screening older women. We can conclude, however, that mammography was not beneficial to women age 50 and younger, because even the three modalities together did not seem to be helpful.

The H.I.P. study used the radiologic techniques of the early 1960s, and significant technical advances have been made since then. The most modern equipment, properly used, can produce distinctly better images now than then so that detection of more lesions at earlier stages is possible. However, no data are available to determine by direct means whether this earlier detection is beneficial for women age 50 and younger. All the evidence is indirect. Much of it depends on the assumption that breast cancer in women over 50, essentially all post-menopause, is the same disease in all important biologic respects as is breast cancer in younger women. This assumption may well be false. Whereas breast cancers in these two age groups tend to have the same morphologic expressions, they differ substantially in epidemiologic features, hormonal and biochemical concomitants, response to treatment and other factors. Thus we cannot ignore the fact that the H.I.P. study, the only reliable source of data on the long-term effects of breast cancer screening, produced entirely negative results for women under age 50. (Large-scale studies with modern mammographic equipment are now or soon will be in progress in the Netherlands, Sweden, and perhaps Canada. Their results, when available, may modify present conclusions.)

With respect to the radiation risks of mammography, again no direct evidence exists. There are simply no data on the long-term follow-up of women exposed to X-radiation of the same dose level, beam quality and fractionation pattern as that used in breast cancer screening. Most of the arguments have centred on whether the dose-response relationship is linear; that is, whether the likelihood of causing breast cancer is in direct proportion to the total amount of radiation absorbed. I believe that the linear model should be used for doses up to several hundred rads, although some people (including many radiologists) believe that it overstates risks, and others (including radiation biologists and others) believe that it understates risks. The linear model for X-ray carcinogenesis in the breast should be regarded as a 'best estimate', not a 'conservative' model, for three reasons: (1) it fits all available data [14–17] very well, (2) it has a direct interpretation in terms of present understanding of cellular and molecular events in radiation carcinogenesis, and (3) it avoids the unnecessary 'looseness' and complexity of models with larger numbers of fitted parameters. That the survivors of the atomic explosions in Japan have had a distinct elevation in the incidence of breast cancer after exposure to just 17 rads is significant.

Application of the linear model requires some knowledge of the radiation doses used in the practice of mammography. These have varied widely, with occasional reports of extremely high doses [2,3]. Radiation doses in mammography need to be quite high (even with 'low'-dose methods) because of the small differences in radiographic density among fat, fibrous and glandular tissue, and masses of malignant cells. In the United States of America, the average midbreast exposure for a complete examination (two films/breast) may have been in the range 3–5 rads at the time of the H.I.P. study. Over time, and with the partial shift from early methods to xeromammography, average doses declined to perhaps 1–2 rads by the summer of 1975. At that time public and professional awareness of the radiation hazards in mammography increased rapidly. As a result, a sharp acceleration occurred in the move toward low-dose methods, and film-screen combinations were much more widely used. Also, the degree of caution and control over the use of existing equipment increased. Average midbreast exposures for a complete examination may now be about 0.5 rads in the United States of America [18], and further significant reductions are likely as more hospitals and clinics adopt improved techniques. This recent rapid drop in average exposure was due mostly to public pressure, and should be regarded as one of several beneficial effects of extensive coverage of the subject by general newspapers, magazines, radio and television.

Radiation risks are not the only health hazards of breast cancer screening. Other authors have commented on the high frequency of negative biopsies, on surgical mortality and on other matters (see, e.g. Refs [19,20], and [21] with following discussion). Some of the research needs on radiation risks have been described by Dethlefsen and co-workers [22].

As discussed above, data on the risks of mammography are not entirely satisfactory, while no data exist to show benefits in women under age 50. Just these two points provide reason to be cautious in the use of mammography to screen asymptomatic young women from the general population. Two additional problems make the broad-scale, indiscriminate, use of mammography before the age of 50 distinctly unwise. These problems are the overdiagnosis of 'cancer', and the likelihood of synergism between radiation and other risk factors.

The first of these problems, overdiagnosis, has also received extensive public exposure in the United States of America, especially during late 1977 and early 1978. A group of 27 large demonstration centres for breast cancer screening had reported a total of 1810 'cancers' found during a series of examinations of about 280 000 women. Five hundred and ninety-two were described as 'minimal cancer' (a term I deplore). A group of eminent pathologists examined slides for 506 of these minimal cancers and concluded that 66 were entirely benign, 22 were non-invasive but could not definitely be classified as benign, and 262 were considered non-invasive neoplasms [23]. Thus there was no evidence that 350 lesions, or 70% of the 'cancers' reviewed by this group, presented any real threat to life and health. This fact is particularly significant because the promoters of mammography have given great emphasis to the 'minimal' cancers as showing that screening can detect cancers at an early stage. Unfortunately, news articles for both public and professional readers failed to distinguish between two distinct kinds of mistakes: whether the pathologist made an error in diagnosis, and whether the surgeon made an error in clinical judgment. The former is most important in evaluating the overall impact of a large public screening programme; the latter is most important in the management of individual patients. Thus statements (see, e.g. Ref.[24]) that there were only three clear errors, not 66, depend on a large number of doubtful assumptions, including the blanket assumption that there was no error in any case in which biopsy and mastectomy were performed as separate surgical procedures. This assumption was presumably

made because a two-stage approach allows examination of permanent as well
as frozen sections, but surely, the same mistake made twice is still a mistake.
The pathology review group stands by its original opinion on each of these
66 benign lesions except for two cases in which the original classification was
ascribed to 'computer error' and 16 in which the classification as 'benign' led
to the submission of additional slides that were claimed to be from the same
patient [25].

This is a serious matter, but more serious is the large group of non-invasive
neoplasms (262 of the 506 lesions reviewed). We simply do not know what proportion, if any, of these neoplasms will ever progress to the more usual forms of
breast cancer that invade, metastasize and kill. That some do is likely, but recent
work indicates that the proportion must be small. For example, Lattes [26] has
reported on a series of 210 patients with lobular non-invasive neoplasms incidentally
detected. Seventeen per cent had developed invasive cancers after an average of
7–8 years of observation, but half were in the breast contralateral to the lobular
lesion. Others [27–30] have also noted a relatively low frequency or rate of
incidence of invasive cancer following the detection of non-invasive neoplasms,
although results have differed on whether lobular or ductal lesions present a greater
long-term hazard. At present we do not know whether and how to treat such
lesions. Answers to these questions will depend in part on the development of a
better understanding of the multicentric origin of many breast cancers, including
those found at early stages by screening [31–32].

With respect to the likelihood of synergism between the carcinogenic effects
of radiation and the effects of other risk factors, we again have no data. However,
the fact that carcinogenic agents are generally synergistic in laboratory animals
is widely accepted, and good evidence demonstrates synergy in some human
cancers. For example, the relation between lung cancer and cigarette smoking
is very much magnified by exposure to either asbestos [33] or radiation [34].
At least two other studies are in progress to determine whether radiation is
synergistic with other causes of cancer in the human female breast, but that
work is not yet complete.[1]

If a significant degree of synergy exists, of course, women at high risk
of breast cancer should be actively excluded from general X-ray screening
programmes. This is contrary to current practice in the United States of
America and elsewhere, and we may in time come to regret the present emphasis
on preferential screening of women who are at especially high risk of developing
breast cancer.

Generally, to assess the impact of risk factors taken one at a time is very
difficult, even without the complications of synergism. Recent work on the

---

[1] See Ref.[35] and BOICE, J.D., Jr., STONE, B.J., "Interaction between radiation and
other breast cancer risk factors", these Proceedings I, IAEA-SM-224/713.

implications of fibrocystic disease has generally suggested a modest elevation
in risk of breast cancer [36,37], family history is important [38], but no good
evidence supports the idea that cancer incidence is correlated with the size
of the breast, which is largely composed of fat and supporting tissues (see,
e.g. Ref. [39]). Suggestions that fibrocystic disease may be associated with
cancers having a favourable prognosis [40] cannot yet be confirmed or denied.
Several authors [41–43] have developed models for estimating the effects of
two or more risk factors in combination, but these models need much testing
and further development before they can be applied with confidence to estimate
risks for specific individuals. Kessler [44] has considered some of the broader
issues in identifying high-risk population segments for special attention in screening
programmes.

An additional point should be considered in discussions of breast cancer
screening for women under age 50, although it is a problem in the use of screening
results instead of in the screening itself. One justification for the periodic examination
of young women has been the value of providing reassurance to most participants that breast cancer is not present. Unfortunately, not all cancers are detectable at screening, and this problem is particularly acute in young women because
the denser breast tissues makes radiologic examination more difficult. Several
reports (see, e.g. Ref. [45]) have shown that mammographic screening of young
women has more often led to a significant delay in diagnosis than it has advanced
the date of cancer detection. To the extent that screening programmes are used
to provide reassurance, this problem of false-negative results will continue to be a
serious one.

In the United States of America, many radiologists would like to give every
woman one or two so-called 'baseline mammography studies' at ages 35–40 [46].
Two reasons have been advanced. The first is to have the films on file for compari
son with later X-rays, if any should be taken. That would be of value only if the
use of baseline films really changes the interpretation of later results in a significan
proportion of cases. Colleagues who are radiologists tell me that baseline films
can provide welcome reassurance that later films have been correctly interpreted,
but that they rarely affect the final diagnosis or the management of patients.

The second reason given for baseline mammography is to identify from the
appearance of the breast parenchyma a small subgroup of women who are at
especially high risk of breast cancer. This argument is based primarily on the work
of John Wolfe [47,48], who has reported very impressive results. However, other
radiologists [49–54] have had very limited success in duplicating these results
in well-controlled studies. Thus, to recommend baseline mammography seems
unwise unless Wolfe's classification can be refined and improved for general
application.

There is a large and expanding literature on newer techniques of mammography, on radiation exposure levels with various techniques, and on methods

of quality control. That literature will not be reviewed here, except for brief comment on a few recent reports that illustrate important points. Several authors (e.g. Refs [55,56]) believe that a single view is sufficient for screening mammography. There is widespread concern, and some evidence, that breast cancer screening often fails to meet minimum quality standards for both radiologic [57,58] and clinical [3] examinations. Much active research is in progress on the development of entirely new imaging systems and on new ways of using present systems (Ref. [59], and several chapters in Ref.[60]).

These and many other questions about breast cancer screening have been examined by a long series of committees. Perhaps it should not be surprising that committees composed primarily or exclusively of radiologists have generally advocated vigorous promotion of mammography with loose control and a low age limit for starting periodic examinations. Committees with a more balanced membership, including surgeons, pathologists, epidemiologists, radiation biologists and persons from other relevant disciplines, in addition to radiologists, have come to different conclusions. Recently, five such committees [4, 23, 61−64] have arrived at nearly identical conclusions with respect to the appropriate role of mammography. The most recent report [64], which drew in part on the others, was summarized by Thier [65] as follows:

It seems reasonable to screen women over 50 years of age with a combination of physical examination and X-ray mammography. Mammographic equipment should be well calibrated, and the dose of radiation should be less than 1 rad. The patient should ask for and keep a record of her radiation exposure. Women under 50 may continue to be screened by physical examination, but should be screened with X-ray mammography only if they have already had breast cancer or if they are between the ages of 40 and 49 and have a mother or sister who has had cancer of the breast. Though the risk from X-ray mammography may be small, it is finite, and must be balanced against the absence of any demonstrable benefit from screening women below 50 years of age. When screening is done, it should probably be on a yearly basis. Lesions of less than 1 cm should be evaluated by more than two pathologists before any definitive operation is performed, and before a firm diagnosis of cancer is reported to the patient.

For reasons implied above, I endorse those guidelines. I do have some reservations about them, also outlined above, but basically I believe these guidelines to be both reasonable and defensible. They were recently adopted as official policy in all agencies of the U.S. Government [66]. In one large screening programme, approximately 17% of women aged 35−49 years actually attending the screening clinic qualified for mammography under guidelines very similar to these [67]. These guidelines apply only to screening, that is, to the examination of women who do not have signs or symptoms that specifically suggest the possibility of breast cancer. Strax [68] and Lester [69] have summarized the views of persons advocating less restrictive guidelines.

I hope that other groups in other countries will examine the matter with equal care before launching breast cancer screening programmes that may be either too broad or too narrow.

REFERENCES

[1]　BAILAR, J.C., Ann. Intern. Med. **84** (1976) 77.

[2]　BAILAR, J.C., Cancer **39** (1977) 2783.

[3]　BAILAR, J.C., Clin. Obstet. Gynecol. **212** (1978) 1.

[4]　UPTON, A.C., et al., J. Natl. Cancer Inst. **59** (1977) 481.

[5]　MORGAN, K.Z., Science **195** (1977) 344.

[6]　BROWN, M., Science **195** (1977) 348.

[7]　ROSSI, H.H., Radiat. Res. **71** (1977) 1.

[8]　ELKIND, M.M., Radiat. Res. **71** (1977) 9.

[9]　WITHERS, H.R., Radiat. Res. **71** (1977) 24.

[10]　BROWN, J.M., Radiat. Res. **71** (1977) 34.

[11]　UPTON, A.C., Radiat. Res. **71** (1977) 51.

[12]　MOLE, R.H., Meeting of British Breast Group, 17 Feb. 1978.

[13]　SHAPIRO, S., Cancer **39** (1977) 2772.

[14]　BOICE, J.D., MONSON, R.R., J. Natl. Cancer Inst. **59** (1977) 823.

[15]　SHORE, R.E., et al., J. Natl. Cancer Inst. **59** (1977) 813.

[16]　MCGREGOR, D.H., et al., J. Natl. Cancer Inst. **59** (1977) 799.

[17]　BARAL, E., Cancer **40** (1977) 2905.

[18]　JANS, R., personal communication, 1 Mar. 1978.

[19]　COATES, M.R., Am. J. Surg. **134** (1977) 77.

[20]　SCHNEIDERMAN, M.A., AXTELL, L.M., Surg. Gynecol. Obstet., in press.

[21]　LEWIS, J.D., Ann. Surg. **184** (1976) 253.

[22]　DETHLEFSEN, L.A., et al., unpublished report, 7 Nov.1977.

[23]　BEAHRS, O.H., Yale Journal, in press.

[24]　Cancer Letter **4** 7 (1978) 2.

[25]　McÐIVITT, R.W., personal communication, 1 Mar. 1978.

[26]　LATTES, R., Cancer, in press.

[27]　FISHER, E.R., FISHER, B., Ann. Surg. **185** (1977) 377.

[28]　PAGE, D.L., submitted for publication, 28 Feb.1978.

[29]　TOKER, C., GOLDBERG, J.D., Pathol. Ann. (Part 1) **12** (1977) 217.

[30]　BETSELL, W.L., et al., presented at Int. Acad. Path. 7 Mar.1978.

[31]　LAGIOS, M.D., Cancer **40** (1977) 1726.

[32]　PATCHEFSKY, A.S., et al., Cancer **40** (1977) 1659.

[33]　SELIKOFF, I.J., et al., J. Am. Med. Assoc. **204** (1968) 106.

[34]　LUNDIN, F.E., et al., Health Phys. **16** (1969) 571.

[35]　MILLER, A., personal communication, 22 Nov. 1977.

[36]　MONSON, R.R., et al., Lancet ii (1976) 224.

[37]　NOMURA, A., Am. J. Epidemiol. **105** (1977) 505.

[38]　ANDERSON, D.E., Cancer **34** (1974) 1090.

[39] ROBERTSON, A.J., Br. Med. J. i (1977) 1283.
[40] BERNSTEIN, T.C., J. Am. Med. Assoc. **238** (1977) 345.
[41] FAREWELL, V.T., Cancer **40** (1977) 931.
[42] DAVIES, D.F., et al., J. Natl. Cancer Inst., to be published.
[43] VAN DER LINDE, F., Schweiz. Med. Wochenschr. **107** (1977) 962.
[44] KESSLER, D.M., J. Commun. Health **1** (1976) 216.
[45] LESNICK, G.J., J. Am. Med. Assoc. **237** (1977) 967.
[46] Am. Coll. Radiol. Bull. **32** 8 (1976) 1.
[47] WOLFE, J.N., Cancer **37** (1976) 2486.
[48] WOLFE, J.N., Radiology **121** (1976) 545.
[49] PEYSTER, R.G., et al., Radiology **125** (1977) 387.
[50] EGAN, R.L., MOSTELLER, R.C., Cancer **40** (1977) 2087.
[51] MENDELL, L., et al., Am. J. Roentgenol., Radium Ther. Nucl. Med. **128** (1977) 547.
[52] WILKINSON, E., et al., J. Natl. Cancer Inst. **59** (1977) 1397.
[53] MOSKOWITZ, M., et al., Breast 3 (1977) 37.
[54] RIDEOUT, D.F., POON,P.Y., Breast Cancer Symposium, Madison, 6 Nov. 1976.
[55] LUNDGREN, B., JAKOBSSON, S., Cancer **38** (1976) 1124.
[56] LUNDGREN, B., Br. J. Radiol. **50** (1977) 626.
[57] HUPPE, J.R., SCHNEIDER, H.-J., Radiologe **17** (1977) 197.
[58] PRESSMAN, P.L., Am. J. Surg. **133** (1977) 702.
[59] SMITH, K.T., et al., Radiology **125** (1977) 383.
[60] LOGAN, W.W., (Ed.), Breast Carcinoma − The Radiologist's Expanded Role,
      Wiley, Toronto (1978).
[61] BRESLOW, L., et al., J. Natl. Cancer Inst. **59** (1977) 467.
[62] BRESLOW, L., et al., J. Natl. Cancer Inst. **59** (1977) 473.
[63] THOMAS, L.B., et al., J. Natl. Cancer Inst. **59** (1977) 495.
[64] THIER, S.O., et al., Yale Journal, in press.
[65] THIER, S.O., New Engl. J. Med. **297** (1977) 1065.
[66] Fed. Regist. (Washington, D.C.) **43** (1978) 4377.
[67] FINK, D.J., personal communication, 1 Dec.1977.
[68] STRAX, P., Consensus meeting, NIH, 14 Sep.1977.
[69] LESTER, R.G., Consensus meeting, NIH, 14 Sep.1977.

DISCUSSION

J. BERGSMA: In most occupational medicine services in the Netherlands
it is common to make mini-X-images of the thorax (ODELCA) by appointment
and as part of periodical medical examinations. This mini-photography is also
commonly used in screening the whole population for tuberculosis and lung
cancer. I think we need to examine whether such irradiations are necessary. An
X-ray of the thorax is pointless, if there is no good indication. Tuberculosis is
rare in Holland, and the prospects of curing lung cancers discovered in the course
of screening are poor. The absorbed dose from a mini-X-ray is 40 millirem in the
bone marrow, and quite a lot of people have more than two such radiographies
a year. My wife was subject to two a year plus an X-mammography. The mean

dose from all sources (natural, medical, etc.) in the Netherlands gives a total of about 160 mrem. A mini-X-ray thus accounts for a quarter of this total. In view of the enhanced leukaemia risk (see the BEIR report) do you think it is wise to continue with these radiographic examinations? The Dutch government medical service is contemplating changing its policy and switching to large-size X-rays (dose a factor of 10−25 smaller). Would the best solution not be to stop these routine X-rays altogether?

J.C. BAILAR: I cannot answer your question without more information on the medical uses of radiation in the Netherlands and on the reasons for the present policy. In general, of course, there should be no deliberate (or accidental) exposure to ionizing radiation unless the chance of a significant benefit justifies the risks and costs. These matters should be evaluated by people who are thoroughly familiar with the situation in your country, but who have no bias for or against any changes in policy.

R.E. LINNEMANN: I am a member of the American College of Radiology Committee on the Exposure of Women. The college does not recommend the routine screening with mammography of women under age 50. The value of routine mammography of women over 50 years has been demonstrated. The college recommends mammography as a useful diagnostic tool for women under 50 who have a strong family history of breast cancer or a history of previous breast cancer, and for women who have clinical conditions indicative of possible breast cancer.

A.M. STEWART: Mr. Bailar, how do you reconcile your advocacy of yearly mammography for women over 50 years of age with the fact that repeated studies of the carcinogenic effects of low-level radiation have shown an increased sensitivity with increase in adult age?

J.C. BAILAR: All available human data show that the sensitivity of the human breast to radiation carcinogenesis decreases with age. See, for example, Upton, A.C., et al., J. Natl. Cancer Inst. 59 (1977) 481.

A.G. LURIE: I am a dental radiologist and concur entirely with your remarks on widespread screening using radiography. In dentistry in the United States of America, patients are routinely screened using films which give a skin entry dose of 600−970 mrem/film. Patients usually receive 15−20 such films in one examination. Cases of malignant disease of the jaws not diagnosable by physical examination and history are extremely rare, making the cost-benefit analysis of such radiographic screening highly dubious. I hope that the long and dubious look already taken at lung and breast radiographic screening will be applied to such use of dental radiology in the future.

J.C. BAILAR: So do I. However, although radiation doses in dental screening are similar to those in mammography, the tissues of the head and neck seem to be much less susceptible to radiation carcinogenesis than those of the breast. Also, there are benefits from dental screening other than the detection of unsuspected malignant neoplasms. Thus both risks and benefits of dental screening would have to be carefully evaluated, paying special attention to its unique features.

A. ARSENAULT: Some years ago, at Michigan, studies were carried out on the impact of certain radiological procedures, such as intravenous pyelography, on the decision-making process of the practitioner as measured by the change in likelihood estimates before and after the result of the procedure was made available. I believe the American College of Radiology was involved in this project. Are there any studies being carried out at present on this particular aspect of mammography from the point of view of validity? Does mammography add a significant amount of information to clinical history and physical examination to the point that the likelihood of the disease is significantly changed?

J.C. BAILAR: I do not know of any studies of precisely the sort you describe, but I believe it is clear from simple observation that positive results from screening examinations do generally make a difference in case management. I believe it is much more doubtful if negative screening results make much difference as to whether other procedures are undertaken or how they are interpreted.

LATE EFFECTS AND TISSUE DOSE IN THOROTRAST PATIENTS
Recent results of the German Thorotrast Study*

G. VAN KAICK
Deutsches Krebsforschungszentrum Heidelberg,
Institut für Nuklearmedizin,
Heidelberg, Federal Republic of Germany

A. KAUL
Klinikum Steglitz der Freien Universität Berlin,
Berlin (West)

D. LORENZ
Deutsches Krebsforschungszentrum Heidelberg,
Institut für Nuklearmedizin,
Heidelberg, Federal Republic of Germany

H. MUTH
Institut für Biophysik,
Universität des Saarlandes,
Homburg/Saar, Federal Republic of Germany

K. WEGENER
Pathologisches Institut der Städtischen Krankenanstalten,
Ludwigshafen, Federal Republic of Germany

H. WESCH
Deutsches Krebsforschungszentrum Heidelberg,
Institut für Nuklearmedizin,
Heidelberg,
Federal Republic of Germany

Abstract

LATE EFFECTS AND TISSUE DOSE IN THOROTRAST PATIENTS: RECENT RESULTS OF THE GERMAN THOROTRAST STUDY.
    The follow-up of German Thorotrast patients was begun in 1968. So far the names of about 5000 patients of the Thorotrast group and 5000 patients of the control group have been

* Work supported by the European Atomic Energy Community (EURATOM) and the Bundesministerium für Forschung und Technologie, Federal Republic of Germany.

obtained from records in various German hospitals. The causes of death of 1257 (926 m; 331 f) patients of the Thorotrast group and 1168 (839 m; 329 f) patients of the control group who died before they could be examined were elucidated in the meantime. The relative risks of the Thorotrast patients concerning neoplastic diseases in the organs of interest were as follows: liver tumour 52, myeloid leukaemia 11.5, lymphatic leukaemia 0.9, lung tumour 0.8. To date we have examined clinically and biophysically 851 Thorotrast patients and 647 control patients. The average age at the time of injection of the Thorotrast patients was 28 years. The mean injected volume of Thorotrast was calculated by the results of whole body counting to be 22 ml. A total of 260 Thorotrast patients and 70 control patients have died since their first examination. Among the causes of death of Thorotrast patients we found a very high number of liver tumours (72) and a relatively large amount of myeloid leukaemia (5). The fraction of liver tumours is so far increasing with the accumulated tissue dose. Absorbed doses to the liver, spleen, red bone-marrow, lungs, kidneys, and to various parts of bone tissue were calculated as mean tissue gamma-ray dose rates for typical injection levels of 10, 30, 50 and 100 ml intravascularly administered Thorotrast. Taking into consideration the variations of the mean Thorotrast tissue distribution and activity ratios between thorium daughters from patient to patient and even on the organ tissue level of one and the same patient, the mean tissue dose rate is associated with a total standard error of at least 150%. If applied to a standard patient with a 30 years Thorotrast burden of 25 ml, the results of tissue dose calculations yield values of the cumulated mean tissue gamma-ray dose that are 750 rads (from 300 to 1880) to the liver, 1800 rads (from 720 to 4500) to the spleen, 240 rads (from 100 to 600) to the red bone-marrow, and 18 rads (from 7 to 45) to bone surface tissue from translocated ^{224}Ra and its daughters. Local gamma-ray dose rates to cells and cellular structures depend on the sizes of the Thorotrast aggregates and the distance of the cells from the aggregates, and may vary between some 10 and 10^4 rads yearly for cells adjacent to 0.1 and about $\leqslant 100\ \mu$m aggregates. The data reported correspond to the actual stage of the study. The incidence of late effects and their dependence on the tissue dose can finally be determined only after the follow-up has finished.

INTRODUCTION

The German Thorotrast study, a supra-regional programme, was begun in 1968. The most important aim of the study is to discover the late effects of incorporated colloidal thorium dioxyd by epidemiological observation and clinical and biophysical examination of the patients, to compare these results with a corresponding control group and to find out the relationship between late effects and radiation dose.

EPIDEMIOLOGICAL STUDIES AND LATE EFFECTS

Material and methods

In about 50 West German hospitals the records were examined to establish the number of Thorotrast patients. The names and addresses were noted of more

TABLE I. THE GERMAN THOROTRAST STUDY

Group of patients	ThO$_2$	Control	Total
Deceased within 3 years	1918	615	2533
Deceased after 3 years (Non-examined)	1257	1168	2425
Examined	851	647	1498
Non-responders	195	1486	1658
Non-traceable	938	1242	2180
Total	5159	5158	10317

than 5000 patients who had received an intravascular injection of contrast medium at the time when Thorotrast was in use (Table I). It was discovered that 70% of the patients were injected with the contrast medium in the A.carotis and 20% of the patients in the A. femoralis.

To calculate the radiation-induced excess rate of neoplasias a pseudo-randomly selected control group of patients from the same hospitals was set up. The control group was drawn from patients whose surnames began with the letter 'B'. Sex and age distribution of the Thorotrast patients were used as a basis for the selection of the control group [1, 2].

The disease that resulted in the hospitalization of the Thorotrast patients was not taken into consideration when the control group was selected. Patients who died from their illness within the first three years after this hospitalization were excluded from the evaluation.

When the study began in 1968 many of the identified Thorotrast carriers and control patients had already died. In such cases we could only establish the cause of death.

All the surviving Thorotrast and control patients were asked to come for examination as out-patients. At these examinations a complete clinical status as well as biophysical measurements (whole body counting) and X-ray examinations were carried out. Depending on the clinical indications, echography of the upper abdomen, radioisotope scanning of the liver or computerized tomography were added to the examination [3–5].

Results

Follow-up of deceased, non-examined patients

Table II gives a summary of this group of patients. The Thorotrast group is divided into the subgroups 'certain' (+) and 'very probable' (?). The follow-up

TABLE II. DECEASED PATIENTS NON-EXAMINED

General data	Thorotrast[a]		Control
	+	?	
Number of patients	607	650	1168
Female patients (%)	29.3	23.4	28.1
Age at injection (a)	40	40	43
Mean survival time (a)	18.1	17.5	17.7
Mean volume Thorotrast (ml)	27.0	?	0
Diseases of interest			
Primary liver tumour	55	49	2
Primary or secondary liver tumour	1	2	3
Tumour of the extrahepatic bile ducts	3	4	6
Myeloid leukaemia	13	4	2
Lymphatic leukaemia	1	1	2
Multiple myeloma	1	1	1
Lymphoreticulosarcoma	3	4	4
Hodgkin's disease	-	-	-
Lung tumour	13	16	28
Mesothelioma of the pleura	2	-	-
Larynx tumour	1	1	1
Bone sarcoma	-	2	-
Cirrhosis of the liver	59	67	37
Aplastic anaemia	3	5	-

[a] +: Certain; ?: very probable.

of these groups is handicapped by the fact that in many hospital records the type
and amount of the contrast medium injected were not documented. However,
by systematic investigation it was possible to establish the time intervals at which
Thorotrast was used in the individual hospitals, so that in these groups of patients
a Thorotrast injection was very probably given. In 157 of these patients we could
later confirm the Thorotrast injection by evaluation of X-ray pictures or by postmortem examinations. For epidemiological reasons, however, the division of the
patients into subgroups remained unchanged even after confirmation of the
Thorotrast injection.

TABLE III. PATIENTS EXAMINED

General data	Thorotrast	Control
Number of patients	851	647
Female patients (%)	25	20
Age at injection (a)	28	28
Interval to first exam (a)	26	26
Mean volume Thorotrast (ml)	22	-
Deceased patients	260	70
Diseases of interest		
Primary liver tumour	72	-
Primary or secondary liver tumour	3	-
Myeloid leukaemia	5	-
Lymphatic leukaemia	-	-
Multiple myeloma	2	-
Lymphoreticulosarcoma	3	-
Hodgkin's disease	-	-
Lung tumour	8	3
Mesothelioma of the pleura	1	-
Larynx tumour	1	-
Bone sarcoma	1	-
Cirrhosis of the liver	56	3
Aplastic anaemia	3	-

The average age at the time of injection was 40 in the Thorotrast group and 43 in the control group. On the average there were more men than women in both groups. The survival time after injection and after hospitalization was 17.5 years in all groups. For the 'certain' Thorotrast group a mean Thorotrast administration of 27 ml according to the hospital records can be assumed.

Of special note among the diseases of interest were neoplastic diseases especially of the organs of the reticulo-endothelial-system (r.e.s.). As can be clearly seen from Table II, a high excess rate of primary liver tumours occurs in the Thorotrast group. The corresponding relative risk for the 'certain' Thorotrast group is about 52.

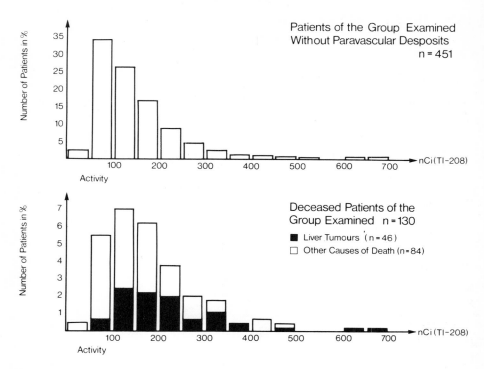

FIG.1.   Thallium-208 activity measured by whole-body counting. Top: activity of patients examined. Bottom: activity of patients examined who have died in the meantime.

The incidence of myeloid leukaemias amongst Thorotrast patients showed a clear increase in contrast to the lymphatic leukaemias, for which no excess rate was established. The figures obtained up to now for multiple myelomas and lymphosarcomas are not definite.

The epithelium of the respiratory tract is subject to constant radiation by the exhaled thoron and daughters. However, the numbers of primary lung tumours are similar in both groups.

Follow-up of examined patients

As can be seen from Table III, since 1968 851 Thorotrast patients and 647 control patients have been examined clinically, radiologically and biophysically. The number of female patients was 25 and 20% respectively. The age of the patients at the time of the Thorotrast injection and hospitalization (with reference to the control group) was 28 years. The interval of time from the injection to the first examination was on average 26 years. The average injected volume of Thorotrast was calculated from the results of whole-body counting to be 22 ml.

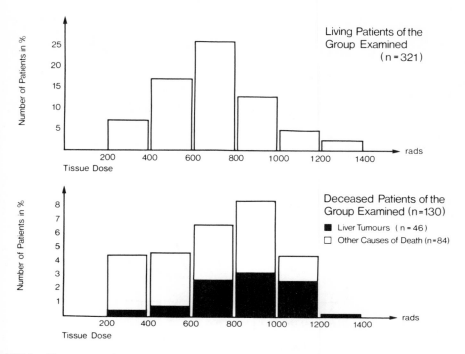

FIG.2.   Mean accumulated tissue dose of the liver in living (top) and deceased (bottom) patients of the group examined.

The number of Thorotrast patients who had died in the time interval since the first examination was 260, and 70 control patients. A high excess rate of primary liver tumours is evident in this Thorotrast subgroup, which is in comparison with the small number of deceased patients larger still than in the group of non-examined Thorotrast carriers. Similarly to the group of non-examined patients, 36% of primary liver tumours developed in a cirrhotic liver [6]. The myelo-proliferative diseases also show an excess in comparison with the control group.

It is too early to state an excess rate for lung tumours, since the number of deceased patients in the control group is comparably smaller.

One remarkable observation was a histologically confirmed osteogenic sarcoma of the humerus in a 59-year old Thorotrast patient 36 years after the injection. At the time of injection the patient was 23 years old.

The upper diagram in Fig. 1 shows the measured activity in patients without paravascular deposits. In about 80% of patients examined the whole-body ^{208}Tl-activity proved to be 50 to 250 nCi. In the lower diagram the activity of the deceased Thorotrast patients is plotted. The black columns represent patients who died from primary liver tumours.

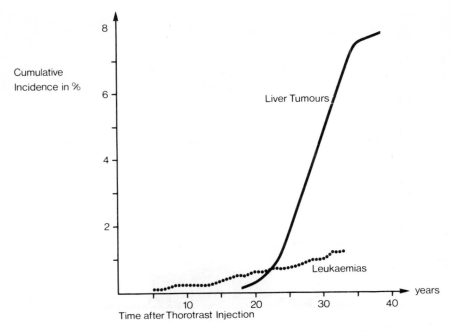

FIG.3.   *Cumulative incidence of liver tumours and leukaemias in German Thorotrast patients (non-examined and examined group).*

Using the dose rates published by Kaul and Noffz [7] for various volumes of Thorotrast, the accumulated tissue dose of the liver was calculated (Fig. 2) for the surviving and deceased Thorotrast patients. It may be seen from the histogram of the surviving patients that the dose values are distributed between 200 and 1400 rads. Corresponding values are found in the deceased patients. The fraction of liver tumours in comparison with other causes of death increases according to the tissue dose.

The cumulative incidence of liver tumours and leukaemias in non-examined and examined Thorotrast patients is illustrated in Fig. 3. From this diagram we see that leukaemias already occur five years after the injection, whereas liver tumours are observed only about 15 years after the injection; thereafter their number increases very rapidly.

The organs of some deceased patients of the examined group were subjected to a detailed patho-anatomical analysis. In the liver, fibroses and cirrhoses with all known actual complications were observed. The liver sarcomas and carcinomas mentioned previously can occur with or without metastases. The tumour cells did not store Thorotrast. There was no difference in the histological typing of the tumours compared with spontaneously occurring liver tumours or those tumour that are induced by arsenic or polyvinyl-chloride.

The histology of the spleen is characterized by a pronounced radiodystrophy with severe fibrosis and atrophy of the organ. Malignant tumours of the spleen were not observed.

A similar patho-anatomical change in the lymph nodes of the upper abdomen is a fibrosis with atrophy of the reticulum and dense Thorotrast concentration. In the bone marrow isolated Thorotrast agglomerates could be identified; however, no fibrosis could be proved [8].

Dose calculations

Mean tissue dose rates

The amount of dose rate delivered to the body tissues of Thorotrast patients depends on:
(1) The volume of administered Thorotrast and the method of administration (e.g. intravascularly, by retrograde pyelography, additional perivascular deposits);
(2) The gross organ distribution of $^{232}ThO_2$ and its daughters;
(3) The activity ratios between ^{232}Th and its daughters in the different organs; and
(4) The average size of the thorium dioxide aggregates in the various body tissues and consequently on the alpha particle self-absorption within the aggregates.

In previous publications [7, 9] and recent [10] results from the literature and from our own investigations on mean Thorotrast tissue distribution, mean steady-state activity ratios between ^{232}Th and daughters, and on self-absorption of alpha energy per disintegration due to agglomeration of Thorotrast particles in the living tissues have been compiled in order to obtain 'best estimates' of data on mean tissue dose rates in patients with long-term Thorotrast burdens.

The results can be summarized as follows: About 95% of intravascularly injected Thorotrast is retained by the organs of the reticulo-endothelial system (r.e.s.) of the 'Standard Thorotrast patient' (liver: 59%; spleen: 26.5%; bone marrow: 9.3%). Only 0.7 and 0.1% are distributed within the lungs and the kidneys respectively. The fractional retention of ^{232}Th in the marrow-free skeleton proved to be 4% on average.

Because of recoil at the moment of their creation by decay, thorium daughters are able to escape from the ThO_2 aggregates in order to be translocated to other organs or to be excreted from the body. Consequently the activity ratios between daughters and ^{232}Th in tissues of Thorotrast patients are quite different from those in sealed Thorotrast ampoules of the same age. Thus, in cases of long-term Thorotrast burdens, ^{228}Ra is only up to about 40% in equilibrium with its parent ^{232}Th in organs of the r.e.s., and in excess to ^{232}Th in marrow-free bone to about 20%. The same is true for ^{224}Ra, which is eliminated from the Thorotrast deposits of

TABLE IV. SELF-ABSORPTION FACTORS, MEAN TISSUE DOSE RATES
AND VARIATION WIDTHS IN PATIENTS WITH LONG-TERM BURDENS
OF INTRAVASCULARLY INJECTED THOROTRAST

Organ	Injected Thorotrast (ml)	Mean self-absorption factor $\bar{F}$	Mean tissue dose rate (rad/year)	Variation width of dose rate (rad/year)
Liver	10	0.85	13	5.0−31
	30	0.65	28	11−71
	50	0.52	38	15−95
	100	0.38	55	22−139
Spleen	10	0.50	42	17−104
	30	0.32	80	32−201
	50	0.29	119	48−297
	100	0.23	189	76−473
Red bone	10	0.97	4	1.5−9.5
marrow	30	0.92	11	4.3−27
	50	0.87	17	6.7−42
	100	0.77	30	12−74
Bone surface	10	1.0	5	2.0−13
Calcified bone		1.0	2.5	1.0−6.3
Kidneys	10	1.0	0.2	0.1−0.4
Main bronchi	10	1.0	5.3	2.1−13
Lobar B.		1.0	2.3	0.9−5.8
Segm. B.		1.0	1.3	0.5−3.3
Subsegm. B.		1.0	1.0	0.4−2.5
Term. B.		1.0	0.8	0.3−2.0
Respiratory zone		1.0	1.5	0.6−3.8

$\bar{F}$ = Fraction of emitted alpha energy escaping the Thorotrast aggregates.

the r.e.s. and translocated in part to the marrow-free skeleton. The corresponding activity ratio between ^{224}Ra and ^{232}Th yielded 0.25—0.36 for the liver, spleen and bone marrow, and was almost 2 for the marrow-free skeleton. In the lungs ^{212}Pb is assumed to be in excess to its parent ^{224}Ra by a factor of nearly 20, from ^{212}Pb bound to the cellular fraction of blood, and the decay of ^{220}Rn having escaped from the r.e.s. into the general circulation.

A study of self-absorption of alpha particles in Thorotrast aggregates according to a method proposed by Kato [11], together with the data on mean Thorotrast tissue distribution and activity ratios, estimated mean alpha-ray dose rates for 10, 30, 50 and 100 ml Thorotrast intravascularly injected 20—25 years previously. The results of the estimations are summarized in Table IV together with the corresponding self-absorption correction factor $\bar{F}$ for alpha particles. For example, in the case of an application of 50 ml Thorotrast the mean alpha-ray dose rate for the liver is only about 50% of that if self-absorption by aggregation of ThO_2 had not to be considered. Because of the high ^{232}Th concentration of the spleen which proved to be approximately 500% of that of the liver [7], self-absorption amounts to 70% so that the mean alpha-ray dose rate of the spleen is only three times that of the liver. According to the lower concentration of ^{232}Th in other tissues, self-absorption of alpha-particle energy is only 13% in red bone marrow and may be neglected for marrow-free skeleton, lungs, and kidneys.

In addition to the 'best estimates' on mean tissue dose rates the variation widths of the given dose values have been calculated from the average standard errors of mean Thorotrast tissue distribution and activity ratios of 150% [10], and are introduced in Table IV. These data, however, do not include variations of dose due to macroscopic inhomogeneities of Thorotrast distribution on the organ level, which may go up by a factor of 100 or occasionally of 1000 [10].

Local and mean aggregate dose rates

Quantitative autoradiography of mouse tissue samples has shown that the process of agglomeration of thorium dioxide colloidal particles in liver tissue is substantially finished at least 20 days after Thorotrast administration [12, 13]. This observation was confirmed by the results of electron microscopically investigated frequency distributions of Thorotrast aggregates in hepatic and Kupfer cells of liver tissue from mice [12, 14]: in contrast to the decrease of the relative number of 0.1 μm-aggregates with time of the Thorotrast burden that of the 0.5 and 2 μm-aggregates increased during the first 5 to 20 days after Thorotrast administration up to approximately 50%. Comparable results were obtained from analysis of liver tissue from the rabbit [15, 16].

The results of earlier [10, 12] local and mean aggregate dose rate calculations are summarized in Table V. According to these results the dose rate at the surface of the aggregates is between 40 rads yearly (0.1 μm-aggregates), and about 40 000

TABLE V. LOCAL AND MEAN AGGREGATE DOSE RATES FROM
THOROTRAST AGGREGATES OF VARIOUS SIZES

Aggregate sizes (μm $\varnothing$)	Dose rate (rad/year)	
	To cells adjacent (0.1 μm) to the aggregates' surface	To cells within the max. range of alpha particles
0.1−4	40− 3500	2×10^{-5} −1.1
5−60	7800−38000	6 −860

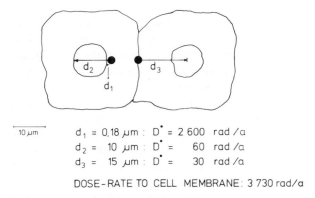

$$d_1 = 0.18 \ \mu m : \dot{D} = 2\,600 \ \text{rad}/a$$
$$d_2 = 10 \ \mu m : \dot{D} = 60 \ \text{rad}/a$$
$$d_3 = 15 \ \mu m : \dot{D} = 30 \ \text{rad}/a$$

DOSE-RATE TO CELL MEMBRANE: 3 730 rad/a

FIG.4. Dose rate to various parts of human liver cells from 3.56 μm Thorotrast aggregates.

rads yearly (60 μm-aggregates), the corresponding mean aggregate dose rate within the maximum range of the alpha particles emitted from the surface of the aggregates is between less than 0.1 mrad yearly and 1000 rads yearly.

With reference to cellular structures of human liver cells the results of local and mean dose calculations can be estimated as follows (see Fig. 4). Nuclei of liver cells of 10 μm in diameter adjacent to thorium dioxide aggregates of about 2 μm in radius at a distance of 0.2 μm will be exposed to alpha rays with dose rates between 2600 (d_1) and 60 (d_2) rads yearly. An aggregate of the same size but located at the cellular membrane will irradiate the membrane with a dose rate of about 3700 rads yearly. The dose rate to the nucleus of a liver cell adjacent to the above aggregate at a distance of 15 μm (d_3) is about 30 rads yearly. The mean aggregate dose rate to cells or cellular structures close to aggregates of about 0.05 to 2 μm radius (between 0 and 16 μm distance from the aggregates' surface) range from 0.02 mrad to about 1 rad yearly. The mean tissue dose rate to liver tissue in the environment of these aggregates is about 30 mrads yearly.

The mean tissue dose rate of 20 rads yearly from large Thorotrast aggregates up to 40 μm in diameter, however, can be expected only in tissue adjacent to these aggregates. They have to be regarded as clusters of smaller aggregates of the order of 1 μm and below according to the results of the electron microscope investigations, so that the inter-aggregate dose rate is more likely that of cellular elements as calculated above. It is not known, however, whether local dose rates of the order of some 10^3 rads yearly can be taken as an index of tumour induction in Thorotrast patients, or whether mean organ dose rates of some 10 to 100 rads yearly are to be taken as a better index of the potential radiation hazard of Thorotrast.

CONCLUSION

The data reported correspond to the actual stage of the study. The incidence of late effects and their dependence on the tissue dose can finally be determined only after the follow-up study has finished. The influence of possible non-radiation effects of the colloid can be considered or estimated only when the final results of our current animal experiments concerning this problem are available.

REFERENCES

[1] IMMICH, H., Statistical problems of Thorotrast studies, Risø Report No. 294 (1973) 148.
[2] SCHMIDLIN, P., WAGNER, G., Development and improvement of the questionnaires, Risø Report No. 294 (1973) 151.
[3] MUTH, H., OBERHAUSEN, E., KUNKEL, R., HERZFELD, M., Expected late effects in Thorotrast patients, Risø Report No. 294 (1973) 320.
[4] LORENZ, D., LORENZ, W.J., VAN KAICK, G., Medical problems concerning the control group, Risø Report No. 294 (1973) 169.
[5] VAN KAICK, G., SCHEER, K.E., Actual status of the German Thorotrast Study, Risø Report No. 294 (1973) 157.
[6] VAN KAICK, G., Thorotrastinduzierte Geschwulsterkrankungen beim Menschen, dargestellt anhand von Untersuchungsergebnissen der Deutschen Thorotraststudie, Habilitationsschrift, Med. Fakultät, Heidelberg (1977).
[7] KAUL, A., NOFFZ, W., "Tissue Dose in Thorotrast Patients", Int. Symposium on Biological Effects of Injected ^{224}Ra (ThX) and Thorotrast, Alta, Utah, United States of America, 21–23 Jul. 1974; to be published in Health Physics.
[8] WEGENER, K., WESCH, H., KAMPMANN, H., ZAHNERT, R., Pathological findings in the RES of Thorotrast patients, Risø Report No. 294 (1973) 248.
[9] KAUL, A., "Tissue distribution and steady state activity ratios of ^{232}Th and daughters in man following intravascular injection of Thorotrast", Proc. Third International Meeting on the Toxicity of Thorotrast, Risø Report No. 294 (1973) 14.
[10] KAUL, A., MUTH, H., "Thorotrast distribution and dose", WHO meeting of a Scientific Group on the Long-Term Effects of Radium and Thorium in Man, Geneva, 12–16 Sep. 1977.

[11] KATO, Y., Determination of thorium amount in Thorotrast patients, Nippon Acta Radiol.
      2b 12 (1967).
[12] KAUL, A., FÖLL, U., HAASE, V.A., PALME, G., RIEDEL, W., STOLPMAN, H.-J.,
      "Microdistribution of Thorotrast and dose to cellular structures"; Int. Meeting on
      Thorotrast and other Alpha-Emitters, Lisbon, 28 Jun.–2 Jul. 1977; to be published
      in Environmental Research.
[13] FÖLL, U., Gammaspektrometrische und histoautoradiographische Untersuchungen zur
      Biokinetik von kolloidalem ThO$_2$ (Thorotrast), M.D. Thesis, Freie Universität Berlin (1978)
[14] HAASE, V.A., Elektronenmikroskopische Untersuchungen über die Konglomerierung
      von kolloidalem ThO$_2$ und Dosisberechnungen, M.D. Thesis, Freie Universität Berlin
      (1977).
[15] HINDRINGER, B., ABMAYR, W., KAUL, A., Erfassung morphologischer Veränderungen
      von Thorotrast-Konglomeraten durch elektronische Bildanalyse (Determination of
      morphological variations of Thorotrast-conglomerates by a picture analysing computer),
      Verh. Dtsch. Ges. Path. **56** (1972) 452.
[16] KAUL, A., ABMAYR, W., HINDRINGER, B., "Mean organ dose rates in man following
      intravascular injection of Thorotrast", Proc. Third Int. Meeting on the Toxity of
      Thorotrast, Risø Report No. 294 (1973) 40.

DISCUSSION

J. BERGSMA: In the records of the Dutch Government Medical Service
(RGD) I came across a case of a patient who had died as a result of bleeding from
the brachial artery due to erosion of the artery. Twenty years earlier the person
concerned had had an examination involving a Thorotrast injection, and it would
seem that a leakage at the point of injection was the cause of death.

A. KAUL: Perivascular deposits are known. In our follow-up study we have
about 70% of patients with Thorotrast injections into the carotid artery and 20%
with administration of the contrast medicine into the femoral artery. In 264 out
of a total of 851 living Thorotrast patients examined, i.e. about 30%, perivascular
deposits have been observed by X-ray analysis.

E. RIKLIS: Whole-body counting for thorium has been described in ICRP,
Vol. 10, as insensitive for low-level measurements, and exhalation measurements
of thoron in breath have been recommended. Have you compared the two
methods, and do you find whole-body counting a sufficiently sensitive method?

A. KAUL: Whole-body counting was found to be sensitive enough in the
measurement of Thorotrast patients. We have compared the results of [208]Tl
whole-body counting and of measurements of exhaled [220]Rn as an index of [224]Ra-
equivalent. Both sets of results agreed within the instrumental limits, but thoron
measurements are greatly affected by physiological factors and the individual
distribution of the thorium colloid, e.g. perivascular deposits. However, in the
case of patients who were not able or willing to come for whole-body measurements, exhalation measurements were performed by means of portable equipment
installed in a car.

HUMAN STUDIES:
OCCUPATIONAL EXPOSURE
Session 5, Part 2, and Session 7

SEGUIMIENTO DE UN CASO DE IRRADIACION HUMANA ACCIDENTAL

J.C. GIMENEZ, G. NOWOTNY
Comisión Nacional de Energía Atómica,
Buenos Aires,
Argentina

Abstract—Resumen

FOLLOW-UP OF A CASE OF ACCIDENTAL EXPOSURE OF A HUMAN SUBJECT.
Between 3 and 4 May 1968 a worker met with an irradiation accident involving strongly inhomogeneous exposure (of the order of 50 rad to 1.7 Mrad) when he carried in his trouser pocket a strong ^{137}Cs source forming part of an industrial gammagraphy device. A previous paper (paper SM-119/35 in IAEA publication STI/PUB/229) gave an estimate of the doses received in the affected areas, described the appearance of radiation-induced somatic effects during the first year and discussed the possible development of the case on the basis of distribution of the radiation dose received. A summary is here given of the most important aspects of the development of the case, taking as reference material the periodic medical examinations carried out in the last ten years. The results of the examinations and analyses performed are discussed, and pictures showing the evolution of the external lesions are presented. A prognosis of future developments in the case is given on the basis of the available data.

SEGUIMIENTO DE UN CASO DE IRRADIACION HUMANA ACCIDENTAL.
Entre los días 3 y 4 de mayo de 1968 un obrero sufrió un accidente de irradiación fuertemente inhomogénea (del orden de 50 rad a 1,7 Mrad) al tener en los bolsillos de su pantalón una fuente de ^{137}Cs, perteneciente a un equipo de gammagrafía industrial. En una publicación anterior del OIEA (STI/PUB/229, memoria SM-119/35) se presentó una estimación de las dosis recibidas en las zonas afectadas, se describió la aparición durante el primer año de efectos somáticos radioinducidos y se comentó la posible evolución del paciente en base a la distribución de la dosis de radiación recibida. En esta memoria se han recopilado los aspectos más importantes de la evolución del caso, tomando como referencia los controles médicos periódicos que se realizaron durante los aproximadamente diez años transcurridos hasta la fecha. Se discuten los resultados de los exámenes y análisis efectuados y se presentan las imágenes que documentan la tendencia evolutiva de las lesiones externas. En base a la información disponible se comenta el pronóstico futuro de la evolución del paciente.

1. INTRODUCCION

En el presente trabajo se describen los aspectos médicos más importantes que durante una década caracterizaron la evolución de un caso severo de radiación humana accidental. El accidente, tal como ha sido descrito por Beninson y colaboradores, ocurrió en una destilería petrolífera situada en la Ciudad de

279

La Plata (Argentina). En el mismo resultó irradiado un obrero soldador de nacionalidad boliviana, que encontró en el suelo una fuente de 13 Ci de cesio-137 extraviada por una empresa subcontratista que realizaba tareas de gammagrafía industrial. Las circunstancias que causaron el accidente fueron motivo de sumario administrativo y proceso judicial. El obrero recogió un objeto metálico brillante sin saber que se trataba de una cápsula radiactiva. El objeto se asemejaba, por su forma y dimensiones, a un perno extraviado de un instrumento y el obrero lo guardó en los bolsillos de su pantalón de trabajo luego de examinarlo brevemente en sus manos. El hecho ocurrió el 3 de mayo de 1968 y desde aquella fecha el irradiado ha estado periódicamente bajo control médico para encontrar un alivio a sus lesiones.

El seguimiento del caso ha permitido incrementar la experiencia en la asistencia médica de las irradiaciones parciales agudas. Más aún, la evolución del caso ha permitido llevar un registro cronológico de los distintos efectos tardíos observados.

2. HALLAZGOS MEDICOS OBSERVADOS DURANTE APROXIMADAMENTE DIEZ AÑOS DE SEGUIMIENTO

Se describen a continuación los eventos médicos observados, sus tiempos de aparición y las dosis asociadas, registrados en los exámenes del estado general del paciente y durante la evolución de las lesiones radioinducidas.

2.1. Estado general del paciente

Se realizaron controles médicos de frecuencia variable. En cada examen se realizó una evaluación clínica global y exámenes complementarios que permitieron en cada circunstancia definir razonablemente el estado de salud del paciente.

El accidente consistió en una irradiación fuertemente inhomogénea, tal como puede observarse en las curvas de isodosis trazadas sobre un corte sagital del accidentado durante la reconstrucción dosimétrica [1], que se presentan en la figura 1.

La información obtenida mediante el interrogatorio del paciente, respecto de ciertas manifestaciones clínicas eventualmente padecidas por el mismo durante los primeros días que siguieron al accidente, permite presumir con cierta incertidumbre la ausencia del síndrome prodromal. Más aún, tal consideración pudo ser confirmada a partir de una estimación de la dosis corporal media en aproximadamente 52 rad, obtenida por la determinación de la frecuencia de aberraciones cromosómicas en linfocitos de sangre periférica.

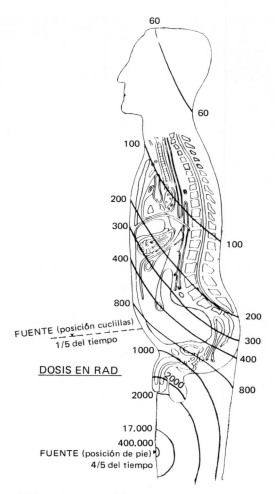

FIG.1. Corte sagital del accidentado (dosis en rad).

Habitualmente, el estado general del paciente fue bueno durante el tiempo del seguimiento, excepto en los primeros meses; particularmente entre el quinto y octavo mes el estado general empeoró debido a la intensificación de un dolor profundo en las lesiones radioinducidas en ambos muslos.

Posteriormente, luego de la amputación de ambas piernas, el paciente evolucionó sin manifestaciones generales hasta 1974, seis años después del accidente. En ese año se le hicieron exámenes de laboratorio previos a una plástica reparadora de una úlcera de postirradiación en la región inguinoescrotal, y se descubrió accidentalmente una glucemia de 204 mg/100 ml acompañada

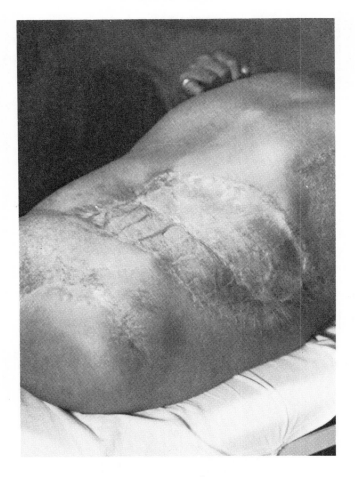

FIG.2. Diez años después del accidente.

de una glucosuria de 20 g/l. Los antecedentes previos, pero posteriores al
accidente permitieron determinar valores de glucemia próximos al límite
superior de variación fisiológica sin glucosuria. Consecuentemente se diagnosticó
diabetes mellitus y se la trató favorablemente por vía oral con antidiabéticos.

Actualmente, diez años después del accidente, el paciente evidencia una
amputación quirúrgica y desarticulación de ambos miembros inferiores, plástica
en manos y periné y recomposición anatómica del canal urinario (fig.2). Su
aspecto es bueno, lúcido, nutrido e hidratado. La piel muestra algunas secuelas
de radiodermitis, hiperpigmentación, fibrosis profunda y vestigios de injertos
cutáneos. Tiene buena perfusión periférica, determinada por pletismografía.

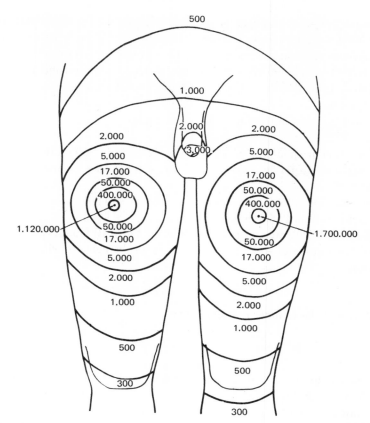

FIG.3. Dosis superficiales en rad. Estimaciones: fuente en muslo izquierdo, 10 h 30 min; fuente en muslo derecho, 7 h.

No se palpa edema sacro, ni adenopatías y esplenomegalia. Se observa buena implantación pilosa en la cabeza de acuerdo al biotipo y la edad. Las mucosas del paciente son húmedas y sanas. Tiene además buena suficiencia respiratoria, que ha sido evaluada por las pruebas funcionales pulmonares (Capacidad Vital, Volumen Espiratorio Forzado, Flujo Espiratorio Forzado y Flujo Medio Espiratorio Forzado) de acuerdo al peso talla y edad. El análisis citológico del esputo ha resultado negativo. Se ha notado un ligero aumento de la silueta cardíaca a expensas del ventrículo izquierdo, sin signos de insuficiencia cardíaca. El electrocardiograma es normal y la tensión arterial registrada es habitualmente del orden de 120/80 mm Hg. No se ha palpado en el abdomen organomegalia alguna. Se registra también ausencia de escroto, con atrofia testicular y de pene. Se ha evaluado el sistema osteomuscular determinando calcio y fósforo en sangre y orina, fosfatasa alcalina, creatina y creatinina. Los valores fluctúan dentro de los límites normales. La punción de hueso en la cresta ilíaca muestra fragmentos óseos esponjosos con intensa osteoporosis. Se determinó una glucemia de 190 mg/100 ml con escapes glucosúricos. Se comprobó además una disminución de la agudez visual (7/10). No se comprobaron eventuales complicaciones de la diabetes.

El análisis de los datos permitiría presumir que:

a)   en el sistema urogenital, situado entre las isodosis de 800 y 2000 rad ha ocurrido una atrofia de genitales externos, esterilidad y ausencia de la líbido;

b)   el páncreas, ubicado entre las isodosis de 100 y 300 rad, se correlaciona con una diabetes franca, sin tendencia a la cetosis;

c)   la cresta ilíaca, incluida entre las isodosis de 200 y 400 rad, evidencia signos anatomopatológicos de osteoporosis, probablemente vinculados a la insuficiencia gonadal.

2.2. Evolución de las lesiones radioinducidas

2.2.1. *En muslos y abdomen*

La desigual distribución de dosis en los muslos cubrió un rango comprendido entre 1,7 Mrad y 1000 rad (fig.3). De acuerdo al trabajo publicado por Beninson y colaboradores, la secuencia de eventos en los muslos, a través de la información aportada por el paciente, por los profesionales que intervinieron durante los primeros días y por observaciones comprobadas directamente por los citados autores, respecto del día de ocurrencia del accidente fueron las siguientes:

1)   A las 24 horas, sensación de pesadez y dolor profundo;

2)   A las 48 horas eritema, tumefacción y ampollas;

3)   A los 23 días la radiodermitis exudativa había alcanzado una extensión de aproximadamente 12 cm de radio en el muslo izquierdo y de 14 cm en el derecho, en la cual una zona de gangrena cubría un radio de 5 cm;

4)   A los 57 días del accidente la radiodermitis húmeda se extendió hasta la región inguinocrural en la isodosis de 1000 rad.

Al mismo tiempo se observó en el abdomen inferior, en un área limitada por la isodosis de 500 rad, una descamación epidérmica seca. Esta zona se reepitelizó entre el tercero y el quinto mes, observándose en ella áreas hipopigmentadas. Durante este tiempo se observó además una progresiva atrofia de piel, músculos y de la intensificación del dolor en profundidad.

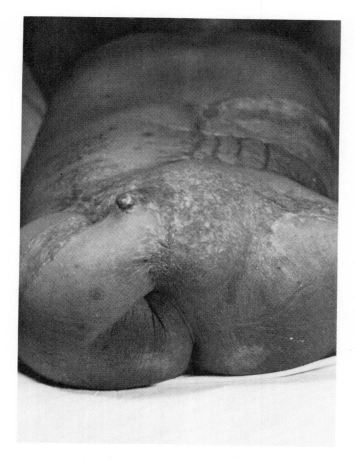

FIG.4. Estado actual de los muñones.

Al sexto mes del accidente se desprendió quirúrgicamente el injerto mediante un colgajo abdominal diferido. Algunos días después se produjeron en el mismo muslo tres hemorragias sucesivas, aparentemente venosas, ante lo cual se ligaron los vasos y se amputó el miembro. A los ocho meses del accidente se produjeron hemorragias similares en la pierna derecha por lo que se decidió igualmente la amputación.

Desde entonces hasta el momento actual se producen en los muñones manifestaciones de hiperemia activa, con prurito, una o dos veces por año, acompañadas de úlceras dérmicas. Se interpretan estos hallazgos muy posiblemente como resultantes del transtorno metabólico vascular, desencadenado por el frío, la acción traumática del peso del cuerpo sobre la piel atrófica y la infección a veces sobreagregada (fig.4).

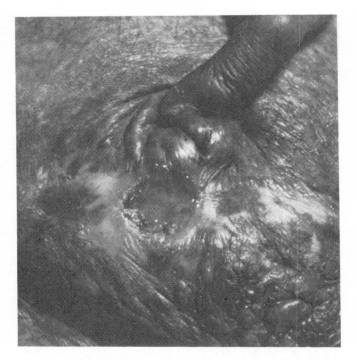

FIG.5.   Ulcera inguinoescrotal seis años después del accidente.

2.2.2. En la región inguinoescrotal

La región inguinoescrotal se estimó limitada entre las isodosis de 3000 rad sobre el glande y 1000 rad sobre el pubis.

Se registraron los siguientes hallazgos a partir de la situación accidental:

1)   A los 7 días el paciente comunicó haber padecido una eritema en bolsas y pene;

2)   A los 14 días se estimó la aparición de la radiodermitis exudativa con un punto necrótico en un borde del meato urinario;

3)   A los 24 días desapareció el vello pubiano y se observó hiperpigmentación de la piel;

4)   A los 40 días la radioepidermitis alcanzó el límite superior del triángulo del pubis;

5)   A los 57 días se observó edema escrotal y parafimosis.

A partir de entonces se evidenció una progresiva atrofia testicular confirmada por punción biopsia, descamación seca y reepitelización de la piel del

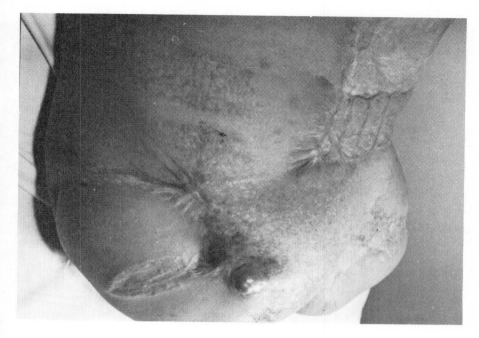

FIG.6.   Favorable evolución de las lesiones.

escroto, proceso que se repitió cíclicamente. Al décimo mes del accidente se produjo una necrosis dermoepidérmica sobre el borde pubiano del arco inguinal derecho, acompañada de intenso dolor. En adelante disminuyó el edema y aumentó la esclerosis escrotal. Se redujó la necrosis alrededor del meato urinario y se evidenció fimosis.

A los seis años del accidente persistía la úlcera inguinoescrotal. Tenía bordes irregulares, tres a cuatro mm de profundidad, base con cierta consistencia, color rojo amarillo, secreción serosa, era dolorosa a veces espontáneamente y tenía moderada repercución ganglionar (fig.5).

Se realizó además un examen anatómico-patológico de la lesión. Este estudio nos permite afirmar que:

a)   En las zonas marginales a la ulceración han aparecido dos tipos de fenó-
     menos; uno degenerativo, con ampollas intraepidérmicas, picnosis y
     glóbulos hialinos en el estrato mucoso; el otro tipo de fenómeno observado
     son lesiones de tipo hiperplásico, en los brotes basales, que protruyen hacia
     la dermis edematosa. Ausencia de reepitelización;
b)   En la dermis papilar se identifican acúmulos de linfocitos subepidérmicos
     y plasmocitos en profundidad;

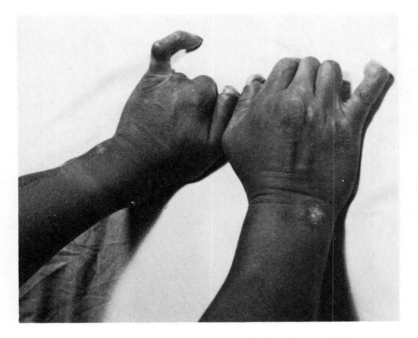

FIG. 7.   Estado actual de las manos (palmas hacia arriba).

c)   En la dermis profunda han aparecido fenómenos fibroesclerosos;
d)   A nivel vascular, las lesiones se gradúan en intensidad en relación inversa al tamaño de los vasos;
e)   La inflamación es más intensa a nivel de las vénulas, con fenómenos de endovascularitis y depósitos de trombos.

Consecuentemente se decidió tratar la lesión mediante una plástica en dos tiempos, con un colgajo que se extiende desde el muñón a la úlcera. La reparación ha evolucionado favorablemente y permite ser optimista respecto del futuro de una lesión potencialmente maligna (fig.6).

2.2.3. En las manos

De acuerdo a la reconstrucción dosimétrica, la dosis en las manos no se ha podido evaluar con precisión. Sin embargo, se pudo estimar que el borde cubital del antebrazo izquierdo, que evidenció una radioepidermitis, recibió una dosis comprendida entre 500 y 1000 rad.

A los siete días del accidente el paciente comunicó la aparición de un discreto eritema en los tres dedos centrales de la mano izquierda, y a los catorce

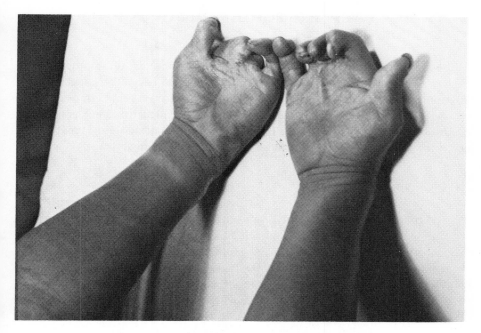

FIG.8.   Estado actual de las manos (palmas hacia abajo).

días una radiodermitis húmeda. Recién a los veinticuatro días el paciente se
quejó de ardor y observó un pequeño eritema en la palma de la mano derecha.
A los cincuenta y siete días se intentó un injerto en la mano izquierda, que
prende parcialmente. A los cuatro meses se notó una mejoría en las lesiones de
ambas manos. La mano izquierda quedó más atrofiada que la derecha. A los
ocho meses el paciente se quejó de prurito y hormigueo en la zona donde se
habían desarrollado previamente las lesiones.

Estas manifestaciones evolucionaron progresivamente, hasta que en agosto
de 1971, a los tres años del accidente, aparece una necrosis e intenso dolor en
los dedos segundo, tercero y cuarto de la mano izquierda. Se procede entonces
a la desarticulación de los mismos a nivel de la articulación metacarpo-falángica.
El estudio anatómico-patológico diagnosticó osteomielitis.

Un mes después, un proceso similar pero menos intenso se presentó en la
mano derecha. Se practicó una plástica en dos tiempos, en el primero de los
cuales se unieron los tres dedos centrales sobre la palma mediante un colgajo.
La operación no ha sido aún completada.

Actualmente ambas manos tienen una intensa retracción fibrosa en flexión,
tal como se presenta en las figuras 7 y 8. Es evidente que las lesiones evolucionan
lentamente a una escleroatrofia que tiende a fijar ambas manos en flexión.

3.   ESTUDIOS ORIENTADOS REALIZADOS DURANTE EL
     SEGUIMIENTO

Se realizaron durante el seguimiento distintos tipos de estudios orientados
a detectar precozmente efectos tardíos radioinducidos, leucemia y cáncer. Con
tal propósito se practicaron durante el seguimiento, entre distintos tipos de
estudios aconsejados [2], los siguientes: recuento de leucocitos, mielogramas,
análisis citogenéticos y del sistema inmune, presuntos indicadores enzimáticos
de enfermedades neoplásicas y estudio del estado sicológico actual.

3.1. Recuento de leucocitos

En todos los controles médicos se realizaron hemogramas, cuyos valores
oscilaron dentro de los límites de variación fisiológica. Los valores del recuento
de leucocitos obtenidos a partir del vigesimoséptimo día de ocurrir el accidente
hasta la fecha han fluctuado entre 12 000 y 6800 leucocitos/mm^3. Los valores
más elevados se determinaron durante los primeros dos años; luego, los recuentos
se aproximaron al valor actual de 6800 leucocitos/mm^3. El recuento diferencial
de leucocitos fue habitualmente normal, excepto durante los primeros dos años
en los que se determinó una eosinofilia comprendida entre el 10% y 20%, tal
como se observa en los quemados convencionales.

3.2. Mielogramas

Se punzó la médual ósea a los cuatro y a los diez años de ocurrir el accidente.
En los dos casos se punzó el esternón, pero en la última oportunidad se hizo
también la punción en la cresta ilíaca. Los mielogramas mostraron una eritro,
gránulo y megacariopoyesis normal, tanto en las proporciones como en la morfo-
logía celular. No se observaron sideroblastos ni otra atipía celular.

3.3. Análisis citogenéticos

Se realizaron estudios sobre cromosomas de linfocitos de sangre periférica
estimulados con fitohemaglutinina [3] aproximadamente al mes y a los diez
años de ocurrir el accidente. En el primer estudio, sobre un total de 226 metafases
analizadas se determinaron 12 deleciones y 11 dicéntricos. En algunos cariotipos
se observó un cromosoma *seudo G,* tal como se registró en otros accidentes radio-
lógicos [4]. A partir de las deleciones se calculó una dosis promedio de 52 rad.
El recuento de 11 dicéntricos permitió calcular una desviación standard de la
distribución espacial de dosis de 86 rad, indicativa de la fuerte inhomogeneidad
de la irradiación [1].

Actualmente, diez años después del accidente, sobre un total de 80 metafaces analizadas se determinaron 2 dicéntricos.

No se observó ningún cromosoma *seudo G.*

3.4. Análisis del sistema inmune

Teniendo en cuenta la alta radiosensibilidad de los linfocitos, así como los antecedentes que vinculan la leucemia y las neoplasias con los procesos inmunológicos [5] se realizaron algunas evaluaciones de la respuesta inmunitaria celular y humoral. Se realizaron pruebas que permiten evaluar la transformación linfocitaria con fitohemaglutinina [6].

La respuesta de los linfocitos cultivados 72 horas respecto de un valor basal es del 56%.

La prueba cutánea a la fitohemaglutinina ha sido negativa en distintas oportunidades.

Se determinaron cuantitativamente inmunoglobulinas, aplicando una técnica de difusión radial. Se halló una deficiencia en la Ig A.

3.5. Análisis de presuntos indicadores enzimáticos de enfermedades neoplásicas

Algunos autores [7, 8] pensaron encontrar espectros enzimáticos asociados a enfermedades neoplásicas. En general, estas esperanzas no se han confirmado. Sin embargo, algunas enzimas pueden evidenciar una variación de su actividad enzimática en estados asintomáticos del cáncer. Se pensó que esta variación de la actividad enzimática podría ser considerada como una alarma, a partir de la cual se profundizase la investigación neoplásica en el paciente. Con este criterio se han determinado en distintos tiempos durante el seguimiento cierto conjunto de enzimas. Las enzimas investigadas fueron: amilasa y lipasa, en suero y orina, relación transaminasa glutámico oxalacética/transaminasa glutámico pirúvica, dehidrogenasa láctica, fosfatasa ácida tartrato débil, fosfatasa alcalina, fosfohexoisomerasa, dehidrogenasa málica, aldolasa, sulfatasa y beta-glucuronidasa, todas ellas en suero. En ningún caso hemos observado variaciones anormales de las actividades enzimáticas.

4.   REPERCUSION SICOLOGICA DEL DAÑO CORPORAL

El accidentado ha sido jubilado como obrero metalúrgico. Cuatro años después del accidente ha iniciado con ciertas interrupciones tareas de vendedor ambulante independiente y trabaja alrededor de doce horas diarias. Separado de su esposa y cuatro hijos, seis años después del accidente, vive habitualmente solo, excepto en ciertas esporádicas circunstancias en las que es acompañado por algún familiar o amigo. Sus actividades recreativas se circunscriben a reuniones con la colectividad boliviana y al cine, cada dos o tres meses. Lee diarios y escucha todo tipo de música.

Tiene dificultades para iniciar el sueño, cuya duración es de tres a cinco horas diarias.

4.1. Estudio del estado sicológico actual

Se realizó un estudio sicológico con el propósito de registrar la posible repercusión síquica de esta severa mutilación física. No ha sido posible conocer el carácter del paciente antes del accidente.

4.1.1. Estudio siquiátrico

En la entrevista siquiátrica, el paciente manifiesta, preocupado, sus dificultades en conciliar el sueño desde que inició la rehabilitación de sus lesiones.

El resumen del diagnóstico siquiátrico indica trastornos de la personalidad, con depresión reactiva y alteraciones electroencefalográficas.

4.2. Síntesis de los test realizados

Se realizaron test sicométricos y proyectivos.

4.2.1. Test sicométrico de Wechsler

Se tomaron los test verbales, cuyos resultados fueron: inteligencia promedio (C.I. 0,91). Se detectan signos de intensa ansiedad y tendencia a la fabulación como actitudes defensivas ante las caídas amnésicas.

4.2.2. Test proyectivos

Se realizaron test proyectivos gráficos y verbales.

4.2.2.1. Test árbol-casa-persona (HTPP)

El diagnóstico indica inseguridad, alteración de la imagen del esquema corporal. Defensas regresivas y fóbicas.

4.2.2.2. Test proyectivos verbales

Se realizan los test de Pigam, Szondi y Rorschach.

4.2.2.2.1. Test de Pigam

Su diagnóstico indica intensa agresividad, que se esfuerza por reprimir. Pánico ante la idea de muerte y destrucción. Estructura básica ansiosofóbica.

4.2.2.2.2. Test de Szondi

Sus resultados son:

Sector sexual:	Opresión, represión y limitación excesiva de su impulso de destrucción.
Sector ético:	Tolerante, con disposición a la religiosidad. Opresión producida por el freno existencial o una excitación erótica.
Vector del ego:	Trabajador, obsesivo, fóbico, con tendencia a la posición paranoide y a la megalomanía.
Vector contacto:	Atención dividida. Falta de madurez sexual con peligro de fijación pregenital.

4.2.2.2.3. Test de Rorschach

Personalidad psicopática histeroepiléptica. Nivel intelectual medio. Disminuido en su productividad creativa por la depresión reactiva. Se defiende con técnicas maníacas negadoras. Autosobrevaloración. Impulsividad.

5. CONCLUSIONES

La coexistencia de mielogramas normales a nivel esternal y de la cresta ilíaca con graves lesiones localizadas en la parte inferior del abdomen y en las manos durante casi diez años de seguimiento confirman la clasificación inicial de este accidente como una fuerte irradiación externa parcial, determinada por la reconstitución dosimétrica.

Se consideran de utilidad, para la vigilancia médica de pacientes expuestos a severas irradiaciones parciales externas, las asociaciones descritas entre eventos clínicos, tiempos de presentación y dosis [9].

Se estima de importancia señalar la mayor vulnerabilidad venosa en el daño tisular, evidenciada en las hemorragias de ambos muslos, así como en el estudio anatómico-patológico de la úlcera inguinoescrotal.

De acuerdo a la evaluación actual, el tratamiento de la úlcera inguino-escrotal, de pronóstico incierto, mediante un colgajo diferido, ha sido satisfactorio.

La esterilidad radioinducida es permanente. La punción biopsia testicular permite observar fibroatrofia tubular y hialinización total.

Las manifestaciones cutáneas de los muñones con úlceras dérmicas pueden ser vinculadas a transtornos de regulación vascular desencadenados por el frío y agravados por la diabetes, la inmunodeficiencia y, eventualmente, la infección sobreagregada.

No es clara la posible interpretación respecto de la aparición de la diabetes. Aparentemente, el paciente no tiene antecedentes hereditarios de diabetes. Además, tanto el tiempo de presentación de la diabetes, respecto de la sobre-exposición accidental, como la edad del paciente son menores que los hallados en estudios epidemiológicos de poblaciones sobreexpuestas [10]. Teniendo en cuenta los elevados valores de glucemia observados después del accidente, se puede suponer que la sobreexposición podría revelar una diabetes preexistente.

La detección de neoplasias asintomatológicas ha sido negativa, aunque la espectativa de estos efectos tardíos es baja para este período de observación.

Las pruebas de hipersensibilidad retardada han sido negativas. Este elemento aislado es el único hallazgo que puede asociar al paciente con poblaciones de probable evolución maligna [11].

De acuerdo al estudio sicológico actual se podría estimar que los transtornos de personalidad con depresión reactiva serían la repercusión de la grave mutilación localizada.

AGRADECIMIENTOS

Los autores agradecen la colaboración recibida por el personal de la División Medicina Radiosanitaria de la Gerencia de Protección Radiológica y Seguridad de la CNEA y del Instituto de Salud Mental Dr. Arturo Ameghino dependiente de la Subsecretaría de Salud Pública del Ministerio de Bienestar Social.

REFERENCIAS

[1] BENINSON, D.J., PLACER, A., VANDER ELST, E., "Estudio de un caso de irradiación humana accidental", Handling of Radiation Accidents (Actas Simp. Viena, 1969), OIEA, Viena (1969) 415.

[2] HUBNER, K.F., ANDREWS, G.A., LUSHBAUGH, C.C., TOMPKINS, E., "A follow-up study program for persons irradiated in radiation accidents", Handling of Radiation Accidents (Actas Simp. Viena, 1977), OIEA, Viena (1977) 57.

[3] VANDER ELST, E., GIMENEZ, J.C., BENINSON, D.J., Comisión Nacional Energía Atómica Argentina, Public. n° SI-1, Buenos Aires (1967).

[4] GOH, K., Radiat. Res. 35 (1968) 155.

[5] KERSEY, J.H., SPECTOR, B.D., GOOD, R.A., Adv. Cancer Res. 18 (1973) 211.

[6] SLATER, J.M., NGO, E., LAU, B.H.S., Radiology 1262 (1976) 313.

[7] SCHAPIRA, F., Adv. Cancer Res. 18 (1973) 77.
[8] ANMAN, A.J., HONG, R., Medicine 50 (1971) 223.
[9] LUSHBAUGH, C.C., Adv. Radiat. Biol. 3 (1969) 277.
[10] SHIMIZU, K., Nagasaki Igakkai Zasshi 40 (1965) 639.
[11] ALLEGRA, M., et al., Cancer Res. 36 (1976) 3225.

DISCUSSION

M. DELPLA: Could you tell us something about the neurological after-effects and the results of psychatric examinations?   Also, what has become of the victim socially, and were those in charge of the radioactive source identified and punished?

J.C. GIMENEZ: There were no neurological manifestations. Psychiatric examinations revealed the following states: (a) reactive depression, (b) panic in the face of apparent approaching death and destruction, and (c) an urge to commit suicide that was gradually overcome. The patient has been paid compensation for his injuries and retired under pension. I have no information as to whether there was any criminal prosecution.

CYTOGENIC FOLLOW-UP STUDIES IN SIX RADIATION ACCIDENT VICTIMS
16 and 17 years post-exposure

L.G. LITTLEFIELD, E.E. JOINER
Medical and Health Sciences Division,
Radiation Emergency Assistance Center
 and Training Site,
Oak Ridge Associated Universities*,
Oak Ridge,
Tennessee,
United States of America

Abstract

CYTOGENIC FOLLOW-UP STUDIES IN SIX RADIATION ACCIDENT VICTIMS (16 AND 17 YEARS POST-EXPOSURE).

Detailed cytogenetic evaluations were recently conducted in cultured lymphocytes from six men accidentally exposed to fission neutron and gamma radiation in 1958 (dose range 22.8—365 rads). Two-day lymphocyte cultures stimulated with phytohaemagglutinin (PHA) and seven-day cultures stimulated with pokeweed mitogen (PWM) were initiated on all six men for routine microscopic and karyotypic analysis. PHA-stimulated cultures from the two men with the highest exposures were also evaluated using Giemsa-banding procedures. Approximately 9% of the metaphases in the PHA cultures and 11% of the metaphases in the PWM cultures were found to have residual radiation-induced aberrations (symmetrical and asymmetrical exchanges and deletions). In both the PHA and PWM cultures the highest frequencies of lesions were observed in preparations from three men with the highest radiation exposures. Likewise, in all cultures, most lesions were of the 'stable' type (abnormal monocentric chromosomes including translocations, inversions and deletions without fragments). Among the abnormal metaphases from the various PHA cultures five possible clones were identified (two or more cells having apparently identical lesions) whereas no stemlines were detected in the PWM cultures. The frequency of stable lesions in 92 banded metaphases from the two men with the highest exposures did not differ significantly from the frequency of lesions detected in 300 metaphases evaluated with routine staining and karyotypic procedures. These data suggest that radiation-damaged lymphocytes responsive to mitogenic stimulation by PHA and PWM may survive for many years following exposure, that the frequency of lymphocytes with persistent aberrations can be roughly correlated with dose, and that in some instances cells bearing 'stable' radiation-induced lesions may propagate in vivo. The findings also show that banding procedures, compared with routine microscopic and karyotypic methods, do not significantly improve the rate of detection of symmetrical lesions in lymphocytes from irradiated persons.

* Operates under contract number EY-76-C-05-0033 with the U.S. Department of Energy. This article is based on work supported by the Division of Biomedical and Environmental Research and NICHHD Grant HD-08828.

In 1962 Buckton and coworkers [1] observed radiation-induced chromosome lesions in cultured lymphocytes from ankylosing spondylitis patients who had been irradiated up to 20 years earlier. Since then several other studies have documented the long-term persistence of chromosomal aberrations in lymphocytes from persons with excessive exposures to ionizing radiation [2-9], and indeed, these cytogenetic sequelae may be considered one of the best biological indicators of previous radiation exposures in man.

We recently conducted detailed cytogenetic evaluations in six men accidently exposed in 1958 to mixed fission neutron and gamma radiation in the Y-12 criticality accident at Oak Ridge, Tennessee [10]. Our objectives were to determine: 1) whether the frequencies of persistent radiation-induced lesions in 1st division T lymphocytes could be correlated with the radiation dose the men had received 17 years earlier; 2) whether those subpopulations of lymphocytes responsive to pokeweed mitogen (PWM) also had residual radiation-induced lesions many years after exposure; and 3) whether chromosome banding techniques improve the rate of detection of symmetrical lesions in cultured lymphocytes from irradiated persons.

1.   MATERIALS AND METHODS

Blood samples were obtained from six of the Y-12 accident victims 16 and 17 years post-exposure. The total gamma radiation and fission neutron doses that these men received was estimated to range from 22.8-365 rads, with fission neutrons contributing 26% of the dose (Table I).

1.1. Culture techniques

In the 16-year study 2-day lymphocyte cultures stimulated with phytohemagglutin (PHA) were initiated on blood samples from all six men. Approximately 1.0ml leucocyte-rich plasma and 2.0ml leucocyte-free plasma were inoculated into 7.0ml culture medium containing antibiotics and 0.1ml reconstituted PHA. After incubation at 37°C for 44-50h, colchicine was added to each culture to arrest mitosis, and 4h later all cultures were harvested by standard procedures.

In the 17-year study a second series of blood samples was obtained from four of the accident victims and 2-day PHA-stimulated cultures initiated and harvested as above. Replicate cultures from each of the men were stimulated with 0.1ml pokeweed mitogen (PWM) and harvested after 7 days of culture.

1.2. Scoring procedures

Metaphases from conventionally stained slides from each of the PHA and PWM cultures were scored for all classes of radiation-induced chromosome aberrations including asymmetric exchanges (rings and dicentrics), symmetric exchanges (translocations and inversions) and deletions. All metaphases were counted and group analyzed by microscopically pairing chromosomes 1, 2, 3 and 16 and by counting the B,

TABLE I. DOSE VALUES FOR EXPOSED PERSONNEL[a]
(Sodium-24 activation analyses)

Patient	Total dose (rads)	Neutron dose (rads)	Gamma dose (rads)	Percentage neutron
A	365	96	269	26.30
D	327	86	241	26.30
B	270	71	199	26.30
E	236	62	174	26.26
F	68.5	18	50.5	26.26
H	22.8	6	16.8	26.32

[a] Data from: United States Atomic Energy Commission, Accidental Radiation Excursion at the Y-12 Plant; Report Y-1234, Office of Technical Services, U.S. Department of Commerce, Washington (1958).

D, E, F and G group chromosomes. Careful note was taken of any apparent nonmatching homologue having an altered centromere index. All metaphases having abnormal monocentric chromosomes were photographed and karyotyped to determine whether the lesion resulted from a translocation, inversion or deletion. Karotypes were carefully compared to determine whether any clones of cells (two or more metaphases having morphologically identical lesions) were present in preparations from any of the men.

1.3. Chromosome banding studies

To determine whether the use of banding techniques would improve the rate of detection of symmetric lesions in preparations from irradiated persons, slides from PHA-stimulated cultures from the two men with the highest exposures were stained using the Giemsa-trypsin technique of Chu [11]. The frequencies of abnormal monocentrics observed in these banded metaphases were compared with the number of lesions noted in conventionally stained slides.

2. RESULTS

2.1. Types and frequencies of persistent chromosome lesions

A minimum of 100 metaphases from conventionally stained slides from each of the PHA cultures were scored for cytogenetic lesions. The frequencies of asymmetrical aberrations observed in the 16- and 17-year PHA-stimulated cultures from each of the men are shown in Table II. Fourteen dicentrics were scored in 1142 metaphases from

TABLE II. FREQUENCY OF DICENTRICS, CENTRIC RINGS AND ACENTRICS IN PHA-STIMULATED LYMPHOCYTES

Subject	Total dose (rads)	Cells scored	Dicentrics	Rings	Acentrics
A (16 years)[a]	365	100	1 (1.0)[b]	0	1 (1.0)[b]
(17 years)		150	5 (3.3)	0	3 (2.0)
D (16 years)	327	125	1 (0.8)	0	3 (2.5)
(17 years)		150	3 (2.0)	0	0
B (16 years)	270	117	2 (1.7)	0	1 (0.9)
(17 years)		100	2 (2.0)	0	3 (3.0)
E (16 years)	236	100	0	0	0
F (16 years)	68.5	100	0	0	2 (2.0)
H (16 years)	22.8	100	0	0	3 (3.0)
(17 years)		100	0	0	0

[a] 16 years post-exposure.
[b] Number of lesions (percentage in brackets).

TABLE III. FREQUENCY OF TRANSLOCATIONS, INVERSIONS AND DELETIONS IN PHA-STIMULATED LYMPHOCYTES

Subject	Total dose (rads)	Cells scored	Translocations	Inversions	Deletions	Possible clones
A (16 years)[a]	365	100	3 (3.0)[b]	1 (1.0)[b]	5 (5.0)[b]	2[c]
(17 years)		150	8 (5.3)	3 (2.0)	2 (1.3)	0
D (16 years)	327	125	10 (8.0)	1 (0.8)	2 (1.6)	0
(17 years)		150	18 (12.0)	3 (2.0)	3 (2.0)	1
B (16 years)	270	117	11 (9.3)	4 (3.4)	4 (3.4)	2
(17 years)		100	2 (2.0)	3 (3.0)	2 (2.0)	0
E (16 years)	236	100	2 (2.0)	0	1 (1.0)	0
F (16 years)	68.5	100	1 (1.0)	0	4 (4.0)	1
H (16 years)	22.8	100	2 (2.0)	0	1 (1.0)	0
		100	1 (1.0)	0	2 (2.0)	0

[a] 16 years post-exposure.
[b] Number of lesions (percentage in brackets).
[c] Two or more metaphases having apparently identical lesions.

the six men, all of these in preparations from the three men with
the highest exposures. No ring chromosomes were observed in any of
the cultures. The most prevalent classes of lesions noted in the PHA
cultures were abnormal monocentric chromosomes including translocations, inversions, and deletions without accompanying fragments. The
frequencies of abnormal monocentrics in cultures from each of the six
men are shown in Table III, and a comparison of the frequencies of
asymmetric lesions versus abnormal monocentrics in pooled data from
all cultures is shown in Table IV. As was the case for dicentrics,
the highest frequencies of translocations and inversions were noted
in preparations from the three men with the highest doses. Karyotypes of the 100 metaphases having translocations, inversions or
deletions were carefully compared to determine whether subpopulations of cells bearing identical lesions were present in cultures
from these six men. Five possible clones of cells were identified.
In preparations from subject A we scored 3 cells having a deletion
of the short arms of a 'C' group chromosome and 2 cells having an
apparent translocation between the long arms of a 'C' and the long
arms of a 'B' chromosomes. In subject B we scored 2 metaphases
with an inversion of a number 2 chromosome and 5 cells with an apparent reciprocal translocation between the long arms of the number
2 chromosomes. In subject F we noted 2 metaphases having a deletion of the short arms of a 'D' chromosome.

2.2. Symmetric aberrations in banded metaphases

In the 17-year cultures from subjects A and D a total of 92
banded metaphases were analyzed for frequencies of abnormal monocentrics; nine translocations, inversions and deletions (10.2%)
were noted in these metaphases compared to a total of 37 abnormal
monocentrics (12.2%) observed in 300 routinely stained metaphases
from the same preparations. Although the number of banded metaphases analyzed in this comparison was considerably smaller than
the number of metaphases scored on conventionally stained slides,
our data show that the more tedious banding analyses did not improve the rate of detection of symmetrical lesions from these two
men.

2.3. Frequency of exchanges in PHA-stimulated lymphocytes in relation to dose

In a recent report on residual lesions in PHA-stimulated
lymphocytes from 130 A-bomb survivors, Awa [5] noted that the average frequencies of asymmetrical + symmetrical exchanges in groups
of persons exposed to 100-199, 200-299, 300-399 and 400-499 rads
could be correlated with dose of radiation these persons received
25 years earlier. We compared the frequencies of exchanges observed in the six Y-12 victims in the same manner, and found that
the mean frequencies of lesions in these men 16 and 17 years after
exposure also showed a good correlation with dose (Table V). A
linear regression line fitted to the Y-12 data points showed good
agreement with the line fitted to Awa's data from the Hiroshima
survivors (Figure 1).

TABLE IV. COMPARISON OF ASYMMETRICAL LESIONS versus ABNORMAL MONOCENTRICS IN PHA-STIMULATED LYMPHOCYTES[a]

Subjects	Dose range (rads)	Total cells scored	Dicentrics	Ring	Acentrics	Trans.	Invers.	Delet.
A, B, C, D, E, F, H	22.8–365	1142	14 (1.23%)	0 0	16 (1.41%)	59 (5.17%)	15 (1.32%)	26 (2.28%)

Total asymmetrical lesions 30 (2.6%)

Total abnormal monocentrics 100 (8.76%)

[a] Pooled data from all cultures.

TABLE V. AVERAGE FREQUENCY OF EXCHANGES IN SUBJECTS RECEIVING DOSES RANGING FROM 0—99 rads, 200—299 rads AND 300—399 rads

Dose range (rads)	Subject	Average dose (rads)	Average frequency cells with exchanges (exchanges/100 cells)
0—99	H[a], F	45.5	1.33
200—299	E, B	253.0	8.20
300—399	D, A	346.0	10.86

[a] Pooled data from 16 and 17 year cultures from subjects H, B, D, and A.

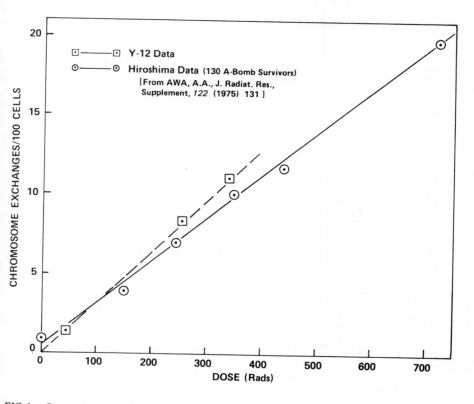

FIG.1. *Comparison of dose response curve for Y-12 patients and the Hiroshima A-Bomb survivors.*

TABLE VI. FREQUENCIES OF LESIONS IN DUPLICATE LYMPHOCYTE CULTURES STIMULATED WITH PHYTOHEMAGGLUTIN OR POKEWEED MITOGEN

(17 year post-exposure)

Subject	Total dose (rads)	Mitogen	Cells scored	Types and numbers of lesions[b]					
				Dicent.	Ring	Delet.	Trans.	Invers.	Delet.
A	365	PHA[a]	150	5	0	3	8	3	2
		PWM	150	0	0	2	14	3	6
D	327	PHA	150	3	0	0	18	3	3
		PWM	150	0	0	1	17	7	6
B	270	PHA	100	2	0	3	2	3	2
		PWM	100	0	0	0	5	1	1
H	22.8	PHA	100	0	0	0	1	0	2
		PWM	100	0	0	0	2	0	2

[a] Cultures stimulated with PHA harvested at 2 days, cultures stimulated with PWM harvested at 7 days.
[b] Dicentric, ring, deletion + fragment, translocation, inversion, deletion −fragment.

2.4. Pokeweed mitogen-stimulated cultures

2.4.1. Types and frequencies of lesions

The types and frequencies of lesions observed in 7-day PWM-stimulated cultures from subjects A, B, D and H are compared with data obtained from replicate 2-day PHA-stimulated cultures in Table VI. As in the PHA cultures, the majority of aberrations in the PWM cultures were abnormal monocentric chromosomes, with the highest frequencies of lesions in the three men with the highest exposures. In karyotypic evaluations of the 64 metaphases with abnormal monocentrics from the PWM cultures, no clones of cells were detected.

3. DISCUSSION

The Y-12 accident victims comprise a unique group of subjects for cytogenetic follow-up studies for the following reasons: 1) the men received an acute, relatively homogeneous exposure; 2) although the radiation was mixed fission neutron and gamma, reconstructions of the accident yielded excellent estimates of the relative contribution of the neutron component and of the total doses the men received; 3) the accident and its immediate effects were extensively documented in the literature, and routine clinical follow-up examinations have been made at intervals of 1-2 years.

Cytogenetic studies in the Y-12 patients were initially conducted by Bender and Gooch two [6] and three and one half years [7] after the accident. Goh subsequently made a cytogenetic evaluation of the men seven [8] and 10 years [9] post-exposure. In each of these evaluations PHA-stimulated lymphocytes were cultured for 72h, a time at which most cells are in the second or third in vitro mitosis. Because of the asynchronous divisions of subpopulations of lymphocytes, and of the possible loss of cells bearing lesions in successive in vitro divisions, aberrations observed in cultures harvested at such late harvest times are now known to underestimate the true frequency of such lesions in vivo. In the present study, PHA-stimulated lymphocytes from the Y-12 accident victims were cultured for 48h-52h to obtain estimates of the types and frequencies of lesions in 1st division metaphases. In these analyses residual radiation-induced lesions were observed in cultures from all six men. The most prevalent classes of aberrations were abnormal monocentric chromosomes, the majority of which were translocations and inversions. These findings are in agreement with data obtained in 2-day PHA-stimulated cultures from the A-Bomb survivors (25-year post-exposure) [5]. In both present and earlier studies, significant numbers of symmetrical lesions were observed after detailed microscopic and karyotypic analyses of conventionally stained slides. Because translocations and inversions are formed by reciprocal exchanges of chromatin material between or within chromosomes, only those lesions involving segments of chromosomes large enough to cause gross alterations in centromere indices can be detected in such analyses. We compared the frequencies of translocations and inversions in banded and conventionally stained material from the two Y-12 victims with the highest exposures to determine whether the use of the more time-con-

suming, but more precise, banding procedures would yield better estimates of the numbers of symmetric exchanges in lymphocytes of exposed persons. No difference in the frequency of lesions was detected
using the two staining techniques, suggesting that detailed karyotypic
analyses of conventionally stained metaphases give reliable estimates
of the numbers of cytogenetically aberrant lymphocytes in persons with
radiation exposures.

In two extensive follow-up studies in the A-Bomb survivors,
Sasaki and Miyata [4] and Awa [5] noted that the frequency of radiation-
induced exchanges persisting in survivors up to 25 years after exposure showed a reasonable correlation with the estimated dose of
radiation that the individuals had received. Dose estimations in the
A-Bomb survivors were complicated by many factors including establishing the exact location of specific survivors in relation to distance from the hypocenter, and elucidating complex shielding situations for each person. Because of the nature of the accident at Oak
Ridge, and the immediate availability of expertise in dosimetry, accurate estimates of doses were made for the Y-12 victims within a few
weeks after exposure. Since these men received a wide range of doses
(from 22.8 - 365 rads) we had an excellent opportunity to evaluate
the dependence of persistent radiation-induced lesions on dose in
these six men. In the present analyses, the highest frequencies of
both symmetric and asymmetric exchanges were noted in the three men
with the highest exposures, although absolute correlations with dose
were not observed in individual cultures from the six men (see Tables
II and III). As in the reported data from the A-Bomb survivors [5],
the frequencies of symmetric exchanges showed better correlations with
dose than the frequencies of asymmetric lesions. To derive points for
dose-response curves for the Hiroshima and Nagasaki survivors, Awa
[5] computed mean doses and the corresponding mean lesion frequencies
for groups of persons having exposure ranges of 100-199, 200-299,
300-399, 400-499, 500-599 and 600+ rads. When data from the Y-12
victims were processed in like manner, a linear dose response was obtained (Figure 1). These data are in good agreement with Awa's findings of the Hiroshima survivors who had radiations of similar quality
to that received by the Y-12 victims (the ratio of neutron to gamma
was estimated to be between 1:3 to 1:5 in Hiroshima [5], while the
ratio in the Y-12 accident was estimated to be 1:3 [10]). Our data
on the Y-12 patients show that the average frequencies of lesions in
PHA-stimulated lymphocytes of exposed persons can be correlated with
dose many years after exposure. However, because of variability in
the frequency of lesions observed in persons having similar doses, our
findings also suggest that data from specific cultures cannot be used
to obtain precise dose estimates for individuals.

In all of the previous studies of persistent chromosome lesions
in irradiated persons, phytohemagglutinin has been used to stimulate
lymphocytes to divide in in vitro culture systems. In animals and
man this mitogen has been shown to stimulate predominately T (thymus-
derived/dependent) lymphocytes [12, 13] which are involved in cellular
immunity. In contrast to PHA, pokeweed mitogen stimulates both human
T and B (bursa equivalent) lymphocytes with maximum mitogenic response
occurring at 5-7 days culture time [14, 15]. B lymphocytes are believed to be progenitors of the antibody-producing plasma cells. In

the present study cultures from four of the Y-12 patients were treated with PWM and harvested after 7 days to determine whether populations of lymphocytes responsive to mitogenic stimulation by PWM also bore residual radiation-induced lesions many years after exposure.

The types and frequencies of lesions in the PWM cultures were similar to those observed in replicate cultures stimulated with PHA, with the exception that no dicentric chromosomes were observed in the 7-day cultures. Because of the complexities of lymphocyte response to stimulation by PWM, and the necessity of using long culture periods with this mitogen to obtain sufficient numbers of mitoses for cytogenetic evaluations, definitive statements regarding the actual percentage of B cells bearing lesions in vivo cannot be made. However, that B cells constituted a significant fraction of the lymphocytes in division at 7 days in the PWM cultures is supported by several earlier observations. In studies in our laboratory [16] in which purified lymphocytes from control persons were stimulated with either PHA or PWM, and harvested after 2, 3, 5 or 7 days, maximum numbers of B cells were observed in 7-day PWM cultures (approximately 56% of the cells bound the B cell specific dye fluorescein labelled goat-antihuman Ig). In contrast to the PHA cultures in which active mitotic proliferation occurred at 2 and 3 days culture time, a major mitotic wave was not observed in the PWM cultures until 5 and 7 days after culture initiation. These data suggest that a subpopulation of lymphocytes different from that responding to PHA enter division after 5-7 days culture time in PWM cultures, and that the cells entering division at the later culture times are primarily B cells. The observation of a significant number of cells with lesions in 7-day PWM-stimulated lymphocyte cultures strongly suggests that human B cells bearing residual radiation-induced abnormalities are also capable of surviving for many years after exposure.

In summary, our 16- and 17-year cytogenetic follow-up studies in the Y-12 patients show: 1) T lymphocytes bearing radiation-induced chromosome lesions are capable of surviving many years after radiation exposure, and the frequency of persistent lesions in previously exposed persons can be roughly correlated with dose; 2) use of chromosome banding techniques does not improve the rate of detection of symmetrical lesions in cultured lymphocytes compared to detailed microscopic and karyotypic analyses of conventionally stained slides; and 3) subpopulations of lymphocytes stimulated to divide with pokeweed mitogen also bear chromosome lesions many years after radiation exposure.

REFERENCES

[1] BUCKTON, K.E., JACOBS, P.A., COURT BROWN, W.M., DOLL, R., A study of chromosome damage persisting after X-ray therapy for ankylosing spondylitis, Lancet ii 7258 (1962) 676.
[2] ISHIHARA, T., KUMATORI, T., "Chromosome studies on Japanese exposed to radiation resulting from nuclear bomb explosions", Human Radiation Cytogenetics (EVANS, H.J., COURT BROWN, W.M., McLEAN, A.S., Eds), North Holland Publishing Company, Amsterdam (1967) 144.

[3] BLOOM, A.D., NERIISHI, S., KAMADA, N., ISEKI, T., KEEHN, R., Cytogenetic
    investigation of survivors of the atomic bombings of Hiroshima and Nagasaki, Lancet ii
    7465 (1966) 672.

[4] SASAKI, M.S., MIYATA, H., Biological dosimetry in atomic bomb survivors, Nature 220
    5173 (1968) 1189.

[5] AWA, A.A., Chromosome aberrations in somatic cells, J. Radiat. Res. 16 Suppl.
    (1975) 122.

[6] BENDER, M.A., GOOCH, P.C., Persistent chromosome aberrations in irradiated human
    subjects, Radiat. Res. 16 1 (1962) 44.

[7] BENDER, M.A., GOOCH, P.C., Persistent chromosome aberrations in irradiated human
    subjects: II. Three and one-half year investigation, Radiat. Res. 18 3 (1963) 389.

[8] GOH, K.O., Total-body irradiation and human chromosomes: cytogenetic studies of
    the peripheral blood and bone marrow leukocytes seven years after total-body irradiation,
    Radiat. Res. 35 1 (1968) 155.

[9] GOH, K.O., Total-body irradiation and human chromosomes: IV. Cytogenetic follow-up
    studies 8 and 10 1/2 years after total-body irradiation, Radiat. Res. 62 2 (1975) 364.

[10] U.S. ATOMIC ENERGY COMMISSION, Accidental Radiation Excursion at the Y-12
    Plant, June 16, 1958, Final Report, U.S. Atomic Energy Commission Report Y-1234,
    Union Carbide Nuclear Company, Y-12 Plant, Oak Ridge, Tennessee (1958).

[11] CHU, E.H.Y., Personal communication.

[12] JANOSSY, G., GREAVES, M.F., Lymphocyte activation. I: Response of T and B
    lymphocytes to phytomitogens, Clin. Exp. Immunol. 9 4 (1971) 483.

[13] HEDFORS, E., Activation of peripheral T cells of sarcoidosis patients and healthy
    controls, Clin. Exp. Immunol. 18 3 (1974) 379.

[14] DOUGLAS, S.D., KAMIN, R.M., FUDENBERG, H.H., Human lymphocyte response to
    phytomitogens in vitro: Normal, agammaglobulinemic and paraproteinemic individuals,
    J. Immunol. 103 6 (1969) 1185.

[15] DOUGLAS, S.D., Electron microscopic and functional aspects of human lymphocyte
    response to mitogens, Transplant. Rev. 11 (1972) 39.

[16] LITTLEFIELD, L.G., JOINER, E.E., Unpublished data.

DISCUSSION

K.E. BUCKTON: I was interested in your finding of clones in these men,
although I am a little concerned at your definition of a clone as two cells alike,
in view of the fact that recent experiments have shown that a number of cells can
be in their second division in culture by 48 hours. Are these men who have the
clones clinically well?

L.G. LITTLEFIELD: I am aware that there is some discussion as to whether
two cells having apparently identical lesions should be considered a clone, and
your objections may have merit. In three of our patients at least three cells had
identical lesions, and these men are clinically well.

CATARACT OF LENS AS LATE EFFECT OF IONIZING RADIATION IN OCCUPATIONALLY EXPOSED PERSONS

I. BENDEL, W. SCHÜTTMANN, D. ARNDT
Staatliches Amt für Atomsicherheit
    und Strahlenschutz der DDR,
Berlin,
German Democratic Republic

Presented by P. Nack

Abstract

CATARACT OF LENS AS LATE EFFECT OF IONIZING RADIATION IN OCCUPATIONALLY EXPOSED PERSONS.

A report is given of ophthalmological observations in occupationally radiation-exposed persons in the German Democratic Republic with cataract of lens at the present time. In the first part a survey is made of casuistic observations in the years 1966 to 1977 which have shown a total of 10 cataracts, exclusively in X-ray-exposed medical personnel. Parallel to this analysis of these cases acknowledged as occupational diseases, in the second part a survey is made on systematic examinations of radiologically working physicians of more than 10 years service. In the Berlin district and surroundings, 53 persons have so far been subjected to a thorough medical examination in the National Board of Nuclear Safety and Radiation Protection. In six persons intensive ophthalmological examination showed suspicious lens opacities which, according to their clinical picture, may have been induced by radiation. As a result of our observations the question arises whether the present proposal by the ICRP (Publication No. 26) can be accepted without reservations.

1. INTRODUCTION

Already only a few years after the discovery of X-rays, observations were reported that the exposure of the human eye to these rays induces a cataract [1–4]. Since that time the cataract has been one of the typical somatic late effects induced by radiation, and has been studied both by ophthalmologists and radio-biologists.

The importance of the cataract as a radiogenic effect has recently been emphasized once more by comments in the ICRP Publication 26 [5]. There, in connection with the 'non-stochastic effects which are specific to particular tissues', the 'cataract of the lens' take first place among the examples.

There is an extensive literature on the subject of radiocataract. It covers mainly studies of animal tests that have been carried out repeatedly from various points of view over the last 50 years [6–13]. The literature is also concerned with experiences in patients undergoing therapy [14–17] after irradiation of tumours near the eye. Further, the experiences in the survivors of Hiroshima and Nagasaki have contributed to the extension of knowledge [18–20]. Finally, publications should be mentioned that are concerned with occupational cataracts after exposure to ionizing radiation [21–25].

The understanding of the importance of radiation protection in the last decades has created the impression, however, that, in view of the protective measures taken, an occupational induction of radiocataract, at least in X-ray application, is excluded. A number of authors have taken this view. Heydenreich [26] formulated that 'since the introduction of various protective measures, cataracts can no longer be observed in employees of X-ray institutes'. This statement can be agreed to in so far as, in the case of occupational handling of ionizing radiation according to instructions, no radiation-induced damage to the eye is to be expected. This does not mean, however, that, in practical work, occupational radiocataracts can still be found today, so that this type of radiation effect is of unchanged relevance for practical radiation protection. In this connection it should be taken into account that, in view of the long latency of fractionated exposure, the causal radiation exposure frequently occurred far back in the past, under conditions that are no longer controllable.

Observations of occupational radiocataract made in the field of practical radiation protection in the last few years are reported below, underlining the importance of this radiogenic late effect. Apart from this importance, the subject of radiocataract has further special aspects:

(1) Without any doubt the lens of the eye is one of the most radiosensitive tissues, and therefore can be damaged by relatively low doses of conventional radiation.

(2) The lens lies on the surface, and thus can be reached by every local penetrating radiation.

(3) The eye lens and its radiogenic changes are a suitable test system for experimental investigations of certain aspects of the effect of ionizing radiation (dose, dose rate, fractionation, radiation quality).

(4) The radiocataract is a radiation effect that can be easily and therefore diagnosed early and also effectively treated, and so does not represent a severe damage.

(5) The main importance of the radiocataract today lies in the field of therapeutic application of ionizing radiation, particularly high LET, in the treatment of tumours in the region of the head.

The development of radiogenic cataract is divided into several stages by various authors. The development of the clinical picture of the radiocataract is described by Wischnewski [27] as follows:

1st stage: Pointlike opacities in the axial range between the posterior capsule and the cortex.

2nd stage: The opacities increase in number and density, are partly interconnected netwise. Individual vacuoles occur. There may be subjective impairments of vision but they are rare in these discrete changes.

3rd stage: The opacities become denser and form an axial thickening in the region of the posterior pole. Vacuoles increase in number and in some cases occur in the subcapsular region of the anterior pole. Impairment of vision increases.

4th stage: The opacities densify to form a circular disc with the axial thickening described above, the paracentral zone being often more transparent than the centre and periphery, so that there may be a ring-like impression. At this stage also the anterior and posterior cortical regions are gradually covered by a diffuse capacity. Because of these changes, vision is considerably reduced.

5th stage: The opacity has spread to all parts of the lens so that there is no longer any difference from the mature cataract of different origin.

Other authors [7, 28, 29] distinguish 3, 4 or 6 stages.

In literature various values are given for the threshold dose. They are listed in Table I. Data on latency contained in Table II vary still more than the values for the threshold dose. After a control covering many years of the history of radiocataracts in 13 radiophysicists, Woods [30] pointed out the reciprocal connection between dose and latency, and the direct connection between dose, extent of lens damage and state of opacity progression. Other authors confirm this connection [14].

In view of the development of the clinical picture described, with special allowance for the first two stages, in which there are usually no disturbances of vision, objections have to be raised against the definition proposed in ICRP Publication No. 14 [31], 'Cataract = Changes in the lens of a degree to impair vision'. 'The phrase "opacity of the lens" will be used to describe changes in the lens detectable by skilled examination but not of a degree sufficient to impair vision' could lead to misunderstandings. From the ophthalmological point of view, a cataract is defined as '*every* inhomogeneity of the lens, whether true opacity or, for example, vacuole formation' [28]. Incidentally, in the summary of this ICRP Publication the definition usual in ophthalmology is also used.

2. PRESENT RESULTS

Our observations are presented below in occupationally radiation-exposed persons on the occurrence of radiocataract at present. The first section presents a

TABLE I. CATARACTOGENIC THRESHOLD DOSES DESCRIBED IN
LITERATURE AT SINGLE TIME AND FRACTIONATED PROTRACTED
IRRADIATION

Ref. Author	Single time radiation exposure (rad)	Fractionated protracted radiation exposure (rad)
[6] ROHRSCHNEIDER	800	
[15] COGAN, DREISLER	100 – 600	600 – 800
[21] HAM	500	
[49] MALBRAN, ALVA		1000
[9] POLITZER	400	
[7] KANDORI	400	1500
[14] MERRIAM, FOCHT	200	1100
[44] KROKOWSKI	200	800 – 1000
[45] HAY, JAMMET, DOLLFUSS	200	
[17] BRITTEN	950	
[38] UPTON	200 – 600	1100 – 1400
[25] PARISOT	300 – 400	
[48] GEERATS	250 – 500	
[47] HANNA	200 – 300	
[39] DONALDSON	600 – 800	
[46] HAGER, LOMMATZSCH	400 – 900	
[51] COGAN	500 – 800	

description of casuistic observations of cataracts of disease rank, and the second
results of systematic examination of exposed persons.

2.1. Casuistic observations of cataracts

Casuistic observations were made in the years 1966 to 1977. The material
was obtained as follows: In the German Democratic Republic all cases in which
a cataract is caused by occupational radiation exposure as well as all other cases of
radiation damage are reported to the National Board of Nuclear Safety and
Radiation Protection. Physicians diagnosing such cataract are bound to report

TABLE II.　LATENCIES DESCRIBED IN LITERATURE UP TO THE MANIFESTATION OF RADIOCATARACT

Ref. Author	Time
[40] JESS	1 — 3 years
[41] KLAUBER	5 — 10 years
[42] SAUTTER	1 — 8 years
[15] COGAN, DREISLER	2 — 3 years
[37] DUKE-ELDER	2 — 12 years
[14] MERRIAM, FOCHT	1 — 20 years
[43] JAENSCH	1 — 2 years
[22] DOLLFUSS	3 years
[38] UPTON	1 — 10 years
[26] HEYDENREICH	2 — 3 years
[39] DONALDSON	6 months — 4 years
[50] WISCHNEWSKI	2 — 7 years
[51] COGAN	6 months — 2 years - - - - - - 8 — 12 years

these cases as occupational disease to certain authorities through prescribed channels. The registration offices have to submit these cases to the Board, where another expert opinion is delivered by an ophthalmologist. In this way all cataracts reported are centrally registered, assessed and analysed. The percentage of undetected occupational radiogenic cataracts that are not registered in this way may be neglected, since both the exposed persons suffering from the disease and the ophthalmologists treating them pay careful attention to observing the prescribed method of registration.

Through this means a total of 10 cataracts have come to our knowledge in the years 1966 to 1977.

The examinations made in the Board for delivering an expert opinion comprise test of vision, visual field control, test of light and colour sense, eye pressure measurement, slit-lamp examination of medicamentally expanded pupil and examination of the posterior of the eye.

At the same time an intensive thorough clinical examination is carried out to exclude other cataractogenic causes and further medical examinations in the field of radiation protection. By means of the patients' data on exposure frequency and time, and on special features of the place of work, the radiation exposure of the eyes is assessed in retrospect.

TABLE III. DATA ON PATIENTS

No.	Year of birth and occupation	Period of occupational radiation exposure	Dose assessment	Period and dose of main radiation exposure	First disturbance of vision	First lens opacity detected	Time of first expert opinion	Cause of increased radiation exposure
1	1913 Surgeon working in X-ray diagnostics	1942–49	40 Gy	1945–49 40 Gy	1959	1965	1970	Cryptoscope
2	1920 X-ray assistant	1936–70			1967	1970	1971	Scattered X-ray radiation, no lateral shielding
3	1920 Male nurse, X-ray assistant	1940–49	(1.2 Gy)	1940–69	1966	1969	1970	Army X-ray device, insufficient supervision and instruction
4	1915 Internist working in X-ray diagnostics	1948–69	70 Gy	1948–50 65 Gy	1960	1962	1971	X-ray screen with lead glass pane
5	1909 Radiologist	1940–42 1946–68	(0.33 Gy)	1950–56	1961	1971	1972	Defective X-ray devices
6	1933 Anaesthetist	1957–70	26 Gy	1957–61 15 Gy	1972	1972	1973	Cryptoscope
7	1920 Radiologist	1946–75	(0.7 Gy)	1946–50 (0.25 Gy)	1970	1970	1972	X-ray screen without lead glass pane?
8	1910 Radiologist	1936–61	(2 Gy)	1946–61	1967	1968	1974	X-ray screen without lead glass pane?
9	1928 X-ray assistant	1951–76	10 Gy	1961–62	1970	1974	1976	Viewing through radiation exit window
10	1925 Surgeon	1950–64	8–10 Gy	1952–57	1973	1974	1977	Cryptoscope

Notes:

1. The dose was retrospectively assessed from data of the insured persons on exposure frequency and time and on special features of the working place.

The 10 cases mentioned are exclusively X-ray radiological medical personnel (3 radiologists, 2 surgeons, 1 internist, 1 anaesthetist, 3 X-ray assistants). The patients' age lies between 44 and 68 years. The duration of occupational radiation exposure lies between 7 and 34 years (see Table III).

The retrospective dose assessment made in 9 cases yielded values in 5 cases that support the diagnosis of radiogenic lens opacity (70 Gy, 40 Gy, 26 Gy, 10 Gy, 10 Gy). In 4 cases values between 0.33 Gy and 2 Gy were assessed. In these 4 cases, however, dose assessment was based on correct protective technique and adequate working behaviour, which, of course, could not be properly checked.

Expert opinions in such cases become difficult because no values of radiation exposure of the eyes of the people concerned are available. The personal dose meter worn under protective clothing obviously gives a measuring value suitable for determining whole-body exposure but does not give any clues for the radiation exposure of the eyes. Therefore the assessment of radiation exposure of eyes, which is important for expert opinions, has in all cases been made on the basis of subjective data of patients.

The period between the main radiation exposure and the first disturbances of vision was between 8 and 20 years in the cases considered. In 7 out of 10 cases, unsatisfactory conditions of radioprotective technique during World War II and in the first postwar years are claimed to be causes of increased radiation exposure. In 4 cases, for example, the lead glass pane of the X-ray screen in the devices used had probably been replaced by a pane of window glass for several years. In 3 cases cryptoscopes were used, the use of which has been prohibited in the German Democratic Republic since 1971 because of well-known deficiencies in the radioprotective technique. In several cases, because of lack of radioprotective measuring devices, the deficiencies mentioned or the results of such deficiencies were often detected only after many years' work. In 1 case it was reported that the radiation exit window was usually looked into to check the working condition of the X-ray tube.

For illustration, extracts from reports on 2 patients of this group of persons are quoted below:

(1)   E.H., born 25 May 1925, surgeon

The patient handled ionizing radiation from 1950 to 1964. He was mainly employed in general and accident surgery. Radiation exposure was particularly from X-ray check-ups using a mobile X-ray device and a cryptoscope for fracture resettings. The radiation exposure of the hands in the same work is assessed to be 45 Gy. Because of radiation damage to the skin of both hands diagnosed in 1963, an occupational disease was officially acknowledged. The eyes were repeatedly examined in 1974, after the patient had noticed subjective disturbances of vision in the right eye since 1973, and 'opacities of cortexes and subcapsular regions of both eye lenses' had been found and reported as suspected occupational diseases. The ophthalmological finding of 1977 runs as follows: Visual faculty to the right 0.1 without correction, to the left 0.8 with correction. Right lens: Numerous pointlike opacities, partly confluent and interspersed with individual vacuoles with axial thickening in the subcapsular region of the posterior pole; paracentral zone with fewer opacities than centre and periphery, ringlike impression. Anterior cortex with individual subcapsular vacuoles in the polar region. Left lens: Few vacuoles and pointlike densities in the subcapsular region of the posterior pole. Anterior polar region free. Cortex and centre free of opacities on both sides. Type of cataract, bilateral nature of lens disease, the case history, patient's age and assessed dose indicate a radiocataract. Other cataractogenic causes could be excluded.

(2)   M.E., born 12 August 1933, anaesthetist

From 1957 to 1961 the patient used X-rays diagnostically in accident surgery with a cryptoscope. The radiation exposure of eyes within this period was retrospectively assessed to be about 15 Gy. From 1961 to 1970 the patient worked in the anaesthetiological department of a surgical institution (bronchographies, cerebral angiographies, serial angiographies according to Seldinger, fracture surgery). This work led to further radiation exposure of the eyes of about 10 Gy. From 1971 to 1974 he worked as an anaesthetist. Radiation exposure within this period is assessed to be around 1.2 Gy. Thus total radiation exposure of the eyes is about 26 Gy. Since 1972 the patient has noticed gradual disturbances of vision. Finding of 1973: Right lens with slight opacities of the posterior cortex in the subcapsular region of the pole. Vision right 6/5, left 6/8. Extraction of left lens in 1975. Finding of 1977: Right lens: Anterior subcapsular region shows individual vacuoles and slight floccular opacities. Disclike subcapsular opacities and opacities of posterior cortex with axial thickening of polar region, individual vacuoles. Vision 0.15. Extraction of lens in 1977. Because of dose assessment, typical clinical picture, latency, bilateral nature, patient's age and exclusion of other cataractogenic causes, an occupational disease was acknowledged according to No. 17 of the list of occupational diseases.

2.2. Systematic observations of physicians working in radiology

Parallel with this analysis of cases acknowledged as occupational diseases [32], systematic examinations of physicians more than 10 years working radiologically were started. In the Berlin district and surroundings, 53 persons have so far been subjected to a thorough medical examination in the field of radiation protection (ophthalmological, dermatological, haematological-cytological). In 6 persons the intensive ophthalmological examination showed suspicious lens opacities (stage 1 and 2) which, according to their clinical picture, may be induced by radiation.

Although, in this group of persons, the retrospective dose assessment did not indicate any excess of the maximum permissible dose equivalent for the eye lens, an intensive check-up was begun, slit-lamp photography and lens photographs in transmittent light (retinal photography) being considered for documentation of lens findings.

Another group of these persons has also had further checkups. They did not exhibit any suspicious changes in terms of a radiogenic cataract but dose assessment has suggested an increased radiation exposure. In addition, the examination showed age-dependent lens changes in 24 persons and hereditary ones in 6 persons which, because of their clinical picture, cannot be classified as radiocataract.

This epidemiological study is to be extended to the entire territory of the German Democratic Republic. At the same time an ophthalmological mass examination of middle-rank medical personnel working in the field of roentgenology is being prepared.

3.   DISCUSSION

Our own experiences and those reported in literature testify that, when ionizing radiation is handled contrary to instructions, cataracts can develop. To avoid such a development, the definition of dose limits for radiation exposure of the eyes is of decisive importance.

Comparative dosimetric studies of the radiation exposure of individual body sections and organs have shown that, at certain radiation-exposed working places, the eye lens is the most exposed tissue apart from the hands. For example Rothe [33] showed that, at angiographic working places, the radiation exposure of the eye is the exposure-limiting factor.

In deriving dose limits we should proceed from the threshold dose from which the occurrence of cataract has to be expected. There is an extensive literature on this problem, especially on the rather contradictory results of animal-test studies (see Table I).

The uncertainty due to these contradictory results also with respect to the definition of dose limits can be clearly seen from their history [34]. In 1954 the ICRP was still recommending for the eye the same dose as for the whole body, gonads and blood-forming organs, namely 0.3 rem weekly. In the reduction of this dose limit in ICRP Publication 1 of 1959 [35] to 5 rem annually, the new value was also recommended for the whole body, gonads, blood-forming organs and eyes. It was only in Publication 6 of 1964 [36] that the ICRP gave up classing the eye and blood-forming organs and gonads on the same level, and recommended a new limit of 15 rem annually for the eye as for other interior organs, although adding a quality factor for particulate radiation with high LET.

Recently the ICRP has recommended another change of the dose limit for the eye in its Publication 26 [5]. There it is stated that, at protracted occupational exposure of the lenses to radiation of high or low LET during the entire working life, an integrated dose equivalent of 15 Sv (1500 rem) would still be below the threshold for causing any lens opacity affecting the vision. The ICRP makes a recommendation that the annual dose-equivalent limit for the lens should be derived from this dose equivalent delivered over the working lifetime. Accordingly the commission proposes to define the limit for the lens with 0.3 Sv (30 rem) yearly, whereas 50 rem yearly are recommended for all other tissues to prevent 'non-stochastic effects'. With this proposal the ICRP corrects its earlier recommendations. In Publication 14 of 1969 [31] it was still stated that 'human evidence suggests that a dose limit of 15 rems per year for both high and low LET radiation would be acceptable without the use of an additional modifying factor of high LET radiation'.

The question arises whether the present proposal by the ICRP can be accepted without any reservations. Further careful clinical checkups are necessary to answer this question after the new dose limits are introduced.

REFERENCES

[1] CHALUPECKY, H., Zentralbl. Prakt. Augenheilkd. 21 (1897) 234.

[2] GUTTMANN, G., Ber. Dtsch. Ophthalm. Gesellsch., Heidelberg (1905) 338.

[3] TREUTLER, B., Ber. Dtsch. Ophthalm. Gesellsch., Heidelberg (1905) 338.

[4] BIRCH-HIRSCHFELD, A., Klin. Monatsbl. Augenheilkd. 46 II (1908) 129.

[5] INTERNATIONAL COMMISSION ON RADIOLOGICAL PROTECTION, ICRP Publication No. 26, Pergamon Press, Oxford, New York, Frankfurt (1977).

[6] ROHRSCHNEIDER, W., Albrecht v. Graefes Arch. Ophthalmol. 122 (1929) 281.

[7] KANDORI, F., Am. J. Ophthalmol. 41 Ser. 3 (1956) 627; 1006.

[8] SALLMANN, L. von, Am. J. Ophthalmol. 44 (1957) 159.

[9] POLITZER, S., Albrecht v. Graefes Arch. Ophthalmol. 157 (1956) 459.

[10] SCHENKEN, L.L., HAGEMANN, R.F., Radiology 117 (1975) 193.

[11] ALTER, A.J., LEINFELDER, P.J., Arch. Ophthalmol. (Chicago) 49 (1953) 257.

[12] LEINFELDER, P.J., RILEY, E.F., Arch. Ophthalmol. (Chicago) 55 (1955) 84.

[13] RICHARDS, R.D., RILEY, E.F., LEINFELDER, P.J., Am. J. Ophthalmol. 42 (1956) 44.

[14] MERRIAM, G.B., Jr., FOCHT, E.F., Am. J. Roentgenol., Radium Ther. Nucl. Med. 77 (1957) 759.

[15] COGAN, D., DREISLER, K., Arch. Ophthalmol. (Chicago) 50 (1953) 30.

[16] PARKER, R.G., et al., Radiology 82 (1964) 794.

[17] BRITTEN, M.J.A., et al., Br. Radiology 39 (1966) 612.

[18] NEFZGER, M.D., MILLER, R.J., et al., Am. J. Epidemiol. 89 (1969) 129.

[19] COGAN, D.G., MARTIN, S.F., KIMARA, I.J., IKUI, H., Trans. Am. Ophthalmol. Soc. 48 (1950) 62.

[20] DODO, T., J. Radiat. Res. 16 Suppl. (1975) 132.

[21] HAM, W.T., Jr., Arch. Ophthalmol. (Chicago) 50 (1953) 618.

[22] DOLLFUSS, M.A., Ophthalmologie 1, 1st Symp. Munich 1966, Karger, Basle, New York (1969) 155.

[23] DOLLFUSS, M.A., Bull. Soc. Ophthalmol. France 5 (1950) 459.

[24] GRÜTZNER, P., Klin. Monatsbl. Augenheilkd. 149 (1966).

[25] PARISOT, H., in Physikalische Strahlenschutzkontrolle nach dem oesterreichischen Strahlenschutzgesetz und der dazugehörigen Strahlenschutzverordnung, Tagungsbericht (1972) 5.

[26] HEYDENREICH, Arbeitsmed. — Sozialmed. — Arbeitshyg. 11 (1969) 280.

[27] WISCHNEWSKI, N.A., Vestn. Oftal'mol. 75 3 (1962) 26.

[28] SAUTTER, H., in Der Augenarzt III (VEHLHAGEN, K., Ed.), Thieme, Leipzig (1975).

[29] KOWALEW, I.F., Vestn. Oftal'mol. 72 6 (1959) 353.

[30] WOODS, A.C., Am. J. Ophthalmol. 47 (1959) 20.

[31] INTERNATIONAL COMMISSION ON RADIOLOGICAL PROTECTION, ICRP Publication No. 14, Pergamon Press, Oxford, New York, Frankfurt (1969).

[32] BENDEL, I., Dipl.-Arbeit, Med. Fak., Humboldt-Univ., Berlin 1977.

[33] ROTHE, W., Radiologia diagnostika 18 1 (1977) 133.

[34] SCHÜTTMANN, W., Report SAAS-201, 3.

[35] INTERNATIONAL COMMISSION ON RADIOLOGICAL PROTECTION, ICRP Publication No. 1, Pergamon Press, London, New York, Paris, Los Angeles (1959).

[36] INTERNATIONAL COMMISSION ON RADIOLOGICAL PROTECTION, ICRP Publication No. 6, Pergamon Press, Oxford, London, Edinburgh, New York, Paris, Frankfurt (1964).

[37] DUKE-ELDER, S., Textbook of Ophthalmology VI, H. Kimpton, London (1954) 6443.

[38] UPTON, A.C., Am. Rev. Nucl. Science 18 (1968) 495.

[39] DONALDSON, D.D., Atlas of Diseases of the Anterior Segment of the Eye V, The Crystalline Lens, Mosby, St. Louis (1976).

[40] JESS, A., Einwirkung der Röntgenstrahlung auf das Auge, Vers. O.G., Heidelberg (1928) 352.

[41] KLAUBER, E., Klin. Monatsbl. Augenheilkd. 97 (1936).

[42] SAUTTER, H., Die Trübungsformen der menschlichen Linse, Thieme, Stuttgart (1951).

[43] JAENSCH, P.A., Augenschädigungen in Industrie und Gewerbe, Wissenschaftl. Verlagsgesellschaft, Stuttgart (1958) 43.

[44] KROKOWSKI, E., Arbeitsmed. Fragen in der Ophthalmologie 1, 1st Symp. Munich 1966, Karger, Basle, New York (1969) 139.

[45] HAY, C., JAMMET, H., DOLLFUSS, M.A., Auge und ionisierende Strahlung, Paris (1965).

[46] HAGER, G., LOMMATZSCH, P., Aktuelle Ophthalmologie (KÜCHLER, H.J., Ed.), Fachalmanach für Augenheilkunde, Lehmann, Munich (1976) 243.

[47] HANNA, C., in "Cataract and Abnormalities of the Lens (BELLOWS, J.G., Ed.), Grune & Stratton, New York, San Francisco, London (1975).

[48] GEERATS, W.J., in Textbook of Ophthalmology VI, H. Kimpton, London (1954).

[49] MALBRAN, J.L., ALVA, O., Prensa med. orgent. (1955) 3224, cited in SCHUMANN, E., "Die Strahlenbehandlung des Auges und seiner Umgebung", in Der Augenarzt 7 (VEHLHAGEN, K., Ed.), Thieme, Leipzig (1967).

[50] WISCHNEWSKI, et al., Vestn. Oftal'mol. (1961) 74 5, 65.

[51] COGAN, D.G., J. Amer. Med. Assoc. 142 3 (1950) 145.

LATE EFFECTS OF IONIZING RADIATION ON THE HUMAN SKIN AFTER OCCUPATIONAL EXPOSURE

U. LENZ, W. SCHÜTTMANN, D. ARNDT
Staatliches Amt für Atomsicherheit
        und Strahlenschutz der DDR,
Berlin

Th. THORMANN
Dermatological Clinic of the
        Medical Faculty (Charité),
Humboldt University,
Berlin,
German Democratic Republic

Presented by P. Nack

Abstract

LATE EFFECTS OF IONIZING RADIATION ON THE HUMAN SKIN AFTER
OCCUPATIONAL EXPOSURE.
    The skin is the organ of the human body that receives the highest dose equivalent at
many work places. Furthermore, the hands are those parts of the body in which the due
limits are very often utilized to the full. At some special places of work they can be even
over-exposed. Therefore, in practice, the most frequently accepted cases of radiation damage
caused by working conditions, and recorded for compensation, refer to skin diseases. A
study of the late effects of low-level irradiation to the skin under working conditions was
therefore performed. A group of occupationally exposed persons were selected who had had
a specially high exposure of the hands (radiochemists, reactor physicists, radiographers, X-ray
technicians). From among these persons 70 who did not show any macroscopically detectable
deviations in the sense of radiation effects were examined by means of the following methods:
Macroscopic evaluation, dactyloscopy, capillary microscopy, thermography, exploratory
excision and histologic investigation. Twenty persons from the study group showed aberrations in capillary microscopy. The histologic investigation of the tissue samples of these
cases disclosed more or less typical findings classifiable in three categories. The earliest
changes occur in the vessels of the corium, aberrations in the epidermis occurring only at a
later stage. The results of the study reveal that a long-term irradiation of the skin in the low-
level region, even below the hitherto valid dose limits, may already cause an effect in the
vessels and the connective tissue of the corium without any macroscopically detectable
deviation of the epidermis. The consequences of this finding are discussed, especially
regarding the equivalent dose limit for the skin.

1.   INTRODUCTION

According to the classification of the detrimental somatic effects of
ionizing radiation in ICRP Publication 26 [1] as stochastic and non-stochastic
effects, the radiation-induced damage to the skin can be both stochastic and
non-stochastic. The stochastic effect to the skin is radiation-induced carcinoma,
the non-stochastic effect is non-malignant damage to the skin.

These two types of radiation effects to the skin are well known. They were
the effects first observed only a short time after the discovery of X-rays in 1895.
Already in 1902, Frieben [2] described the first radiation-induced neoplasm of
the skin which had developed from a radiation dermatitis.

In the most recent comment on the detrimental effects of ionizing radiation, the ICRP [1] states in the section dealing with tissues at risk that the skin
is thought to be much less liable to develop fatal cancer after irradiation than
other tissues and organs such as red bone marrow, bone, lung, thyroid and
breast. On the other hand, the ICRP [1] mentions that cosmetically unacceptable
changes in the skin may occur after irradiation with absorbed doses of 20 Gy
or more.

Other publications listing radiation-induced somatic changes do not at all
mention skin damage, e.g. the Beir Report [3] quotes as possible somatic effects
of low-level irradiation neoplasms, opacities of the lens, impairment of fertility
and shortening of life. Effects to the skin are not specified. Such an estimation might give rise to the opinion that low-level irradiation may be without
importance to the skin.

This idea must be rejected for several reasons. One of the most important
is the circumstance that the hitherto valid maximum permissible dose for hands,
fore-arms, feet and ankles and also for the skin of these parts according to the
earlier recommendations of the ICRP [4] was 75 rem in a year, an even somewhat
higher value in comparison with the then tolerance dose recommended for the first
time in the 1920s [5]. In practice, the hands are those parts of the body in
which the due limits are frequently utilized to the full. Frequently they are over-
exposed at some work places. In these conditions the accumulated working
lifetime dose at the hands may easily reach the value of 2000–3000 rem.

This dose is already within the range of the carcinogenic effects of ionizing
radiation with regard to the human skin [6–10]. In agreement with several
authors we have also observed skin cancers in persons occupationally exposed
to X-rays in the range mentioned [11]. In some cases, the carcinomas were
situated in areas of skin without signs of typical radio-dermatitis, in agreement
with similar observations published by other authors [3, 7].

On the basis of the statement that the skin belongs to the organs most
exposed to ionizing radiation we have directed our attention again to the late
effects of low-level irradiation to the skin under working conditions. We studied

that problem by means of clinical methods in contrast to those authors who tried to answer this question by way of questionnaires [12].

2.   MATERIALS

Among some 40 000 occupationally exposed and medically supervised persons in the German Democratic Republic, a group of persons has been selected which has had a specially high exposure of the hands. These persons have been working as radiochemists, reactor physicists, radiographers and X-ray technicians. From among these selected persons, 70 who did not show any macro-scopically detectable deviations in the sense of radiation effects to the skin have been examined by the same examiners at the Dermatological Unit in the Medical Department of the National Board of Nuclear Safety and Radiation Protection by means of the methods described below.

3.   METHODS

3.1. Macroscopic-dermatological diagnostics

The dermatological findings were obtained by macrovisual and diascopic examination including documentary photomacrography. Special attention was paid to rarefaction of the epidermis, to deviations of pigmentation and hairi-ness, to teleangiectasis and to anomalies of the finger-nails. By definition, only persons without any of these findings were included in the study, so that only early changes in the irradiated skin would be detected.

3.2. Dactyloscopy

To disclose radiation-induced rarefaction of the papillary pattern of the finger-tips, two methods were used: (1) a printing method as a special modi-fication of one's own and (2) a special macrophotography of the finger-tips. Persons with findings by dactyloscopy were also excluded from the study.

3.3. Capillary microscopy

The microscopic examination of capillaries is particularly successful in the region of the perionychium for their suitable, palisade-like arrangement of the vessels with a well-distinguishable arterial and venous branch. The examination was carried out by a stereo-microscopic technique including documentary photomicrography. The evaluation of the changes of the capillaries in their distal row or in the proximal region of the perionychium took place according to the qualitative deviations and the quantitative findings (number of capillaries per millimetre and length of the arterial and venous branches).

To evaluate the early effects of irradiation to the capillaries, the following criterions were used:

(1) Decrease of the contrasting appearance of the capillaries.
(2) Disarrangement of the palisade-like pattern of the capillary loop in the distal row.
(3) Shortening of the capillary branches.
(4) Rarefaction of the capillaries.
(5) Partial shooting up of capillaries in the proximal region of the perionychium.

3.4. Thermography of the hands by means of liquid crystals (contact thermography)

Thermography is a suitable method to examine the functional behaviour of the skin's vascular system. We apply the surface technique by means of liquid crystals [13]. The skin of the hands is painted with a special preparation of soot, the dried black layer being coated with the solution of the thermographic crystals. To assess the kinetic behaviour of the vessels, the hands are cooled in a standardized manner and then the time for recalefaction is measured. Such dynamic function tests have been found to be very informative regarding the effects of ionizing radiation to the vascular system of the skin, and also in cases of acute radiation damage.

3.5. Exploratory excision and histologic investigation

In cases with conspicuous findings in capillary microscopy an exploratory excision in the most affected region of the perionychium was performed. The ovular samples of tissue comprise material sufficient for investigating the epidermis and corium. The samples extend to the level of the sudoriferous glands in the middle of the corium. For the histologic examination, the slices of the formalin-treated samples were stained by haematoxylin-eosin, and sometimes by PAS.

4.   RESULTS

Among the 70 persons examined with a relatively high exposure of the hands but without any macroscopically (including dactyloscopy) detectable deviations of the skin, 20 (= 29% of the study group) were discovered with findings in capillary microscopy. The duration of occupational exposure of these 20 persons was between 8 and 25 years. Radiation accidents were not reported in their case histories. Some of the persons, working with unsealed radionuclides, gave an account of occasional or frequent contaminations of the hands, always easily removed. In some cases an estimation of the accumulated total dose could be made on the basis of sampling measurements by means of a finger-ring dose meter. The doses established in this way range from about 1000 to 3000 rads. In the other cases pertinent inquiries did not yield any hints of much higher doses.

Among the 20 persons the capillary changes detected at the perionychium were somewhat different. Mostly, the more developed deviations were found on the right hand, which is usually more exposed than the left one, especially in radiochemical work. With regard to the fingers, almost regularly the second and third ones were the most afflicted. The changes in the vessels were poor contouring of the capillaries, disintegration of their palisade-like arrangement, shortening of the arterial and venous branches of the vessels, and slight ectasias or obliteration of some vessels in the middle of a rarefied capillary network. The most frequent and almost constant findings were grouped capillary buds and thickened vascular sections in the proximal region of the perionychium.

The thermographic investigation of the 20 persons with capillary anomalies revealed in 16 cases remarkable deviations. The distal phalanxes of the fingers with capillary changes showed distinct hyperthermic regions, in particular in the dynamic function tests. In these regions the recalefaction time after standardized cooling of the hands was distinctly shortened. This surprising finding corresponds with similar pictures seen by us in the early stage of acute radiation damage of the skin. Perhaps it represents the early vascular response to irradiation preceding the definite involution of the vascular network. This response, taking place with the vessels of the corium, affects the thermoregulation and becomes therefore detectable by means of thermography. In the course of the early reaction to ionizing radiation the vascular supply in the region of the terminal vessels is increased, and is recognizable as a hyperthermic dysfunction.

The histologic investigation was aimed at changes in the epidermis and at deviations in the vessels and in the connective tissue in the corium. It must be pointed out that the samples were taken from the most affected region according to the capillary microscopic findings. Therefore they represent the most advanced alterations of the respective case. All 20 samples yielded more or less typical findings. The following alterations in the vessels were in the first place: swelling or hyperplasia of the endothelium; swelling of the vessels' walls; hyaline-fibrous thickening of the walls; and constricted or dilated lumina. Sometimes the detectable perivascular infiltrations were on a small scale. In addition to the changes in the vessels the corium repeatedly showed swollen, frequently clumsy and partially degenerated fibres. Only in four of the 20 cases, were deviations of the epidermis detected apart from the described changes of the corium. These four persons had the most developed aberrations observed by capillary microscopic and thermographic methods. In one of these cases, also without any macroscopically detectable finding, the histologic examination disclosed thickened epidermis cells with hyperchromatic nuclei and also intercellular oedema besides marked wall fibrosis and lumen narrowing of the corium vessels. These findings represented a clear alteration in the basal layers of the epidermis, suspicious of passing into malignant transformation.

The results of our histologic investigation enable us to classify the changes in three categories, corresponding to their extent:

I: Changes only of vessels in the upper corium.
II: Changes both of vessels and connective tissue in the corium.
III: Changes both in the epidermis and the corium.

So far, our results indicate that the earliest response of the skin to low-level irradiation is to be seen in the alterations in the vessels in the corium. Typical changes in the epidermis cells are to be found only at a later stage or after a greater exposure.

5.   DISCUSSION AND CONCLUSIONS

The results of our study may contribute to the discussion of several problems regarding the late effects to the skin. Within this discussion, the following points appear important.

Our experience suggests that slight effects to the skin may occur as a result of an occupational exposure to ionizing radiation, even within the hitherto valid limits. It is evident that in most of our cases an exact correlation between effect and accumulated dose equivalent cannot be made. Nevertheless, the circumstances argue in favour of the statement that at some work places with a special exposure to the hands or other parts of the skin a damaging effect of ionizing radiation may be possible, more than for other parts or organs of the body. Therefore, the supervision of radiation workers at such work places should include measures to detect effects to the skin as early as possible.

Besides the dosimetric control of exposure by means of a finger-ring dose meter, a regular medical supervision with special attention to the hands should be performed. In addition to a careful inspection of the hands, the methods described should be used in all cases with a special risk. We found a good correlation between the capillary microscopic and the histologic findings. Therefore capillary microscopy seems a suitable screening method for detecting early radiation-induced skin reactions. In relevant cases, this method should be performed every two or three years. If suspicious findings are detected, an additional examination should be carried out, and a decision should be made regarding the further work of the person.

Another problem concerns the recommendations for the maximum permissible dose to the skin. The history of these recommendations has recently

been described in detail [5]. The most recent recommendations are given in
ICRP Publication 26 [1]. They are derived from the statement that non-
stochastic changes in the skin may occur after irradiation with absorbed doses
of 20 Gy or more, delivered over weeks or months to limited portions of skin.
It is accepted that the use of this value, as a limit for exposure over the whole
occupational lifetime, should prevent the occurrence of such non-stochastic
changes. The ICRP believes that the changes will be prevented by applying
a dose-equivalent limit of 0.5 Sv (50 rem) in a year to all tissues, including the
skin, apart from the lens.

With this, the earlier distinction made by the ICRP [4] between the limit
of 30 rem annually for exposure of the whole skin and the limit of 75 rem
annually for exposure of the hands, fore-arms, feet and ankles is discarded.

The changes found in our study have been caused by chronic long-term
exposure with a total dose in a range that could be achieved by a long-life
exposure within the hitherto recommended limit of 75 rem in a year. Therefore,
this earlier limit value was the only one allowing somatic damage to develop. It
was high time to revise this limit. Already in 1971, a British forum of experts [14]
concluded a discussion on this problem with the statement that the dose limit
of 75 rem in a year was unacceptable, and that the lower limit then given by
ICRP for the whole skin, namely 30 rem in a year, should apply to all parts of
the body.

Now, the new recommendations of the ICRP propose a dose-equivalent
limit of 50 rem in a year likewise to all regions of the skin. Assuming that at
many work places some parts of the skin, e.g. the hands, will be exposed up to
that limit, an occupational lifetime dose of 2000 to 2500 rem will be possible.

According to our experience the first radiation-induced changes in the
tissues of the skin detectable by specialized methods may occur even in the
range of the recently recommended limit. Therefore, careful observation must
be made in cases of skin exposure, equivalent to that limit, to recognize early
changes. The comparatively high limit of 50 rem in a year will remain the
continual subject of criticism, not least for the carcinogenic effects of ionizing
radiation.

In practice, radiation-induced skin diseases represent one of the most frequently accepted categories of radiation effects caused by working conditions
and recorded for compensation. For instance, in the years 1970–77 the
following numbers of cases were recognized for compensation in the German
Democratic Republic:

Year	1970	1971	1972	1973	1974	1975	1976	1977
Radiodermatitis	1	2	6	1	2	2	3	2
Skin carcinoma	–	1	–	2	–	–	1	–

Finally, the results of our study may contribute to the discussion on the carcinogenic effects of ionizing radiation to the skin. These effects can occur within the total dose equivalent obtained during a life-long occupational exposure up to the relevant limit. This statement is valid although some authors [15, 16] underline the obviously low frequency of skin carcinomas after therapeutic irradiation. Hulse and co-workers [17] have pointed out that this phenomenon may depend on an especially large radiosensitivity of the transformed cells to the cell-killing effects of radiation which may be higher in the skin than in other organs. Also other authors [10] call attention to the paradox that high doses of, for instance, 5000 or 6000 rads cause fewer carcinomas of the skin than lower doses.

In this connection the fact must be emphasized that, also according to our study, the most sensitive tissue of the skin is the vessels of the corium. The question arises whether there may be an interrelation between the changes in the epidermis and the alterations in the corium, especially with respect to the carcinogenic effects of ionizing radiation. For further investigation, a study should be made on a possible relation between a stochastic and a non-stochastic effect. Moreover, the prevalence of the vascular aberrations described in the early radiation effects to the skin corresponds with the attention that the radiation damage of the vessels has found recently [18]. According to the literature, during recent years there has been an increasing interest in the specific role that radiation damage to the blood vessels may play in causing serious late radiation sequelae.

REFERENCES

[1] INTERNATIONAL COMMISSION ON RADIATION PROTECTION, Recommendations of the International Commission on Radiological Protection, ICRP Publication 26, Pergamon Press, Oxford, New York, Frankfurt (1977).

[2] FRIEBEN, A., Cancroid nach langdauernder Einwirkung von Röntgenstrahlen, Fortschr. Röntgenstr. 6 (1902) 106.

[3] NATIONAL RESEARCH COUNCIL, Report of the Biological Effects of Ionizing Radiations, National Research Council (1972).

[4] INTERNATIONAL COMMISSION ON RADIATION PROTECTION, Recommendations of the International Commission on Radiation Protection, ICRP Publication 9, Pergamon Press, Oxford (1966).

[5] SCHÜTTMANN, W., Zur Geschichte der Strahlenschutzgrenzwerte, Report SAAS 201 (1976).

[6] MOLE, R.H., Radiation induced tumours – human experience, Br. J. Radiol. 45 (1972) 613.

[7] PEGUM, J.S., Radiation induced skin cancer, Br. J. Radiol. 45 (1972) 613.

[8] ROWELL, N.R., Discussion remarks, Br. J. Radiol. 45 (1972) 610.

[9] EMMET, E.A., Occupational skin cancer: a review, J. Occup. Med. 17 (1975) 44.

[10] Medical News, J. Am. Med. Assoc. 235 (1976) 1823.

[11] ARNDT, D., et al., Plattenepithelkarzinom der Haut mit Todesfolge bei einem beruflich
      strahlenexponierten Stomatologen, Berufsdermatosen 23 (1976) 201.
[12] ELLIS, R.E., Radiation dose and minimal reactions in chronically irradiated skin,
      Br. J. Radiol. 45 (1972) 612.
[13] LENZ, U., SCHMIDT, P., Thermographie mit kristallinen Flüssigkeiten bei Strahlen-
      schäden der Haut, Radiobiol. Radiother. 17 3 (1976) 329.
[14] Special Report No.6, Radiobiology forum on radiological protection and the skin,
      Br. J. Radiol. 45 (1972) 617.
[15] ALBERT, R.E., OMRAN, A.R., Follow-up study of patients treated by X-ray epilation
      for tinea capitis, Arch. Environ. Health 17 (1968) 899.
[16] MODAN, B., et al., Radiation-induced head and neck tumours, Lancet i (1974) 277.
[17] HULSE, E.V., MOLE, R.H., PAPWORTH, D.G., Radiosensitivities of cells from which
      radiation-induced skin tumours are derived, Int. J. Radiat. Biol. 14 (1968) 437.
[18] EBERT, M., HOWARD, A. (Eds), Current Topics in Radiation Research X, The
      Influence of Radiation on Blood Vessels and Circulation, North-Holland Publishing
      Company, Amsterdam, New York, Oxford (1977).

DISCUSSION

(on the previous two papers)

G.B. SCHOFIELD: I should be interested to hear whether you have considered whether other causes than radiation are likely to have affected the capillary tufts in the skin. It is my experience that the application of a wide variety of skin decontamination agents causes greater damage to the skin than the irradiation from the contamination.

P. NACK: This question can be answered properly only by a dermatologist. I think that damage to the skin from decontamination agents can be observed macroscopically if it includes the capillary system. Besides, some of our cases were subject to external exposure without possibility of contamination, e.g. radiographers and their assistants.

A. ARSENAULT: It appears that the populations of workers most adequately surveyed are employed in the medical environment. There is another group at risk that we have great difficulty in monitoring in Canada, namely teaching and research personnel in laboratories using radiation sources in, say, X-ray fluorescence analysis or crystallography. Do you meet the same difficulty in your country?

P. NACK: In the German Democratic Republic all radiation-exposed persons are medically surveyed on a uniform basis. The monitoring of external exposure is centralized at the Board of Nuclear Safety where all dose meters are analysed. For work places where there is the possibility of incorporation of radioactive materials, a special control programme is operated by the Board, independently of monitoring at the work place. Nevertheless, we do sometimes experience difficulty with dose estimation, particularly in cases involving contamination.

G. COWPER: Since there are many uncertainties in the determination of beta doses received by the skin of the hands of workers, it may be well worthwhile examining those radiation workers whose skin doses can be predicted from the type of work they carry out routinely. I refer to workers in nuclear fuel fabrication facilities where unclad pellets of UO_2 are handled using gloves of known thickness. In these cases the actual doses to the finger tips can be determined with some confidence, and it may be useful to look for the presence of radiation effects in these workers.

P. NACK: In the field of radionuclide production the doses were estimated in some cases by means of thermoluminescence tablets at the finger tips and in the palm of the hands. No signs of excessive doses were detected by this procedure.

R.E. LINNEMANN: In your follow-up of skin exposures of radiation workers, have you ever seen a skin cancer that was not preceded by a chronic radiodermatitis?

P. NACK: Yes, in some of our patients we have seen skin cancers in areas without any signs of typical radiodermatitis. This condition has also been reported by other authors named in the references of our paper.

A.F. STEHNEY: What information do you have on the age dependence of cataracts in the population as a whole (that is, in non-exposed persons)?

P. NACK: The age dependence of cataracts has been recorded and documented in the German Democratic Republic, but I do not have any data with me. In our cases the typical form of the cataracts observed indicated that they were caused by radiation. In these cataracts the development of opacities is found at the posterior pole of the lens.

SURVIVAL TIMES OF
WOMEN RADIUM DIAL WORKERS
FIRST EXPOSED BEFORE 1930*

A.F. STEHNEY, H.F. LUCAS, Jr.,
R.E. ROWLAND
Center for Human Radiobiology,
Argonne National Laboratory,
Argonne,
Illinois,
United States of America

Abstract

SURVIVAL TIMES OF WOMEN RADIUM DIAL WORKERS FIRST EXPOSED BEFORE 1930.
Life table methods were applied to survival data on U.S. women radium dial workers in
order to compare observed and expected deaths as a function of time after exposure to radium.
The study population consisted of 1235 workers employed in the industry before 1930 for
whom age and year of death, withdrawal or loss from the study were known. Expected deaths
were estimated from age- and time-specific death rates for U.S. white females. The closing
year for analysis was 1976, so observation times of 45 to 60 years were possible. For all causes,
529 deaths before age 85 were observed versus 461 expected, and the cumulative survival of the
population was significantly less than expected at 10 and more years after first employment.
Estimates were made of the net survival probabilities after elimination of risk due to the well-
known radium-related malignancies, i.e. bone sarcomas and carcinomas of the paranasal sinuses
and the mastoid air cells. There were 455 observed deaths from other causes versus 460 expected,
and there was no significant difference between observed and expected cumulative net survival
at one-year intervals from zero to 59 years after first employment. These findings indicate that
only the known radium-related malignancies contributed significantly to life shortening of the
exposed population as a whole, but the presence of other radium-related causes of death may
yet be detectable by examination of specific risks as a function of dose.

INTRODUCTION

The possible biological effects of internal deposits of radium in
humans have been described in various reports [1—9]. Among radium dial
workers, the most significant effects are neoplasms arising in bone
('bone sarcomas') and carcinomas originating in the paranasal sinuses and
the mastoid air cells ('head carcinomas'). Reports of early deaths from
acute anemias and from possible leukemias [6] indicate that these were

---

* Work performed under the auspices of the U.S. Department of Energy.

also radium related, and greater than expected numbers of cancer of the brain and of the large intestine have been observed [9], but a causal association with radium has not been established. A debilitating effect of radium is extensive skeletal damage, such as bone necrosis and coarsening of bone trabeculation [4].

In view of the above, the life-shortening effects of radium may be ascribed to deaths from bone sarcomas and head carcinomas, to deaths from other specific causes which are not well established as radium related, and to generally reduced viability because of skeletal damage and other morbid effects. In this paper, we examine the survival times of women first employed in the U. S. radium dial industry before 1930. The purpose is to determine the average life shortening in this population and to determine whether there is detectable life shortening which can be ascribed to risks other than bone sarcomas and head carcinomas. This study, which is not yet completed, utilizes life-table methods and compares observed mortality rates with age- and time-specific mortality rates for U. S. white females.

METHODS AND MATERIALS

The study population

The study population was derived from women employed in the U. S. radium dial-painting industry before 1930. The U. S. Bureau of Labor Statistics estimated that 'not more than 2000 individuals' had worked in the luminous paint industry up to 1929 [10]. We have identified about 1600 individuals who started work in the industry before 1930, 1474 of whom were female. From this group of (white) women, 1235 cases were left for analysis after elimination of 212 unlocated cases and 27 cases for whom no year of birth was available.

Table I summarizes our follow-up of these 1235 women by period of entry into the industry. Regardless of the date of first employment, the average age at employment was about the same; for the entire group the average age was 20.0 years with a standard deviation (S.D.) of 5.9 years and a distribution somewhat skewed toward the greater ages. The deceased cases (as of 12/31/76) are also summarized by period of entry; about 44% of this study group are deceased.

These women, for the most part, worked in luminous dial-painting plants located in Connecticut, New Jersey and Illinois. Most of the identification and follow-up of these dial painters has been through studies conducted at Argonne National Laboratory and at the Massachusetts Institute of Technology from the 1950's to the present, and studies done as part of the New Jersey Radium Research Project from 1957 to 1967. Records of all dial workers in these studies are centralized at Argonne.

TABLE I. STUDY POPULATION OF WOMEN FIRST EMPLOYED IN THE
U.S. RADIUM DIAL INDUSTRY BEFORE 1930

Year of first exposure	All cases				Deceased cases		
	Number of cases	Age at first exposure			Number dead	Age at death	
		Mean	S.D.	Range		Mean	Range
1912−14	14	20.5	6.2	14−38	8	62.6	36−76
1915−19	369	20.0	5.3	12−50	214	59.5	16−91
1920−24	471	20.2	6.7	12−64	221	55.3	17−92
1925−29	381	19.5	5.2	12−56	97	55.0	18−90
Total	1235	20.0	5.9	12−64	540	57.0	16−92

Radium exposures

The paint used in the luminous-dial industry contained varying
proportions of ^{226}Ra (half life ∼1600 y), and ^{228}Ra (half-life 5.75 y) as
activators. The proportion of these isotopes varied with time and between
the various companies using luminous compounds. For example, the paint
used in Illinois appears to have contained predominantly ^{226}Ra, whereas the
plants on the East coast often employed paint rich in ^{228}Ra.

Of this study group of 1235 women, some 759 have had their radium
body content measured. From this measurement the 'initial systemic intake'
for each woman has been calculated. This is the quantity of radium,
expressed in microcuries, that entered the blood during the period of exposure.
It is calculated by extrapolating the measured body content back to the time
of exposure utilizing the radium retention function of Norris et al. [11].
This measure of internal exposure allows the cases to be grouped by intake
level. Because this parameter is time invariant [12] and does not specify
a critical organ, it seems more appropriate for a study of life shortening than
another frequently used parameter, the average skeletal dose [4]. For the
present analysis, we have used the sum of the initial systemic intakes of
^{226}Ra and ^{228}Ra in order to indicate the level of radium intake by means of
a single parameter.

Survival calculations

Life-table methods [13, 14] were used to record the time sequence of
events and to obtain estimates of survival probabilities and survival times.
Counting of person-years of follow-up was done by methods described by
Monson [15]. For some of the life tables, the year of entry was the year of
first employment in the radium dial industry, and in others it was the year of
first measurement of radium burden. Events were entered into the table in

one-year intervals, with the first interval (Year 0) being the year of entry. Since the data for each person were comprised of the calendar years of birth, employment and death or withdrawal while living, events were assumed to occur on the average at mid-year, except for those withdrawn on the common closing date, December 31, 1976. Thus, a woman born in 1900 and first employed in 1920 would be given 0.5 year of follow-up at age 20 in the first interval and 0.5 year at age 20 plus 0.5 year at age 21 in the next interval (Year 1). If she died or was lost from follow-up in 1960, the death or loss would be entered in the 41st interval after exactly 40 years of follow-up in ages 20 through 59. If she survived until the end of 1976, she would be counted as withdrawn alive at age 76 after 56.5 years of follow-up.

Expected numbers of deaths were calculated by multiplying age-time-specific U. S. mortality rates for white females [15] by age-time-specific person-years of follow-up and entered into the intervals in which the corresponding follow-up time had been counted. Because age-time-specific mortality rates were not available for women age 85 and older, those who survived to age 85 were withdrawn while living, and follow-up time and deaths after age 84 were not counted.

The primary quantities[1] calculated for each interval were p_i, the observed probability that a person alive at the start of the ith interval would survive to the end of the interval, and r_i, the ratio of observed to expected survival probabilities. The probability of surviving from entry to the end of the ith interval was calculated as the product $p_1, p_2, \cdots p_i$ and designated as P_i, the cumulative survival. The corresponding cumulative relative survival, R_i, was calculated as the product $r_1, r_2, \cdots r_i$. The mean survival time from entry to the end of the ith interval was calculated as

$$\mu_i = \sum_{j=1}^{i} \frac{P_{(j-1)} + P_j}{2} \tau_j$$

where $P_o = 1$ and the τ_j are the time durations of the intervals.

Also estimated were the survival probabilities and mean survival time that would have been observed in the absence of the known radium-related tumors. This was done with the following formula, which includes a correction for deaths from other causes that might have occurred if not precluded by death from radium-related tumors [14]:

$$p_{i \cdot a} = p_i^{(D_i - A_i)/D_i}$$

where $p_{i \cdot a}$ is the net probability that a person alive at the start of interval i will die in the interval if cause 'a' is eliminated as a risk of death, D_i is the total number of deaths observed in the interval and A_i is the number of

---

[1] Formulas for calculation of the quantities and standard errors are given in the appendix.

deaths from cause a. An adequate approximation to the net expected survival probability was obtained from the net expected deaths calculated from the differences between the all causes rates and the rates for those tumors. The values of $p_{i.a}$ and $r_{i.a}$ were then used to calculate the cumulative net survival, the cumulative net relative survival, and the mean net survival time, where 'net' designates the values obtained after elimination of risk of death due to the radium-related tumors.

RESULTS

Deaths from all causes

The numbers of persons under observation, observed deaths and expected deaths are shown in Table II as a function of time after first exposure. It may be noted that 590 of the 1235 women were known to be alive at the end of 1976. Of the 116 women withdrawn earlier, 28 were withdrawn at age 85, with the consequence that 11 deaths during 80.5 person-years of subsequent follow-up were not counted. The difference between the number of observed deaths and the number expected is statistically significant ($P < 0.005$, by Mantel-Haenszel chi-square test) [15,16], and most of the excess deaths occurred within 25 years after first exposure.

The same relative trend of mortality was evident in the survival probabilities. These were calculated in one-year intervals, and the cumulative values at an average of 4.5, 9.5, 14.5, etc., years after first exposure are plotted in Fig. 1. The cumulative survival probability at 59.5 years was 0.445 with a binomial standard error (S.E.) of 0.022. The lower than expected survival for about 25 years after first exposure is seen in the downward trend of the cumulative relative survival ratios (upper points). The ratios show a much smaller downward trend for the next 25 years, and this trend apparently continues into the final 10-year period in which the ratios have large standard errors.

Deaths after elimination of risk of radium-related tumors

The major causes of excess deaths are indicated in Table III which shows the time distribution of persons who died with diagnosed bone sarcomas or head carcinomas or, for two persons, both. We use the word 'with' because the ultimate cause of death was not necessarily the radium-related tumor in each case [9,17]. However, the average time from diagnosis to death was 1.2 years for the bone sarcoma cases and 1.1 years for the head carcinoma cases, so we shall consider these cases as deaths caused by the tumor. Although analysis of the tumor rates is not the subject of this paper, it is of interest to note that cases of bone sarcoma began to appear earlier and are three times more numerous than the head carcinomas. Both types have a wide distribution of occurrence times and occurred as late as the 50 to 54 year interval in which one case of bone sarcoma and three cases of head

TABLE II. OBSERVED AND EXPECTED DEATHS FROM ALL CAUSES BY
CALENDAR YEAR AFTER YEAR OF FIRST EXPOSURE

Interval since year of entry (years)	Number of persons at start of interval	During interval				
		Live withdrawals		Observed deaths	Expected deaths	Obs./Exp.
		End 1976	Earlier			
0−4	1235	0	0	23	17.4	1.32
5−9	1212	0	0	33	20.2	1.64**
10−14	1179	0	0	31	21.3	1.46*
15−19	1148	0	0	30	21.1	1.42
20−24	1118	0	0	37	23.1	1.60**
25−29	1081	0	1	25	27.7	0.90
30−34	1055	0	0	38	34.5	1.10
35−39	1017	0	0	49	45.7	1.07
40−44	968	0	7	66	61.5	1.07
45−49	895	127	33	86	80.3	1.07
50−54	649	293	34	79	69.0	1.14
55−59	243	144	31	31	37.2	0.83
60−61	37	26	10	1	2.4	0.42
Total	1235	590	116[a]	529	461.2	1.15***

[a] Includes only 5 cases that were not withdrawn at age 85 or within 5 years of the common
   closing date of December 31, 1976.
  *   P < 0.05 (Mantel-Haenszel chi-square).
  **   P < 0.01.
*** P < 0.005.

carcinoma were diagnosed. The number of other deaths observed was obtained
by subtracting the number of persons who died with these tumors from the
number of observed deaths in each interval.

The mortality rates that were used to calculate the number of other
deaths expected in Table III were obtained by subtracting the mortality rates
for bone sarcomas and head carcinomas from the mortality rates for all causes.
Age-time-specific rates for U. S. white females were used for the bone
sarcomas [15] and the current age-specific rates for the combined categories
160 and 163 for U. S. white females [18] were used as the closest
approximation available for the head carcinomas. (In categories 160 and
163 are deaths caused by malignant neoplasms of the respiratory system,
excluding larynx, trachea, bronchus and lungs.) As indicated by comparison

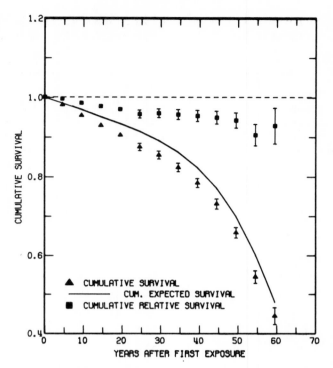

FIG.1. Observed and expected probabilities of survival versus time (years) after first employment as a radium dial worker. Error bars represent one standard error and are not shown if they tend to merge with the symbols.

with Table II, the total number of 461.2 expected deaths was reduced by only 0.9 death by correction for expected bone sarcoma deaths (0.6) and deaths in categories 160 and 163 (0.3).

The ratios of other deaths observed to other deaths expected are given in the last column of Table III, and it may be noted that there is no significant difference at the 5% level in the total nor in any of the time intervals. Assuming independence among the causes of death, this comparison is not much affected by deaths that might have occurred if not precluded by death from radium-related tumor, because the probability of any death is small in each interval. If the tumor cases were not removed from the study by death, observed deaths from other causes would be more numerous, but expected deaths from other causes would also increase because of the greater number of person-years.

A correction for the effect of competing risks was made by calculating for each one-year interval the net survival probability [14] after elimination of the risk of the radium-related tumors. This method assumes independence

TABLE III. NET OBSERVED AND NET EXPECTED DEATHS AFTER
REMOVAL OF DEATHS WITH TUMOR TYPES KNOWN TO BE RADIUM
RELATED

Interval since year of entry (years)	Number of persons at start of interval[a]	During interval				
		Deaths with bone sarcoma	Deaths with head carcinoma	Other deaths observed	Other deaths expected	Obs./Exp.
0−4	1235	0	0	23	17.4	1.32
5−9	1212	8	0	25	20.1	1.24
10−14	1179	9	0	22	21.2	1.04
15−19	1148	6	1	23	21.0	1.09
20−24	1118	13	2	22	23.0	0.96
25−29	1081	2	1	22	27.6	0.80
30−34	1055	6	5	28	34.4	0.81
35−39	1017	3	2	44	45.5	0.97
40−44	968	3	3	60	61.4	0.98
45−49	895	6	1	79	80.1	0.99
50−54	649	2	3	75	68.9	1.09
55−59	243	0	0	31	37.2	0.83
60−61	37	0	0	1	2.4	0.42
Total	1235	58	18	455[b]	460.3	0.99

[a] The numbers of live withdrawals and observed deaths are those shown in Table II.

[b] Two women died with both types of tumors, so the total number of 'Other Deaths Observed'
is 74 less than the total number of observed deaths in Table II.

among the causes of death and constant risk of specific causes relative to
the total risk during the interval. The cumulative net survival probabilities
are shown graphically in Fig. 2. The cumulative net relative survival ratios,
also plotted in Fig. 2, give some indication of less than expected net surviva
in the early period and more than expected in the late intervals, but the
differences are not statistically significant.

Expectation of life

        The cumulative survival probabilities (Fig. 1) and the cumulative net
survival probabilities (Fig. 2) were used to calculate mean survival times of
the radium dial workers. These are shown in Table IV as estimates of
expectation of life to age 85 limited to 59.5 years after first exposure, the

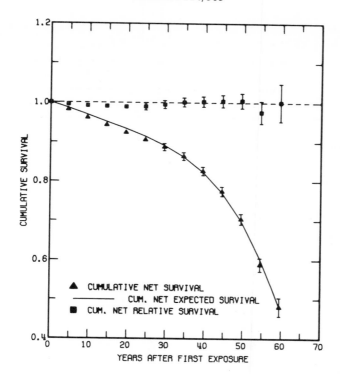

FIG.2. Observed and expected net probabilities of survival versus time (years) after first employment as a radium dial worker, when risk of radium-related tumors is eliminated. Error bars represent one standard error and are not shown if they tend to merge with the symbol.

time period in which sufficient women were under observation. It should be noted that these expectancies are the combined result of the natural determinants of remaining life, chiefly the age distribution of the group of women under study, and the consequences, if any, of the common experience of employment as radium dial workers. The years of life remaining to 59.5 years at the various times T after entry are independent of the mortality experience at times less than T, but include the experience (and statistical errors) of all the succeeding years.

The observed expectation at entry was 48.5 years of life remaining when deaths from all causes were considered and 50.3 years when risk of the radium-related tumors was eliminated. The difference of 1.8 years is an average for the entire study population, and it reflects the number of tumor deaths and the times at which they occurred. The second and fifth columns of Table IV show the expected years of life at natural rates; these were calculated from age-time-specific mortality rates for U. S. white women with the same distribution of age and year of birth as the radium workers under observation at one-year intervals from entry to 59.5 years later. The close

TABLE IV. ESTIMATES OF EXPECTATION OF LIFE TO AGE 85, LIMITED TO 59.5 YEARS AFTER AGE AT FIRST EXPOSURE

| Time since first exposure T (years) | Mean survival time (years) from T to 59.5 years | | | | | |
| | All causes | | | Net (Ra-tumor risk removed) | | |
	Expected	Observed	S.E.	Expected	Observed	S.E.
0	50.28	48.48	0.46	50.29	50.14	0.43
4.5	46.47	44.86	0.43	46.48	46.56	0.39
9.5	42.21	41.05	0.39	42.23	42.50	0.36
14.5	37.95	37.09	0.35	37.96	38.25	0.32
19.5	33.61	33.01	0.31	33.62	33.98	0.29
24.5	29.27	29.06	0.27	29.28	29.62	0.26
29.5	24.97	24.67	0.25	24.98	25.18	0.24
34.5	20.73	20.50	0.22	20.73	20.79	0.22
39.5	16.58	16.39	0.19	16.58	16.60	0.19
44.5	12.53	12.41	0.16	12.54	12.54	0.16
49.5	8.54	8.48	0.13	8.54	8.53	0.13
54.5	4.50	4.60	0.07	4.50	4.60	0.07
—	0.479[a]	0.445[a]	0.022[b]	0.480[a]	0.481[a]	0.023[b]

[a] Cumulative survival probability from 0.0 to 59.5 years after first exposure.

[b] Standard error of observed cumulative survival probability.

agreement at all times after entry between expected years at natural rates and expected years observed after elimination of risk of the known radium-related tumors leads to the conclusion that no life-shortening effect due to early deaths from other radium-related causes was detectable when the population as a whole was considered.

Dose groups

The most sensitive procedure would be search for excess deaths by examination of subgroups based on radium dose. Unfortunately, an analysis of this type cannot be done with entry at the time of first exposure, because measurements of radium burden have not been made for all of the radium dial painters, and there is a preponderance of deaths among the unmeasured. The reason is that intensive efforts to measure all radium dial workers did not begin until about 1955 and few of those who died earlier were measured.

TABLE V. NET OBSERVED AND NET EXPECTED DEATHS BY SUBGROUP WHEN ENTRY IS AT YEAR OF FIRST EXPOSURE

Group	Persons with a measurement of radium burden	Persons unmeasured	Total
Number of persons	759	476	1 235
Mean date of entry	1922.7	1922.1	1922.5
Mean age at entry	19.0	21.5	20.0
Person-years	37 756	18 307	56 063
Deaths	235	294	529
Deaths with bone sarcoma	35	23	58
Deaths with head carcinoma	14	4	18
Other deaths observed	188	267	455
Other deaths expected	308.5	151.8	460.3
Observed/Expected	0.61	1.76	0.99

This effect is illustrated by the comparison of measured and unmeasured persons in Table V. For deaths other than those with radium-related tumors, the ratio of observed to expected is 1.76 for the unmeasured and 0.61 for the measured.

Since it appears that the persons measured are largely those who survived until measurement, we have examined the time distribution of deaths after entry at first measurement while living. There were 41 persons for whom measurements have been obtained after death by analysis of exhumed remains, autopsy material or surgical specimens. For the 718 persons measured while living, there were 8707 person-years of follow-up after first measurement, starting, on the average, at about 40 years after first exposure and at age 58 (Table VI). There were 21 deaths with bone sarcoma and 12 deaths with head carcinoma in this group after first measurement, and the ratio of other deaths observed to other deaths expected was 0.98.

Table VI also shows the results when the 718 persons are separated into dose groups based on initial systemic intake of radium. Only one death with radium-related tumor occurred at initial intake of less than 50 µCi radium, whereas in the highest dose group (≥500 µCi) 14 of the 16 deaths before age 85 were with radium-related tumors. The difference between other deaths observed and expected was not statistically significant at the 5% level (Mantel-Haenszel chi-square test) for any of the dose groups, but comparison of the ratio of observed to expected deaths for the 50—500 µCi group with the ratio for the lowest dose group suggests a dose effect.

TABLE VI. NET OBSERVED AND NET EXPECTED DEATHS BY RADIUM DOSE GROUP WHEN ENTRY IS AT FIRST MEASUREMENT WHILE LIVING

Dose range (μCi intake)	<0.5	0.5–5	5–50	50–500	≥500	Total
Number of persons	202	265	152	80	19	718
Mean date of entry	1965.4	1962.5	1961.0	1957.7	1950.4	1962.2
Mean age at entry	61.1	58.3	57.4	54.3	50.3	58.2
Person-years	2062	3328	2100	1073	144	8707
Deaths	39	63	37	40	16	195
Deaths with						
Bone sarcoma	0	0	0	11	10	21
Head carcinoma	0	0	1	6	5	12
Other deaths observed	39	63	36	24	2	164
Other deaths expected	44.8	64.2	38.8	16.9	2.2	166.9
Observed/Expected	0.87	0.98	0.93	1.42	0.91	0.98

DISCUSSION

The relationship of radium to total deaths and to specific causes of death is discussed in some detail in a recent report on mortality studies of women radium dial painters ascertained from employment lists [9]. The discussion here is restricted to the significance of the life-span findings of the present work.

The workers in the dial industry constitute a unique and valuable population for study of the effects of internally deposited, alpha-emitting bone-seeking isotopes. The major exposure took place more than 50 years ago, before the hazards of radium began to be recognized in 1925. The simple precautions that were subsequently taken proved to be adequate, for no radium-related malignancies have been observed in workers who entered this industry after 1925. Thus this population provides a long observation time of persons presumably in normal health at entry. The quantity of radium acquired varied widely, and has been shown to be independent of the length of time an individual was employed [19]; apparently the individual techniques used by the dial painters accounted for the wide range of levels of radium acquired. The measured radium body burdens varied from a lower detection limit equivalent to about 0.5 μCi initial systemic intake to the equivalent of more than 4400 μCi. Moreover, these individuals were subject to inhalation of radon and to whole-body irradiation (from radium in paint) of probably not insignificant magnitude. This wide range of exposures, observed in the measured portion of the group and assumed to exist in the unmeasured cases, resulted in an exposed population in which 74 individuals have died with 76 malignancies attributed to radium.

In the present work, the average survival times of this population were determined by actuarial methods. Although actuarial methods are patently approximate, a recent review indicates that they provide estimates of survival and of standard errors that are similar to those obtained by other interval methods that invoke more rigorous treatment of the statistical problems of withdrawals and losses [20]. The conditions stated were that the q_i's be less than 0.3 and the L_i's be 'fairly large' (as small as 158 in the review); these conditions were easily met in obtaining the results of Figs 1 and 2 (and Table IV) shown above. Of more concern to us is the assumption that the q_i's are the same for withdrawn persons as for those not withdrawn during an interval. This is a poor assumption for a population of mixed ages and mixed radium doses. However, the corrections for withdrawals could hardly have introduced appreciable error, because persons withdrawn on the closing date were withdrawn at the ends of intervals, and the early withdrawals were not a large fraction of the L_i's.

This study has demonstrated that when the radium tumor deaths are removed, the average survival of the dial-worker population is indistinguishable from estimates of the survival of contemporary white females of the same age. This is a remarkable result, for it implies that, to the precision obtainable with a population of some 1000 persons, the life expectancy of the remaining population was unaffected by radium burden. However, it is known that some of the early dial workers died with blood dyscrasias at relatively short times after entry into dial work. There is good reason to believe that these individuals acquired very high radium burdens, and they may account for the slight excess of deaths noted in Fig. 2 during the first 25 years after exposure to radium. Further, there is an indication in Table VI that those with high levels of radium did experience more net deaths than expected, although the numbers are not highly significant. Thus the finding that there was no difference between observed and expected survival after removal of the radium-related malignancies was not anticipated. The excess early deaths seem to have been off-set by greater than expected net survival at older ages. Discussion of possible reasons for the apparently favorable longevity during a period of late life can only be speculative at this time. More detailed study of the radium workers by dose group, by age, and by year of entry is needed, and comparison with the survival times of other occupational groups of women would be desirable.

ACKNOWLEDGMENTS

The authors are grateful to Dr. Richard R. Monson for providing a computer tape of abstracted U. S. death rates and a program for calculating person-years and expected deaths. Follow-up data on the dial workers were obtained by the dedicated efforts of several persons, for which we especially thank Betty C. Patten and Carol Daun Croft at Argonne and Mary Margaret Shanahan at M. I. T. We also thank Frances R. Clark for preparing the manuscript.

Appendix

FORMULAS FOR CALCULATION OF
QUANTITIES AND STANDARD ERRORS

The closing date of the study is December 31, 1976. Those known to be alive on the closing date or later are counted as withdrawn while living, W, after a full year of observation in the year of withdrawal. For those who died, the fraction lived of the last year of life is assumed to be 0.5. Those not dead or withdrawn on the closing date are designated as lost while living, U, and the fraction observed of the last year they were known to be alive is also assumed to be 0.5. Since date of first employment for most of the dial painters is known only by calendar year, entry is assumed to be at mid-year on the average. The number of person-years in the ith interval is then equal to $L_i - \frac{1}{2}U_i - \frac{1}{2}D_i$, except in the first interval (Year 0, the year of entry) for which $PY_1 = \frac{1}{2}(L_1 - \frac{1}{2}U_1 - \frac{1}{2}D_1)$. Of course, $L_{i+1} = L_i - W_i - U_i - D_i$.

The probability that a person living and under observation at the start of an interval will die during the interval is given by $q_i = D_i/L_i'$, where L_i' is the effective number of persons living at the start of interval i. The total number of person-years during the interval is the sum of the years lived by those who survive the entire year plus the sum of the years lived before death by those who died. Therefore,

$$PY_i' = (L_i' - D_i + a_i D_i)h_i$$

where $h_i = 1$ year, except for $h_1 = 0.5$ year, and a_i is the fraction lived of the last year of life, which we have already assumed to be 0.5. We then find L_i' from the equality of PY_i' and PY_i:

$$L_i' - \tfrac{1}{2}D_i = L_i - \tfrac{1}{2}U_i - \tfrac{1}{2}D_i$$

$$L_i' = L_i - \tfrac{1}{2}U_i$$

Thus,

$$q_i = \frac{D_i}{L_i - \tfrac{1}{2}U_i}$$

The probability that a person alive at the start of a year will survive to the end of the year is the survival probability,

$$p_i = 1 - q_i = 1 - \frac{D_i}{L_i - \tfrac{1}{2}U_i}$$

and the binomial variance of p_i is given approximately by:

$$[S.E.(p_i)]^2 = \frac{p_i(1 - p_i)}{L_i - \frac{1}{2}U_i}$$

The number of expected deaths during interval i, E_i, is obtained by summing the age-time specific standard mortality rates for the PY_i person-years. We then write the expected probability of death during interval i as $eq_i = E_i/L_i'$, where L_i' is the effective number of persons at the start of the interval for the calculation of the expected probability of death. We derive L_i' in the same way as for the observed probabilities:

$$PY'' = (L_i'' - \tfrac{1}{2}E_i)h_i \qquad \text{and} \qquad L_i'' - \tfrac{1}{2}E_i = L_i - \tfrac{1}{2}U_i - \tfrac{1}{2}D_i$$

so $\qquad L_i'' = L_i - \tfrac{1}{2}U_i - \tfrac{1}{2}D_i + \tfrac{1}{2}E_i$

Therefore, the expected survival probability is

$$ep_i = 1 - \frac{E_i}{L_i - \frac{1}{2}U_i - \frac{1}{2}D_i + \frac{1}{2}E_i}$$

The relative survival ratio is $r_i = p_i/ep_i$ and the fractional standard error of r_i is equal to the fractional standard error of p_i.

The net survival probability, $p_{i \cdot a}$, is the probability of surviving interval i if risk 'a' is eliminated. When the risks are independent and the force of mortality from risk a relative to the total force of mortality is constant during the interval, the following formula holds [14] :

$$p_{i \cdot a} = p_i^{(D_i - A_i)/D_i}$$

where A_i is the observed number of deaths from cause a and D_i is the total number of deaths observed. Series expansion provides the result that

$$p_{i \cdot a} \cong 1 - \left(1 + \frac{A_i}{2L_i'}\right)\frac{D_i - A_i}{L_i'}$$

Thus, when $A_i/2L_i$ is small, the value of $p_{i \cdot a}$ is approximately equal to the value obtained by substituting $D_i - A_i$ for D_i in the expression for p_i.

The standard error of $p_{i \cdot a}$ is obtained by propagation of errors, using the binomial variances of A_i and B_i, the number of deaths from other causes.

Omitting subscript i for convenience and writing $p_{i \cdot a}$ as an explicit function of A and B, we have

$$p_{i \cdot a} = \left(1 - \frac{A + B}{L'}\right)^{B/(A + B)}$$

and

$$[S.E.(p_{i \cdot a})]^2 = \frac{p_{i \cdot a}}{L' p_i (1 - p_i)} \; (I + II)$$

where $\;\; L' = L - \tfrac{1}{2}U$,

$$I = \frac{B(L' - B)}{L'} \left(\frac{A}{A + B} \; p_i \log p_i - \frac{B}{L'}\right)^2$$

and $\quad II = \dfrac{A(L' - A)}{L'} \left(\dfrac{A}{A + B} \; p_i \log p_i + \dfrac{B}{L'}\right)^2$

The net expected survival probability, $ep_{i \cdot a}$, is the probability of surviving interval i at standard mortality rates if risk a is eliminated:

$$ep_{i \cdot a} = ep_i^{\,(d_i - a_i)/d_i}$$

where d_i and a_i are total expected deaths and expected deaths from cause a, respectively.

The various other life-table parameters are obtained from the p_i's, $p_{i \cdot a}$'s, r_i's or $r_{i \cdot a}$'s which are assumed to be independent. The standard error of each function, F, is then calculated from the usual differential equation for the propagation of errors [21]. For example, for $F(p_i)$:

$$[S.E.(F)]^2 = \sum_{i=1}^{n} \left[\left(\frac{\partial F}{\partial p_i}\right)^2 [S.E.(p_i)]^2\right]$$

The life-table functions and binomial variances are listed below:

1. Cumulative survival probability from the start of the first interval to the end of the jth interval:

$$P_j = p_1 p_2 \cdots p_j = \prod_{i=1}^{j} p_i$$

$$[S.E.(P_j)]^2 = P_j^2 \sum_{i=1}^{j} \left[\frac{S.E.(p_i)}{p_i}\right]^2$$

2. Cumulative relative survival probability:

$$R_j = \prod_{i=1}^{j} r_i \qquad \text{and} \qquad S.E.(R_j) = \frac{R_j}{P_j} \, S.E.(P_j)$$

3. The mean lifetime is given by the time integral of P(t) [22]. The mean survival time from time zero ($P_O = 1$) to the end of interval n is approximately

$$\mu = \tfrac{1}{2} \sum_{j=1}^{n} (P_{(j-1)} h_j + P_j h_j)$$

$$[S.E.(\mu)]^2 = \tfrac{1}{4} \sum_{i=1}^{n} \left\{ \left[\sum_{j=i}^{n} (P_{(j-1)} h_j + P_j h_j) - P_{(i-1)} h_i \right] \left[\frac{S.E.(p_i)}{p_i} \right] \right\}^2$$

REFERENCES

[1]   MARTLAND, H.S., The occurrence of malignancy in radioactive persons, Am. J. Cancer **15** (1931) 2435.

[2]   AUB, J.C., EVANS, R.D., HEMPELMANN, L.H., MARTLAND, H.S., The late effects of internally-deposited radioactive materials in man, Medicine **31** (1952) 221.

[3]   LOONEY, W.B., HASTERLIK, R.J., BRUES, A.M., et al., A clinical investigation of the chronic effects of radium salt administered therapeutically, Am. J. Roentgenol., Radium Ther. Nucl. Med. **73** (1955) 1006.

[4]   EVANS, R.D., The effect of skeletally deposited alpha-ray emitters in man, Br. J. Radiol. **39** (1966) 881.

[5]   FINKEL, A.J., MILLER, C.E., HASTERLIK, R.J., "Radium-induced malignant tumors in man", Delayed Effects of Bone-Seeking Radionuclides (MAYS, C.W., JEE, W.S.S., LLOYD, R.D., Eds), University of Utah Press, Salt Lake City (1969) 195.

[6]   LOUTIT, J.F., Malignancy from radium, Br. J. Cancer **24** (1970) 195.

[7]   SPIESS, H., MAYS, C.W., Bone cancers induced by ^{224}Ra (ThX) in children and adults, Health Phys. **19** (1970) 713.

[8]   SHARPE, W.D., Chronic radium intoxication: Clinical and autopsy findings in long-term New Jersey survivors, Environ. Res. 8 (1974) 243.

[9]   POLEDNAK, A.P., STEHNEY, A.F., ROWLAND, R.E., Mortality among women first employed before 1930 in the U.S. radium dial-painting industry, Am.J. Epidemiol. **107** (1978) 179.

[10] U.S. BUREAU OF LABOR STATISTICS, Radium poisoning, Monthly Labor Rev. **28** (1929) 1200.

[11] NORRIS, W.P., SPECKMAN, T.W., GUSTAFSON, P.F., Studies of the metabolism of radium in man, Am. J. Roentgenol., Radium Ther. Nucl. Med. **73** (1955) 785.

[12] STEHNEY, A.F., "A time-invariant dose parameter for radium cases", Radiological
      Physics Division 1971 Annual Report, Argonne National Laboratory, ANL-7860,
      Part II (1971) 9.

[13] CUTLER, S.J., EDERER, F., Maximum utilization of the life table method in analyzing
      survival, J. Chronic Dis. 8 (1958) 699.

[14] CHIANG, C.L., Introduction to Stochastic Processes in Biostatistics, John Wiley and
      Sons, New York (1968).

[15] MONSON, R.R., Analysis of relative survival and proportional mortality, Comput.
      Biomed. Res. 7 (1974) 325.

[16] MANTEL, N., HAENSZEL, W., Statistical aspects of the analysis of data from retro-
      spective studies of disease, J. Natl. Cancer Inst. 22 (1959) 719.

[17] POLEDNAK, A.P., Bone cancers among female radium dial workers: Latency periods
      and incidence rates by time after exposure, J. Natl. Cancer Inst., in press.

[18] U.S. PUBLIC HEALTH SERVICE, Vital Statistics of the United States, 1968–73,
      Vol.II, part A, National Center for Health Statistics, Rockville, Maryland (1972–77).

[19] ROWLAND, R.E., et al., Current status of the study of ^{226}Ra and ^{228}Ra in humans at
      the Center for Human Radiobiology, Health Phys., in press.

[20] ELANDT-JOHNSON, R.C., Various estimators of conditional probabilities of death in
      follow-up studies: Summary of results, J. Chronic Dis. 30 (1977) 247.

[21] BEVINGTON, P.R., Data Reduction and Error Analysis for the Physical Sciences,
      McGraw-Hill, New York (1969).

[22] KAPLAN, E.L., MEIER, P., Nonparametric estimation from incomplete observations,
      J. Am. Stat. Assoc. 53 (1958) 457.

DISCUSSION

A.F. STEHNEY: If I may, I should like to supply some additional data
before the discussion on my paper begins.

While I believe that there is good reason to use initial radium intake as a
dose parameter for a time analysis, I presume that you would like some indication
of what the rad doses were. The following are approximations of the alpha-
particle doses only.

The average bone dose for the 759 measured women was about 1200 rads.
If we assume that the bone dose was the same for the unmeasured women, then
the life-shortening per person was 1.8 years per 1200 rads or 0.15 years per
100 rads to the skeleton.

For evaluation of the finding of no life-shortening when risk of radium
tumours is removed, the dose to persons in dose groups without the tumour
should be considered. For those with less than 50 μCi radium intake, the average
bone dose was about 60 rads. The corresponding soft tissue dose, very approximately, was about 1 rad. The weighted average whole-body dose is then about 6 rads
These numbers can be compared with the standard error of about 0.5 year for
our estimates of life expectancy. I might add that the 1972 BEIR report estimated
life-shortening at about one year per 100 rem whole body.

K.F. BAVERSTOCK: Have you observed an excess in breast cancer deaths in this population? I ask this because in the United Kingdom we have a population of luminizers numbering some 1500 persons who worked between 1940 and 1950. Among a sub-population of about 800 young females at the time of occupation we find an excess of breast cancer when comparison is made with national statistics (14 cases observed, 8.5 expected). This sub-population worked for two or more years as luminizers and it is estimated that they may have received whole-body doses of up to 15 rads per year of occupation from radium paint pots and luminized articles. Since there are several complicating factors to be taken into account when comparing breast cancer incidence in a small population with national statistics, any conclusions regarding radiation association with this excess must be provisional at the moment. In view of the small size of our population I should be interested in any similar effects observed in related populations.

A.F. STEHNEY: We did not find breast cancer associated with radium burden in the early United States dial painters. Follow-up data are still being compiled for a mortality study of about 1000 women dial workers of the 1940s.

W.A. MÜLLER: Did you see differences in the incidence of osteosarcomas and in life-shortening according to whether radium intake took place over a short or long period of time?

A.F. STEHNEY: No, but we have not yet fully examined this possible relationship.

V. KLENER: May I comment briefly on the occurrence of other types of cancer among dial painters. In Czechoslovakia we have a small group of about 60 dial painters with fairly low body burdens of ^{226}Ra and ^{90}Sr. In a long-term follow-up we found seven cancers of different parts of the body (two of the skin and one each of the lower large intestine, urinary bladder, lungs, mammary gland and a lymphoreticular cancer) compared with about 1.5 expected. We cannot, as yet, offer any explanation for these findings, however. If radiation contributes to these effects at all, we are inclined to suspect rather the external component of the exposure.

A.F. STEHNEY: We have not found an elevated incidence of these tumours associated with radium dose in the United States dial painters. It would be of interest to see a full report on your cases.

G.W. BEEBE: I seem to recall a paper in which a non-specific life-shortening effect was claimed for this sample. If in fact my recollection is correct, is the explanation for the change in findings a matter of method?

A.F. STEHNEY: On this particular point, I know only of a paper by P.G. Failla and R.E. Rowland that was given at the 1972 meeting of the Radiation Research Society (Portland, Oregon). But they did not find a non-specific life-shortening effect. The authors of that paper did not use interval methods or standardized mortality ratios.

STUDIES ON PERSONS EXPOSED TO PLUTONIUM*

G.L. VOELZ, J.H. STEBBINGS,
L.H. HEMPELMANN, L.K. HAXTON,
D.A. YORK
Los Alamos Scientific Laboratory,
University of California,
Los Alamos,
New Mexico,
United States of America

Abstract

STUDIES ON PERSONS EXPOSED TO PLUTONIUM.

The results of four studies of persons exposed, or potentially exposed, to plutonium are summarized. The studies are: (1) a five-year update on clinical examinations and health experience of 26 Manhattan District workers heavily exposed at Los Alamos in 1944–45; (2) a 30-year mortality follow-up of 224 white male workers with plutonium body burdens of 10 nCi or more; (3) a review of cancer mortality rates between 1950 and 1969 among Los Alamos County, New Mexico, male residents, all of whom have worked in or have lived within a few kilometres of a major plutonium plant and other nuclear facilities; and (4) a review of cancer incidence rates between 1969 and 1974 in male residents of Los Alamos County. No excess of mortality due to any cause was observed in the 224 male subjects with the highest plutonium exposures at Los Alamos. The total cancer and cardiovascular mortality rates were lower than expected based on age and year-specific rates for United States white males. Lung cancer mortality was lower than expected and no bone or liver cancer was experienced. Clinical examinations of the Manhattan District workers, whose average age in 1976 was 56 years, show them to be active persons with diseases that are not unusual for their ages. The two deaths in this group over the past 30 years have not been due to cancer. The mortality study of Los Alamos male residents showed a possible excess of cancers of the combined lymphatic and haematopoietic tissues, but the incidence data suggest this excess, if real, is no longer occurring. Higher than expected incidence of cancers of the digestive tract in Los Alamos males and females is more likely to be due to socio-economic and cultural factors than to occupational exposures. Mortality and incidence data indicate no excess of lung cancer in Los Alamos males.

INTRODUCTION

Research and development work on plutonium has played an important role throughout the entire history of Los Alamos, New Mexico. It began during World War II when Los Alamos, the isolated mountain location of a small private

---

* Work performed under the auspices of the USERDA, Contract W-7405-ENG. 36.

boys' school, was selected as the site for the Manhattan Engineer District's laboratory that was to develop the first atomic bomb.. One of the tasks for the scientists, technicians and craftsmen assigned to the Los Alamos project in 1943–45 was to develop methods to process and fabricate the newly discovered element, plutonium. Other workers were engaged in chemistry, physics and metallurgy research. These workers and their families lived in wartime accommodation located close to the laboratories.

From this unusual beginning, Los Alamos has grown to a community of over 15 000 persons in the 1970s. It is still a one-industry town in which the principal employer is the Los Alamos Scientific Laboratory. Laboratory personnel continue to conduct research in nuclear and particle physics, plasma physics, nuclear chemistry, analytical and physical chemistry, materials science and many other areas of advanced science and technology. Throughout the years, hundreds of persons have continued to work with transuranic elements, especially plutonium. The community residents have been closely associated with Laboratory activities, both as employees in the Laboratory and as neighbours. Some residential areas of the town are still located within a few hundred metres of chemical laboratories and radiation areas, including major plutonium facilities. Probably this community has been more intimately associated with the plutonium industry than has any other community.

Since the early 1950s, 26 Los Alamos workers with high plutonium body burdens received in 1944–45 have been studied clinically for evidence of adverse health effects from internally deposited plutonium. In the 1973 reports on this clinical study [1, 2] no medical findings were reported that could be attributed definitely to plutonium. The study of this small group, although providing valuable clinical information, could not provide the extensive information on late health effects that epidemiologic studies can provide. In 1974, we extended our programme to include a mortality study of all Los Alamos workers with high body burdens of plutonium as a preliminary effort to provide information on an expanded number of workers.

It was also recognized that the cancer incidence and mortality experience of the population of Los Alamos County might provide useful and important information. This population has lived close enough to the Laboratory facilities to make it useful to attempt to detect potential effects of Laboratory operations, including effects of possible exposures to low environmental levels of chemical or radioactive effluents. Furthermore, as we have seen, a large proportion of the adult population works at the Laboratory and has a potential for occupational exposures to chemicals, radiation and other hazards. Epidemiologic studies on the Los Alamos County population serve as a screening mechanism for possible health effects.

We have here summarized the methods and results of our four studies on plutonium workers and the general population of Los Alamos County.

METHODS AND RESULTS

Clinical study of early Los Alamos plutonium workers

A group of 26 persons, who had worked with plutonium for the Manhattan Engineer District project at Los Alamos in 1944 and 1945, has been followed with medical examinations periodically since 1953. The subjects were selected for this study based on their exposure history and relatively high plutonium excretion values in urine. The principal mode of exposure was by inhalation. Five of these individuals had contaminated wounds that were excised surgically; only one of these wounds contained a significant amount of plutonium.

Current plutonium body burden estimates on these persons range from 6 to 230 nCi, or 15 to 575% of the 40 nCi maximum permissible body burden for lifetime occupational exposure [3, 4]. Eleven persons in the group are estimated currently to have body burdens in excess of 40 nCi.

The latest medical re-examinations of the 24 living subjects in the study were completed in 1976 and 1977. Two deaths have occurred in the group: one in 1959 due to myocardial infarction in a 36-year-old male and the second in 1975 in a 50-year-old male due to an auto-pedestrian accident.

The latest examinations included complete medical history, physical examination, blood chemistry profiles, haematologic studies, including chromosome analysis of peripheral lymphocytes, sputum cytology, radioanalysis for plutonium in urine, blood and faeces samples, and X-ray studies of the chest, pelvis, femur and teeth. All but two persons were counted with phoswich detectors for plutonium in the chest, liver and hands, and with a large, NaI(Tl) detector for other radionuclides. No unusual radioactivity was found in the 22 subjects, except for 5 ± 2 nCi of plutonium detected in a wound site that was excised in 1944. The two persons who did not have in-vivo measurements made did not travel to Los Alamos for their medical examinations, and the only plutonium measurements on them at this time were made on urine samples.

The mean age of the group in 1976 was 56 years. The current examinations have shown these individuals to be active persons with diseases that are not unusual for their ages. The most significant diagnoses were one case each of coronary heart disease, total blindness due to glaucoma, hypertension with electrocardiographic evidence of left ventricular hypertrophy, and bronchitis and early emphysema in a heavy smoker. This last person had marked atypia of exfoliated cells in sputum in the 1971—72 studies, but subsequent sputum examinations have shown less severe changes. No subjects were found to have abnormal lung cytology in the latest samples. X-ray evidence of bone changes was discovered in two individuals. Neither has had symptoms due to these bone lesions nor have they required treatment. One individual, a 63-year-old male with a plutonium body burden above 40 nCi, has slowly progressive Paget's

Disease (osteitis deformans) which, in retrospect, can be seen on previous X-rays dating back to 1965. The second individual, 54-years-old with a body burden less than 40 nCi, has developed a small area of bone sclerosis in the pelvis since the last X-rays were taken in 1960. These findings are probably not unexpected in a group of this age. For example, X-ray studies show that about 3% of persons over age 40 have Paget's disease; the prevalence increases to about 10% of persons in their 80s [5]. It affects men more often than women, and the pelvis is the bone most commonly affected.

Histories of two skin cancers, a localized melanoma of the anterior chest and an epithelioma on the back of the hand, have been noted in the study. Both lesions were treated with local surgical excision over five years ago and neither has recurred. No other cancers have occurred in the group. Three benign tumours have been noted: a haemartoma of the lung, a tumour of the nerve sheath, possibly a neurilemoma, located in a tooth, and a small transient thyroid nodule that is no longer evident.

Mortality study of 224 Los Alamos plutonium workers

A study of the mortality experience of all Los Alamos area plutonium workers with estimated body burdens of 10 nCi or more has been completed. Selection of persons for this study was done by review of the health physics records at the Los Alamos Scientific Laboratory. All persons with plutonium burdens equal to or greater than 10 nCi by urine assay as of 1 January 1974 according to the version of the PUQFUA Code [6] then in use were identified. That Code incorporated assumptions that, for the radiological protection of workers, overestimated plutonium body burdens in some cases [7]. An update of that Code is now used which is designed to give an estimate closer to actual deposition values. Had the current version of PUQFUA been in use, the subjects would have been classified only slightly differently but there would have been fewer in the study. Body burdens for the clinical study group discussed above were from the current PUQFUA version.

All 241 Anglo-white[1] and Spanish or Spanish-surnamed subjects were followed, but we report here only on the 224 male subjects, 173 Anglo-white and 51 Spanish. Study subjects were individually followed through 30 June 1976 to determine mortality status. Follow-up was 100% complete through June 1976; there were no untraceable individuals with burdens above 10 nCi despite the thirty-year period of follow-up on most subjects.

---

[1] In New Mexico the term Anglo is used in some state statistics to designate white persons not of Spanish heritage. There are some differences in disease morbidity and mortality rates between the Anglo-white and Spanish populations in New Mexico.

TABLE I.   30-YEAR MORTALITY IN 224 WHITE MALE PLUTONIUM
WORKERS

	Observed	Expected	Obs./Exp.
All causes of death	33	61.3	0.54
All malignant neoplasms	7	10.9	0.64
All diseases of circulatory system	12	31.8	0.38
All respiratory diseases	3	3.3	0.92
All external causes	8	6.9	1.16
Other	3	8.4	0.36

Average year of entry: 1947.4

Average age of entry: 30.9

Total person-years of survival: 6205

Subjects were entered into the study cohort mid-year of the year of their
first recorded urine test or of the recorded accident by which they presumably
were first exposed. Most subjects would not have received their current or final
body burden until some time after entry into the cohort. Because exposure
protection was less in earlier years, during and shortly after World War II, and
because most of the subjects were young when exposed and are only now
incurring significant risk of mortality, the precise timing of the major exposure
would not significantly affect either observed or expected mortality.

Mortality analysis was carried out using a computer program developed and
described by Monson [8]. Age and calendar-year adjusted expected numbers of
deaths, based on United States white male rates, were generated and compared
with observed numbers of deaths for each cause as coded (ICDA 8) from the
death certificates obtained on deceased subjects. Coding of death certificates
has not yet been reviewed by an experienced nosologist, but the very few
problematic certificates would not significantly affect the conclusions reported
in this paper.

Table I describes some characteristics of the cohort of 224 white male
plutonium workers and the standardized mortality ratios (SMRs) for broad
categories of deaths. Nearly all subjects entered the cohort in the middle or
late 1940s, as shown by the average year of entry, 1947.4. The cohort was
young at entry, the mean age being 30.9.

The SMR for total mortality was 0.54 ($p < 0.001$), for all malignant
neoplasms 0.64 (not significant), and for diseases of the circulatory system

TABLE II.   30-YEAR CANCER MORTALITY IN 224 WHITE MALE
PLUTONIUM WORKERS

	Observed	Expected
Buccal cavity and pharynx	1	0.39
Stomach	1	0.67
Large intestine	1	0.96
Rectum	1	0.39
Lung	1	3.20
Bladder	1	0.31
Lymphosarcoma, etc.	1	0.29
All digestive organs	3	3.20
All respiratory system	1	3.44
All lymphopoietic	1	1.17

0.38 (p < 0.001). SMRs for respiratory diseases and external causes were near
unity. Results when Anglo-white and Spanish subjects are analysed separately
are consistent with the results presented above.

Cancer is an outcome of special interest in studies of plutonium, and Table II
shows observed and expected numbers of cancer for all sites for which a cancer
was observed. For no site was there a clear excess; for lung cancer there is an
observed deficit. Tests of statistical significance are not useful when observed
and expected numbers are as small as this.

Cancer mortality in Los Alamos County male residents

The portion of the Los Alamos County mortality study reported here
concerns only cancer mortality in males. Demographic data are from the
1970 United States Census published in the *City and County Data Book* [9].
Cancer rates are from Mason and McKay's *U.S. Cancer Mortality by County:
1950–1969* [10], and some data on statistical significance are taken from
Mason and co-workers' *Atlas of Cancer Mortality for U.S. Counties: 1950–1969*
[11].

Published cancer rates for white males in Los Alamos County are compared
with rates for the State of New Mexico and for the United States of America.
In addition, Los Alamos County white male cancer rates are compared with
rates in five socio-economic and occupational control counties and in five high
education Western control counties.

From all U.S. counties with a population above 5000 and a median income rank $\leqslant 1000$, the two counties in the United States of America most closely bracketing Los Alamos County were selected with respect to four criteria: median education, median family income, percentage professional and managerial, and percentage government employees. This process, because of correlation among attributes, yields five rather than eight counties: Pitkin, Colorado; Montgomery, Maryland; Mineral, Nevada; Tooele, Utah; and Fairfax, Virginia.

From the remaining counties we selected all Western counties with a median education $\geqslant 12.8$ years for persons aged 25 and above. These were: Marin, California; Boulder, Colorado; Benton, Oregon; Whitman, Washington; and Albany, Wyoming. In this report only summary data for the control counties will be given.

Tests of significance for cancer mortality data are based either on a method given by Chiang [12] for age-adjusted rates or, when small observed numbers are involved, on a method given by Haenszel and co-workers [13] based on the Poisson distribution.

Table III shows cancer death rates in Los Alamos County of white males between 1950 and 1969. Most of the male residents were employed by one of two Atomic Energy Commission contractors at Los Alamos or by the Atomic Energy Commission directly. Interpretation is made difficult by the small number of observed and expected deaths. The county population was young in 1950 and has been aging in the same way as the occupational cohort. Mortality due to all cancer was low compared with that in the United States of America as a whole, and is almost identical with that in the State of New Mexico.

In general, deaths from cancer of the digestive tract were significantly less common in Los Alamos males between 1950 and 1969 than in United States males; only liver cancer did not differ significantly according to Mason and McKay [9]. Lung cancer has been notably and significantly low during this period. Bladder and prostatic cancer have been high, but the number of deaths involved is too small to draw any conclusion.

Lymphosarcoma and leukaemia have been high, but not statistically significantly high when looked at separately. Because of the respectable number of deaths involved, ten, it was decided to look at all cancer of lymphatic and haematopoietic tissue. A total of 15 were observed: 2 Hodgkin's, 4 lymphosarcoma, 3 multiple myeloma and 6 leukaemia. The total expected was computed from available published data as the sum of: (the observed deaths, for each specific cause) $\times$ (U.S. age-adjusted rate)/(Los Alamos County age-adjusted rate). A standardized mortality ratio of 1.63 (15 observed, 9.2 expected) was obtained; by the method of Haenszel [13] the lower limit of its 95% confidence interval is 0.913. The excess of cancers of the lymphatic and haematopoietic tissues is, then, not statistically significant at the 5% level but is a borderline finding.

TABLE III. CANCER MORTALITY RATES[a] IN LOS ALAMOS COUNTY, NEW MEXICO, AND UNITED STATES WHITE MALES, 1950–69

	Los Alamos County	New Mexico	United States	Significance[b] of difference between Los Alamos Co. & U.S. White cancer rates		
	Rate Cases	Rate	Rate	Direction	Mason & McKay[c]	Poisson[d]
Stomach	3.5 (3)	17.96	15.22	Low	p < 0.05	p < 0.05
Large intestine	8.8 (4)	9.15	16.54	Low	p < 0.05	NS
Rectum	2.8 (2)	3.39	7.65	Low	p < 0.05	NS
Biliary passages & liver	6.3 (2)	5.33	5.16	High	NS	NS
Pancreas	1.0 (1)	8.79	9.63	Low	p < 0.05	p < 0.05
Trachea, bronchus & lung	12.0 (8)	24.71	37.98	Low	p < 0.05	p < 0.05
Prostate	30.3 (3)	15.87	17.84	High	–[e]	NS
Bladder	15.7 (3)	3.97	6.78	High	NS	NS
Brain and . . . nervous system	4.9 (5)	3.30	4.42	High	NS	NS
Lymphosarcoma and reticulosarcoma, etc.	7.1 (4)	3.64	4.89	High	NT	NS
Leukaemia	16.3 (6)	7.71	8.81	High	NT	NS
All malignant neoplasms	142.6 (54)	136.30	174.04	Low	NS	NS

[a] Direct age-adjusted average annual rates per 100 000 population, 1950–69; from *U.S. Cancer Mortality by County: 1950–1969* (Ref. [10]).

[b] Two-sided probability (p); NS means not significant, NT means not tested.

[c] The 95% confidence intervals for the local and national rates do not overlap; from maps in Ref. [11]. Confidence intervals by method of Chiang (Ref. [12]).

[d] National rate outside 95% confidence limits for estimate of a Poisson-distributed variable (Ref. [13]).

[e] Ref. [11] appears to be in error.

Cancer mortality rates in Los Alamos County males are also compared with rates in two groups of control counties in Table IV. Results are very similar to those in the previous analysis, but the frequency with which rates in Los Alamos were highest or lowest emphasizes the unique character of the Los Alamos County male population. Again digestive cancer rates were very low, lung cancer was very low, and lymphosarcoma and leukaemia were highest. Liver, prostate and bladder cancer, whose rates are all based on very small numbers, showed the same pattern as previously.

Close control, then, of the socio-economic characteristics of Los Alamos County does not change the conclusions drawn concerning cancer mortality based on national and state comparisons.

Cancer incidence in Anglo-white males, 1969–74

A study of cancer incidence rates in Los Alamos County residents in recent years supplements the above mortality study. Data on cancer incidence in Los Alamos County were obtained from the New Mexico Tumor Registry of the Cancer Research and Treatment Center at the University of New Mexico. Data are from the registry data base as of October 1976 for the years 1969 through 1974. The data for Anglo-white males are presented in Table V and compared with data from Albuquerque (the largest urban area in New Mexico) and from the entire State of New Mexico for Anglo-white males. Again only small numbers are available for comparison.

Incidence rates for cancers of the digestive tract are high compared with rates in either Albuquerque or the entire state. The standardized morbidity ratio for cancer of the large intestine is 2.35 relative to New Mexico, 2.02 relative to Albuquerque. Lower 95% confidence limits are 1.17 and 1.01, suggesting statistically significantly elevated rates. For all cancer of the digestive tract the corresponding standardized morbidity ratios are 2.33 and 2.02 (lower 95% confidence limits 1.48 and 1.28).

Lung cancer incidence rates were not low, as were mortality rates, but there is no suggestion they were above average during this 1969 to 1974 period. There is also no suggestion that leukaemia and lymphoma incidence rates were above average during this period.

DISCUSSION

These studies provide some insight into the incidence and mortality rates of cancer in persons who have lived and worked in close association with the nuclear industry, especially plutonium research and development. The findings on the individuals with highest occupational exposures to plutonium are of

TABLE IV. CANCER MORTALITY RATES[a] IN LOS ALAMOS COUNTY AND CONTROL COUNTY WHITE MALES, 1950–69

	Los Alamos County	Socio-economic control counties	High education Western control counties	Rank[b] of cancer rates in Los Alamos Co. relative to		
				Socio-economic & occupational controls	High education Western controls	All controls combined
	Rate (Cases)	(range of five)	(range of five)	(rank n = 6)	(rank n = 6)	(rank n = 11)
Stomach	3.5 (3)	7.0 – 13.7	10.9 – 13.8	6	6	11
Large intestine	8.8 (4)	6.4 – 25.5	10.2 – 16.4	5	6	10
Rectum	2.8 (2)	0.0 – 6.5	4.7 – 8.4	5	6	10
Biliary passages & liver	6.3 (2)	0.0 – 4.2	3.7 – 4.3	1	1	1
Pancreas	1.0 (1)	8.9 – 10.5	7.0 – 12.0	6	6	11
Trachea, bronchus & lung	12.0 (8)	36.8 – 45.0	18.6 – 37.5	6	6	11
Prostate	30.3 (3)	17.2 – 25.8	16.8 – 22.8	1	1	1
Bladder	15.7 (3)	0.0 – 12.7	5.5 – 8.0	1	1	1
Brain and . . . nervous system	4.9 (5)	0.0 – 5.8	2.3 – 7.9	2	2	3
Lymphosarcoma & reticulosarcoma, etc.	7.1 (4)	1.6 – 6.0	1.3 – 6.2	1	1	1
Leukaemia	16.3 (6)	3.8 – 9.2	9.0 – 11.4	1	1	1
All malignant neoplasms	142.6 (54)	159.4 – 175.0	134.7 – 173.9	6	3	8

[a] Direct age-adjusted average annual rates per 100 000 population, 1950–69, from U.S. Cancer Mortality by County: 1950–1969 (Ref.[11]).
[b] Rank 1 is highest rate of group, 6 or 11 lowest.

TABLE V.   ANGLO-WHITE MALE CANCER INCIDENCE RATES IN
NEW MEXICO, 1969—74[a]

Neoplasms	Los Alamos Co.		Bernalillo County (Albuquerque)	New Mexico
	Cases	Rate	Rate	Rate
Stomach	3	28.4	8.1	8.8
Large intestine	11	60.7	30.0	25.8
Rectum	3	38.2	15.1	11.7
Biliary passages & liver	2	5.7	6.2	5.6
Pancreas	4	29.3	12.5	10.0
Trachea, bronchus & lung	5	72.4	69.7	63.9
Prostate	6	47.2	80.7	60.0
Bladder	4	61.9	32.2	20.7
Brain and . . . nervous system	2	3.7	7.7	6.4
Lymphosarcoma & reticulosarcoma, etc.	3	6.5	6.6	7.1
Leukaemia	5	12.7	15.2	13.1
All malignant neoplasms Rate		420.2	380.0	311.0
Cases	62	1739	4696	

[a]   Rates are per 100 000, age-adjusted to U.S. 1970 population. Source is New Mexico
Tumor Registry of October 1976 for years 1969—74. Rates are based on ICDA 8
classification but may be compared with rates based on ICD 6.

special interest. In 26 workers heavily exposed 32 years ago, and followed by
periodic medical examinations since 1953, only two cancers, both of the skin,
have been recorded. No excess of cancer mortality was noted after a 30-year
follow-up period among the 224 white male plutonium workers whose body
burdens in 1974 were estimated to be above 10 nCi. Their cardiovascular disease
death rates were also notably low. Cancers of bone and liver were absent in
these occupational groups, and lung cancer was less than expected based on
United States white male mortality rates.
     Interpretation of cancer mortality and morbidity data on male residents
of Los Alamos is complicated by a lack of consistency among some findings.
The findings are also based upon small numbers, and are thus subject to
proportionately large random errors. It should also be noted that incidence

rates do not necessarily show the same detailed patterns as mortality rates, especially in the case of cancers with significant five-year survival.

The highly unusual characteristics of Los Alamos community residents could affect expected cancer rates in unpredictable ways. These characteristics include a security clearance required for employment, a high educational level compared even with university communities, a socio-economic status ranking with the highest counties in the United States of America, and an isolated non-urban residence. Further, government housing policy linked eligibility for government housing, the only housing available in the county until about 1960, to active employment in the community. This policy could conceivably have led seriously ill persons to move elsewhere; that the policy was never enforced on seriously ill residents was not generally known. Also, because Los Alamos was a newly created community, a tendency for seriously ill persons to return to home communities and be certified at death as residents there might be expected.

No attempt will be made to give all possible explanations for the results presented, but we shall set forth a set of hypotheses which seem reasonable to us.

A borderline excess of deaths due to the combined cancers of the lymphatic and haematopoietic tissues did appear in Los Alamos male residents between 1950 and 1969. Neither mortality rates in females from 1950 to 1969 nor incidence rates in males from 1969 to 1974 were high. This suggests that any excess, if real, was probably occupationally induced prior to employment at Los Alamos or during early years when controls of all hazards, including chemicals, in the work place were not up to current standards. Tumours of lymphatic and haematopoietic tissue differ in aetiology, and it is not suggested that any one factor could be expected to be responsible. Before and during Los Alamos employment some workers could be expected to have been exposed to various hazards of modern technology, including radiation in all its forms and organic and inorganic chemicals.

High incidence rates of cancers of the digestive tract in white males were noted from 1969 to 1974, although mortality from these cancers was significantly low between 1950 and 1969. Digestive cancer mortality rates in females were significantly high from 1950 through 1969, and the incidence rates in females remained above average from 1969 to 1974. No simple explanation is possible, but occupational exposures seem a less likely explanation than socio-economic and cultural factors, counteracted at first by an exaggerated healthy worker effect. Males were selected for active military service originally, and since 1945 for active employment in a demanding industry and for regional geographic mobility. Females were subject to selection in most cases only by marriage to such males. Both sexes could share the same white-ethnic, social or behavioural risk factors, counteracted in the males during the first years by the strong healthy worker, healthy migrant, and/or healthy military effects.

It should be noted that neither mortality nor incidence data suggest an excess of cancer of the lung in the male population of Los Alamos County.

Future studies

Whereas the present study has yielded no evidence of excessive mortality among 224 male plutonium workers, a more extensive study is required. We are currently undertaking a follow-up study of all plutonium workers at Los Alamos; Rocky Flats, Colorado; Mound, Ohio; Savannah River, South Carolina; Hanford, Washington; and Oak Ridge, Tennessee. These plutonium workers, both with and without measurable plutonium burdens, plus unexposed controls, will total about 20 000 study subjects.

Case-control studies of individuals with cancer in Los Alamos County since 1950 are also under way. These studies will investigate Los Alamos employment and past job histories, known radiation exposures, neighbourhood of residence, and any other factors that can be determined from existing records. We believe these studies will shed needed light on the observations in this paper.

ACKNOWLEDGEMENTS

The authors would like to thank C.R. Key and R.W. Buechley of the New Mexico Tumor Registry for furnishing data on Los Alamos County from their data base.

REFERENCES

[1] HEMPELMANN, L.H., LANGHAM, W.H., RICHMOND, C.R., VOELZ, G.L., Manhattan Project plutonium workers: A twenty-seven year follow-up study of selected cases. Health Phys. 25 (1973) 461.
[2] HEMPELMANN, L.H., RICHMOND, C.R., VOELZ, G.L., A Twenty-seven Year Study of Selected Los Alamos Plutonium Workers, USAEC, Los Alamos Scientific Laboratory Rep. LA-5148-MS (1973).
[3] NATIONAL COUNCIL ON RADIATION PROTECTION, Maximum Permissible Body Burdens and Maximum Permissible Concentrations of Radionuclides in Air and in Water for Occupational Exposure [Includes Addendum 1 issued in August 1963], NCRP Report No. 22, Washington, D.C. (1959).
[4] Report of ICRP Committee II on Permissible Dose for Internal Radiation (1959), Health Phys. 3 (1960) 1.
[5] BERKOW, R. (Ed.), The Merck Manual of Diagnosis and Therapy, 13th Ed., Merck Sharp and Dohme Research Laboratories, Rahway, New Jersey (1977) 1363.
[6] LAWRENCE, J.N.P., PUQFUA, an IBM 704 code for computing plutonium body burdens, Health Phys. 8 (1962) 61.

[7]   VOELZ, G., UMBARGER, J., McINROY, J., HEALY, J., "Considerations in the
      assessment of plutonium deposition in man", Diagnosis and Treatment of Incorporated
      Radionuclides (Proc. Seminar Vienna, 1975), IAEA, Vienna (1976) 163.
[8]   MONSON, R.R., Analysis of relative survival and proportional mortality, Comput.
      Biomed. Res. 7 (1974) 325.
[9]   U.S. BUREAU OF THE CENSUS, City and County Data Book, 1972, U.S. Government
      Printing Office, Washington, D.C. (1973).
[10] MASON, T.J., McKAY, F.W., U.S. Cancer Mortality by County: 1950–1969, DHEW
      Publication No. (NIH) 74-615 (1974).
[11] MASON, T.J., McKAY, F.W., HOOVER, R., BLOT, W.J., FRAUMENI, J.F., Jr., Atlas
      of Cancer Mortality for U.S. Counties: 1950–1969, DHEW Publication No. (NIH)
      75–780 (1975).
[12] CHIANG, C.L., Standard Error of the Age-Adjusted Death Rate, Vital Statistics —
      Selected Reports 47 9 (1961), U.S. Government Printing Office, Washington, D.C.
[13] HAENSZEL, W., LOVELAND, D.B., SIRKEN, M.G., Lung-cancer mortality as related
      to residence and smoking histories: I. White males., J. Natl. Cancer Inst. 28 (1962) 947.

DISCUSSION

A.F. STEHNEY: I noticed that your table showed an elevated incidence of cancers of the pancreas. Are there any environmental and/or industrial factors that may have had an influence here?

J.H. STEBBINGS: There is reason to believe that cancer of the pancreas is frequently induced by environmental factors and is becoming much more frequent in highly industrialized societies. I am not aware of any specific environmental agents which have been identified. In our study pancreatic cancer, as far as can be determined from the very small number of observed cases, behaves like other cancers of the digestive tract. Mortality was very low from 1950 to 1969 but incidence rates from 1969 to 1974 have been high.

P.G. SMITH: You report some excess of deaths from leukaemia and lymphoma in Los Alamos County in the period 1950–69. Was it possible for you to look at the occupational histories of these patients at the Los Alamos facility, to determine if they had had any unusual exposure to radiation compared with other workers?

J.H. STEBBINGS: Case-control studies of residents of Los Alamos County who have died of cancer, or who have developed it in recent years, are being carried out. These will include subjects with leukaemia and lymphoma. Investigations of plutonium body burden and external radiation exposures will be included in these studies.

V. VOLF: Did you obtain any data on hepatic and pancreatic morbidity in Los Alamos?

J.H. STEBBINGS: We did not, but even if we had tried we would not have been able to obtain reliable and epidemiologically useful data.

A.M. STEWART: You quoted 2% as the expected incidence of Paget's disease but this figure relates to a special X-ray study, and the spontaneous incidence is much lower. Were the plutonium workers screened for bone diseases or not?

J.H. STEBBINGS: It is the prevalence, not incidence, of Paget's disease which is about 3% in persons in their 40s. This prevalence is of disease seen in X-ray series, not the frequency of reported clinical diagnoses of disease. X-ray screening for bone disease is part of the routine follow-up physical examinations in this clinical study.

CANCER MORTALITY IN
HANFORD WORKERS*

S. MARKS, E.S. GILBERT
Battelle, Pacific Northwest Laboratory,
Richland

B.D. BREITENSTEIN
Hanford Environmental Health Foundation,
Richland,
Washington,
United States of America

Abstract

CANCER MORTALITY IN HANFORD WORKERS.

Personnel and radiation exposure data for past and present employees of the Hanford plant have been collected and analysed for a possible relationship of exposure to mortality. The occurrence of death in workers was established by the Social Security Administration and the cause of death obtained from death certificates. Mortality from all causes, all cancer cases and specific cancer types was related to the population at risk. Standardized mortality ratios were calculated for white males, using age- and calendar year-specific mortality rates for the U.S. population in the calculation of expected deaths. This analysis showed a substantial 'healthy worker effect' and no significantly high standardized mortality ratios for specific disease categories. A test for association of mortality with levels of radiation exposure revealed no correlation for all causes and all cancer. In carrying out this test, adjustment was made for age and calendar year of death, length of employment and occupational category. A statistically significant test for trend was obtained for multiple myeloma and carcinoma of the pancreas. However, in view of the absence of such a correlation for diseases more commonly associated with radiation exposure such as myeloid leukaemia, as well as the small number of deaths in higher exposure groups, the results cannot be considered definitive. Any conclusions based on these associations should be viewed in relation to the results of other studies. These results are compared with those of other investigators who have analysed the Hanford data.

INTRODUCTION

A study of the mortality of workers at the Hanford plant, located at Richland in the southeastern part of the State of Washington in the United States, has been in progress since 1964. The initial purpose of the plant was the manufacture, chemical separation and purification of plutonium. In addition, supporting research of a diverse character and, more recently, power generation have been conducted at the facility. The study was

---

* Work performed for the U.S. Department of Energy under Contract E(45−1)−1830.

initiated by the U.S. Atomic Energy Commission and then sponsored succes-
sively by the Energy Research and Development Administration and now the
Department of Energy. In addition to the study of Hanford workers, data
have been collected at the Oak Ridge, Mound Laboratories, and several
uranium feed plants for the investigation of the health of workers. As in
many occupational epidemiologic studies, mortality was selected as the
most reliable and feasible measure of health. The principal investigator
for the study was Dr. Thomas F. Mancuso of the University of Pittsburgh
Graduate School of Public Health. Data for the Hanford and Oak Ridge
plants were collected and processed on site. The Hanford Environmental
Health Foundation, the contractor for occupational health services at the
Hanford plant, collected data for the Hanford facility.

Hanford mortality data have been analyzed by Dr. Barkev Sanders, who
was associated with the study as Dr. Mancuso's statistician from 1964 to
1976 [1-4]; by Dr. Samuel Milham, Jr., of the Department of Social and
Health Services of the State of Washington in 1974 [5]; by one of the
authors of this paper (E.S.G.) since 1975 at the Pacific Northwest
Laboratories (PNL) in Richland (operated for the Department of Energy by
Battelle Memorial Institute)[6]; by Drs Alice Stewart and George Kneale,
who have conducted analyses for Dr. Mancuso since 1976 [7]; and by
Dr. Charles E. Land since 1976[8]. This report will present the PNL
results based on currently available data and will provide comments on
the other studies.

EMPLOYEE DATA

Employment and radiation exposure records have been kept on all
employees since the plant was built. The employment records include data
on age, sex, race, dates of employment and termination, and job classification. In defining a study population, we excluded persons hired after
1965[1], leaving 20 842 white males, 7 721 white females, 185 nonwhite males
and 63 nonwhite females. In the analysis we focused our attention on
the largest group, the white males.

Life status was established by a Social Security Administration (SSA)
search of their files. The SSA search fails to discover the deaths of a
limited number of individuals for whom no death claims are filed. One
available estimate of the percentage of deaths missed in this manner is
6% [9]. Death certificates were obtained from the states where deaths
occurred, and the cause of death was coded according to the eighth revision
of the International Classification of Diseases (ICD). Among deaths
reported by the SSA, death certificates were obtained for 96.8% of the
white males who died before April 1, 1974, the cutoff date for this study.[2]
For men employed two or more years at Hanford, the group of greater interest in the analysis, certificates were obtained for 97.7%

Our analysis is limited to the consideration of exposure to whole
body, penetrating radiation. The data, consisting of cumulative annual
doses expressed in rem, are obtained primarily from measurements of
personnel dosimeters worn by employees. Although internal exposure data
have been collected on Hanford employees, the number of cases of internal

---

[1] This eliminated only 20 white male deaths for which we had death certificates; of
those only one had a cumulative radiation exposure greater than 1 rem.

[2] Data on deaths occurring after April 1, 1974, are not yet available.

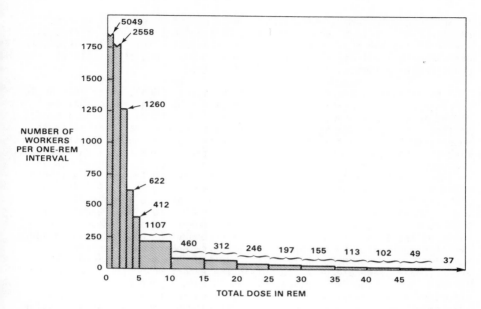

FIG.1. Distribution of cumulative doses for white male workers employed at least two years.

deposition is too small to influence the analysis. Only about 450 veri-
fied cases of internal deposition have occurred in the entire employee
population, including all survivors.

The distribution of cumulative doses through 1973 is presented in
Figure 1. The distribution is highly skewed because the predominant
exposure of most Hanford employees is to natural background radiation
(typically about .1 rem per year), while only a smaller number (perhaps
5 to 10% of the work force) receive annual whole body doses in excess of
1 rem with a very small number of those exceeding 4 rem per year. Because
of the skewed nature of the distribution and the lesser likelihood of
demonstrating effects at low levels, we have chosen to present many of
our results in terms of the number (or percent) of workers with doses
exceeding 5 rem. In general, cumulative radiation exposure is correlated
with length of employment. For example, a breakdown by duration of employment discloses that radiation doses of 5 rem or more were accumulated
by 2 of 7767 (.03%) workers employed <2 years, by 339 of 5470 (6.2%)
employed 2-9 years, by 998 of 3353 (25.9%) employed 9-19 years and by
1439 of 3752 (38.4%) employed 20 or more years.

METHODS OF ANALYSIS

In view of the availability of a defined population base to which
the deaths due to any specific cause can be related, the analysis included
the calculation of population-based mortality ratios and testing for a
possible correlation between mortality and the level of radiation exposure.

In epidemiologic terms, this study is of a cohort or prospective type despite the fact that much of the data were collected from past records. When data for the population at risk are available, this method is usually preferred to a retrospective or case-control approach, especially if quantitative estimates of risk are desired [10].

We calculated standardized mortality ratios (SMRs), which provide in percentage form the ratio of the number of deaths observed to that expected in the same population or subgroup (100 x observed deaths ÷ expected deaths). Expected deaths, corrected for age and calendar year of death, were based on U.S. vital statistics for deaths occurring in the same five-year age and calendar year group. In the application of this method, the years of observation are allocated to the appropriate categories as in the following example. A person who initiates employment on his 26th birthday at the beginning of 1953 and survives until April 1974 (the cut-off date for the study) will have 2 years allocated to the age 25-29, year 1950-54 category; 2 years to the age 25-29, year 1955-59 category; 3 years to the age 30-34, year 1955-59 category; and so forth. For any disease, the total person-years in each category in the study population are then multiplied by the appropriate age-calendar year-specific mortality rates for U.S. white males, and the results are summed over age-calendar year categories to obtain the expected number of deaths due to that cause. The SMRs are calculated in this manner by means of a computer program developed by Monson [11], which provides SMRs for 23 categories of cancer and 34 other disease categories. The cause-specific SMRs are corrected for the 2-4% of deaths with no certificates on the reasonable assumption that the distribution of causes is similar for identified deaths with and without death certificates. Statistical significance of the SMRs was tested by a continuity corrected chi-square test.

The interpretation of SMRs is conditioned by the 'healthy worker effect', which is the reduction in the values of SMRs that is observed frequently in the case of workers in industries free of serious life threatening hazards [12]. The health of employees may be favorably influenced by pre-employment screening, health insurance and medical surveillance programs and by the socioeconomic benefits of steady employment. For these reasons, SMRs below 100 are not interpreted to signify protective effects of exposure factors. On the other hand, low SMRs are not compatible with important adverse effects but, instead, may reflect a favorable health experience under the conditions of employment. More importantly, in our results as in other studies, the magnitude of the healthy worker effect varies with the disease category. The SMRs are likely to be higher for cancer than for most other diseases because the factors responsible for the healthy worker effect are less likely to be effective for most cancer types than for other causes of death, such as cardiovascular disease [13]. This differential effect tends to bias proportional mortality analyses toward falsely indicating an excess of cancer [14].

In our analysis for a possible relationship of radiation exposure to mortality rates, we categorized the workers with respect to their cumulative exposure at a given time and then compared the subsequent mortality experience of the various exposure groups. Only past exposure to radiation is included for a stated time since future exposure would be correlated with survival. Four groups were selected with arbitrary cutpoints at <2, 2-5, 5-15 and >15 rem. Since these analyses are concerned with com-

parisons between workers grouped according to exposure, expected deaths
are calculated from the combined experience of the groups under consideration, using the Mantel-Haenszel method [15]. Such expected values should
not be confused with those calculated previously on the basis of U.S.
vital statistics mortality rates. To illustrate this method of calculating expected rates, assume that there are P person-years and d deaths from
all causes for a particular age group. If, in exposure category i, there
are P_i person-years for that age group, the value for expected deaths in
group i will be $\frac{P_i}{P}$ x d. Similar calculations can be made for all age
groups and the results summed to obtain the total number of deaths that
would be expected in group i if mortality rates are not affected by
exposure. The total number of deaths expected for a given exposure
category can then be compared with the number actually observed.

The possibility of a relationship between mortality and radiation
exposure was analyzed by means of a statistical test for trend. The population defined for this analysis included only white males employed at
least two years and excluded those who had terminated employment before
January 1, 1960. Of the 2278 men with total doses exceeding 5 rem, only
77 (2.8%) fail to meet these criteria while only 3 (0.2%) of the 1211
men with total doses exceeding 15 rem are excluded from this group. The
population was grouped according to exposure categories of <2, 2-5, 5-15
and >15 rem. In order to avoid biases in the comparison, the groups were
adjusted for age (in 5 year intervals), occupational category (craftsmen
and operators vs. others) and calendar year combined with employment
status in three strata.[3] Mantel's single degree of freedom chi-square test
for trend, which accounts for the influence of the above factors, was
used [16]. The test requires the assignment of scores to each group; we
selected the median of each of the four groups as its score, i.e. 0.80,
3.21, 7.85 and 21.32. For a few causes of death, an exact permutation
test was used in place of the chi-square because of the small number of
deaths and the severely skewed nature of the distribution of radiation
exposures in the worker population.

RESULTS

Standardized mortality ratios are presented for a variety of causes
of death for white males grouped according to length of employment
(<2, 2+ years) in Tables I and II. The reader may wish to adjust the SMRs
for missing deaths by adding an increment of 6% in accordance with the
estimate cited above. The SMR for deaths from all causes among workers
employed at least two years is 75, which may be interpreted to mean that
the number of observed deaths is 75% of that expected on the basis of
age-calendar year-specific rates for U.S. white males. In the case of
workers employed less than two years, the SMR is 86. These low values are
compatible with the healthy worker effect discussed above [13]. The SMRs
for all cancer cases are 85 for 2+ years and 88 for <2 years, which are

---

[3] Stratum 1 — employed 2 years and working on January 1, 1960; stratum 2 — those
of stratum 1 who terminate employment before January 1, 1965 but are alive on that date;
stratum 3 — employed 2 years and working on January 1, 1965 (mostly derived from stratum 1).
The three strata, which are not mutually exclusive, account for employment period (termination
before or after 1965) and time of death (before or after 1965). Cumulative exposure is calculated to 1960 or 1965, depending upon the stratum.

TABLE I. OBSERVED DEATHS, EXPECTED DEATHS AND STANDARDIZED MORTALITY RATIOS (SMRs) FOR MAJOR CAUSES OF DEATH IN WHITE MALES GROUPED BY LENGTH OF EMPLOYMENT

	Length of employment					
	< 2 Years			2 + Years		
Population at risk	7767			13 075		
Number with 5+ rem cumulative dose	2			2 778		
Cause of death	Obs.	Exp.[a]	SMR	Obs.	Exp.	SMR
All causes	1905	2216.6	86	2089	2796.8	75
All malignant neoplasms (140–209)[b]	319	363.0	88	414	487.7	85
Diseases of the circulatory system (390–429, 440–458)	839	965.4	87	955	1254.2	76
Accidents, poisonings and violence (800–999)	243	222.9	109	216	288.8	75
All other causes	423	568.1	74	455	700.8	65
No death certificate[c]	81			49		

[a] Expected deaths are calculated from age-calendar year-specific U.S. mortality rates for white males, 1945–1967.

[b] International Classification of Diseases (ICD) codes.

[c] Expected deaths and SMRs are corrected for those deaths with no crtificates on the assumption that the distribution of causes is similar for those with and without certificates.

greater than the SMRs for all causes. The less marked healthy worker effect for cancer than for other diseases in those employed at least two years is attributed to a lesser impact of the benefits of employee selection and prolonged employment on cancer than on most other diseases as discussed previously. For specific cancer types the distribution of SMRs in Table II is more or less random relative to the reference value of 100; there are more SMRs below than above 100. The only statistically significant SMRs are those for all malignant neoplasms, carcinoma of the lung and leukemia, all of which are low. SMRs below 100 should not be interpreted as evidence that environmental factors such as radiation are protective. It is equally misleading to conclude that SMRs above 100 are representative of radiation effects while those below 100 are due to random variation. Random variation will account for SMRs both above and below 100. In addition, biases must be considered along with causative factors to account for SMRs that are statistically significantly low or high

Since myeloid leukemia is a cause of death for which an association with radiation exposure has been demonstrated consistently [17, 18], additional detail for this disease and for other neoplasms of lymphatic and hematopoietic tissue is presented in Tables III and IV. Table III shows the relevant cause of death categories for which published U.S. vital statistics are available prior to 1968 while Table IV shows a more detailed breakdown based on vital statistics available since 1968 when the eighth revision of the ICD was implemented. Table IV includes deaths occurring from 1965 to 1974. Only about half the expected number of leukemia deaths are observed in Table III. This deficiency is still present to a lesser extent in Table IV where only experience and deaths from 1965 to 1974 are considered. For the latter period the deficiency in leukemia deaths is confined to the lymphatic type; observed and expected deaths are approximately equal for other types, including myeloid leukemia, which is most likely to be influenced by radiation exposure.

In Table V, the observed and expected deaths for the four exposure categories and results of the test for trend are presented for all causes of death, all cancer, and several specific cancer types. A significant test for trend is determined by a generally increasing ratio of observed over expected deaths with increasing exposure. The categories of all causes and all malignant neoplasms do not show a significant trend with increasing radiation exposure. For all malignant neoplasms 26 deaths are observed in comparison with 29.8 expected. Among the individual cancer types, only multiple myeloma ($p = .01$) and carcinoma of the pancreas ($p = .03$) are statistically significant. The numbers of deaths in the higher exposure categories are small for the individual cancer types. For multiple myeloma, there is 1 observed vs. 0.8 expected in the 5-15 rem group and 2 observed vs. 0.4 expected in the 15+ rem group. For carcinoma of the pancreas, 1 death is observed vs. 2 expected in the 5-15 rem group and 3 observed vs. 1 expected in the 15+ rem group. The highest two exposure groups showed no excess of observed over expected deaths for lung cancer; leukemia and brain are not noteworthy; prostate and the category of other digestive organs are examples of types for which fewer deaths are observed than expected.

As an additional means of summarizing our data, mortality rates for white males, aged 25-70, included in the exposure analysis discussed above, were calculated. The rates, expressed in deaths per 1000 and adjusted for age, occupational category and calendar year, are presented in Table VI. U.S. mortality rates as applied to this population are included for comparison.

DISCUSSION

Neither the SMRs nor the analysis of trend relative to exposure levels indicate an association of radiation with overall mortality or with malignant neoplasms as a group. The only statistically significant tests for trend were obtained with multiple myeloma and carcinoma of the pancreas. However, these diseases are not typically associated with radiation exposure. Myeloid leukemia and carcinoma of the lung, which have been identified as associated with radiation exposure in several studies [17,18], were not present in excess in this population and failed to show a correlation of mortality with level of exposure.

TABLE II. OBSERVED DEATHS, EXPECTED DEATHS AND STANDARDIZED MORTALITY RATIOS (SMRs) FOR SPECIFIC CANCER TYPES IN WHITE MALES GROUPED BY LENGTH OF EMPLOYMENT

| | Length of employment | | | | | |
| | < 2 Years | | | 2 + Years | | |
	Obs.	Exp.[a]	SMR	Obs.	Exp.	SMR
All malignant neoplasms (M.N.) (140–209)[b]	319	363.0	88	414	487.7	85
M.N. of buccal cavity and pharynx (140–149)	6	12.6	48	18	17.0	106
M.N. of esophagus (150)	8	8.7	92	11	11.9	93
M.N. of stomach (151)	17	27.8	61	23	33.3	69
M.N. of large intestine (153)	23	33.5	69	44	43.6	101
M.N. of rectum (154)	6	15.0	40	13	19.0	68
M.N. of liver (155, 156)	12	10.7	112	7	13.6	51
M.N. of pancreas (157)	27	20.7	130	28	28.1	100
M.N. of larynx (161)	5	8.8	57	5	7.9	63
M.N. of lung (162)	93	101.5	92	115	147.7	78
M.N. of prostate (185)	24	24.0	100	25	27.8	90
M.N. of kidney (189.0)	9	9.0	100	13	12.5	104
M.N. of bladder (188, 189.1 – 189.9)	5	11.9	42	10	14.9	67
M.N. of skin (172, 173)	5	6.7	75	8	9.5	84
M.N. of brain (191, 192)	11	11.5	96	17	16.7	102

M.N. of thyroid (193)	(2)^c	(0.8)	250	(0)	(1.3)	0
M.N. of bone (170)	(0)	(2.5)	0	(2)	(3.1)	65
Leukemia (204–207)	9	16.1	56	10	21.6	46
M.N. of other lymphatic and hematopoietic tissue (200–203, 208, 209)	18	22.2	81	33	31.5	105
Other M.N. (residual)	51	44.3	115	47	60.0	78

a   Expected deaths are calculated from age-calendar year-specific U.S. mortality rates for white males, 1945–1967. For cancer of the lung, leukemia and M.N. of other lymphatic and hematopoietic tissue, U.S. data for 1945–1973 are used.

b   ICD codes.

c   Observed or expected death values less than 5 are enclosed in brackets.

MARKS et al.

TABLE III. OBSERVED DEATHS, EXPECTED DEATHS AND
STANDARDIZED MORTALITY RATIOS FOR MALIGNANT NEOPLASMS
OF LYMPHATIC AND HEMATOPOIETIC TISSUE FOR WHITE MALES
GROUPED BY LENGTH OF EMPLOYMENT

| | Length of employment | | | | | |
| | < 2 Years | | | 2+ Years | | |
	Obs.	Exp.[a]	SMR	Obs.	Exp.	SMR
Lymphosarcoma and reticulosarcoma (200)[b]	6	8.4	71	13	12.4	105
Hodgkin's disease (201)	6	6.1	98	7	8.1	86
All leukemia (204–207)	9	16.1	56	10	21.6	46
Other (202, 203, 208, 209)	6	7.7	78	13	11.0	118

[a] Expected deaths are calculated from age-calendar year-specific U.S. mortality rates for white males, 1945–1973.
[b] ICD codes.

    Prior consideration of a relationship of multiple myeloma to radia-
tion exposure rests upon evidence from studies of radiologists and of the
Japanese survivors of the atomic bombings. Matanoski et al. have reported
higher mortality from multiple myeloma in a particular cohort of radiologists when compared with the control groups of internists, ophthalmologists
and otolaryngologists [19] but, on the basis of more recent data, he
finds no important difference between radiologists and the ophthalmologists
and otolaryngologists [20]. These medical specialists, and internists to
a lesser extent, have high relative risks for multiple myeloma, but
Matanoski suspects that an unidentified common factor rather than radiation
is responsible. In the Japanese atomic bomb survivors, one death due to
multiple myeloma was recorded for the group exposed to 100 rad or more and
5 for exposures between 1 and 99 rad [21]. The Japanese results have been
variously interpreted as supporting a relationship between radiation and
multiple myeloma [21] and, on the other hand, providing no evidence for
such a relationship [22].

    An excess of cancer of the pancreas as well as excess cancer of the
pharynx, esophagus, stomach and large intestine have been described in
patients heavily irradiated for the treatment of ankylosing spondylitis
[17,23]. The dosimetry to the abdominal organs has not been published
yet, but the radiation exposures are known to have been well into the

TABLE IV. OBSERVED AND EXPECTED DEATHS DUE TO SPECIFIC
LEUKEMIA TYPES, MULTIPLE MYELOMA AND CERTAIN OTHER
NEOPLASMS OF LYMPHATIC AND HEMATOPOIETIC TISSUE FOR
DEATHS OCCURRING IN WHITE MALES DURING AND AFTER 1965

	Length of employment			
	< 2 Years		2 + Years	
	Obs.	Exp.[a]	Obs.	Exp.
All leukemia	5	7.6	9	11.4
Lymphatic (204)[b]	1	2.4	1	3.4
Myeloid (205)	3	3.3	5	5.1
Monocytic (206)	0	0.4	1	0.6
Other and unspecified (207)	1	1.5	2	2.3
Certain other neoplasms of lymphatic and hematopoietic tissue	4	5.1	10	7.8
Multiple myeloma (203)	4	2.5	5	3.8
Other (202, 208, 209)	0	2.6	5	4.0

[a] Expected deaths are calculated from age-calendar year-specific U.S. mortality rates for white males, 1968–1973.
[b] ICD codes.

therapeutic range (probably hundreds of rad). In the study of medical specialists by Matanoski, radiologists, internists, ophthalmologists and otolaryngologists had roughly comparable SMRs for carcinoma of the pancreas, which are all less than 100 [20]. Among the Japanese survivors, no excess of pancreatic cancer was detected in the life span study, using customary follow-up procedures. However, tumor registry data indicated excess mortality in Nagasaki but not in Hiroshima. The report of these findings warned against possibilities of bias in the use of tumor registry data [17]. In general, the epidemiologic study of mortality due to pancreatic cancer may be complicated by variation in the reliability of diagnosis of this disease.

We have not yet had the opportunity to consider the exposure of Hanford workers to agents other than radiation. Some manufacturing, such as chemical processing, and research activities at the plant do involve important exposure to chemicals. Furthermore, the first prime contractor

TABLE V. OBSERVED AND EXPECTED DEATHS DUE TO SELECTED CAUSES BY EXPOSURE CATEGORY FOR WHITE MALES INCLUDED IN EXPOSURE STUDY (SEE TEXT)

Cause of death	Exposure category								Probability of trend arising due to chance [b]
	0 – 2 rem		2 – 5 rem		5 – 15 rem		15 + rem		
	Obs.	Exp.[a]	Obs.	Exp.[a]	Obs.	Exp.[a]	Obs.	Exp.[a]	
All causes	587	578.5	122	113.1	84	96.3	44	49.1	> 0.5
All malignant neoplasms (M.N.)	112	117.9	33	23.3	15	19.5	11	10.3	> 0.5
M.N. of buccal cavity	4	3.3	0	0.7	1	0.6	0	0.4	> 0.5
M.N. of colon	11	12.5	4	1.8	0	1.2	1	0.5	> 0.5
M.N. of pancreas	7	8.8	3	2.2	1	2.0	3	1.0	0.03
M.N. of other digestive organs	11	10.9	3	1.9	1	1.6	0	0.7	> 0.5
M.N. of lung	34	39.1	14	8.2	7	7.0	3	3.8	> 0.5
M.N. of prostate	10	7.4	1	1.5	0	1.3	0	0.9	> 0.5
M.N. of brain	4	6.3	3	1.2	1	0.9	1	0.7	0.18
Lymphosarcoma and reticulum cell sarcoma	2	1.5	0	0.5	1	0.6	0	0.4	> 0.5
Hodgkin's disease	2	2.1	1	0.5	0	0.4	0	0.0	> 0.5
Leukemia	3	2.9	0	0.6	1	0.3	0	0.2	> 0.5
Multiple myeloma	1	2.3	0	0.6	1	0.8	2	0.4	0.01
Other neoplasms of lymphatic and hematopoietic tissue	2	1.6	0	0.3	0	0.1	0	0.0	> 0.5
All other cancers	21	19.3	4	3.4	1	2.8	1	1.4	> 0.5

All noncancer causes	461	449.2	89	87.3	66	74.9	33	37.6
No death certificate	14	11.4	0	0	3	1.9	0	1.2

a Expected deaths are calculated from the experience of all workers in the exposure study, allowing for age, occupation, and follow-up stratum.

b The significance levels are for a one-tailed test.

TABLE VI. AGE-, CALENDAR YEAR- AND OCCUPATION-ADJUSTED
MORTALITY RATES BY EXPOSURE CATEGORY FOR WHITE MALES
AGED 25 TO 70 INCLUDED IN EXPOSURE STUDY (SEE TEXT); RATES
PER 1000 PERSON-YEARS (APPROXIMATE 95% CONFIDENCE LIMITS
ARE GIVEN IN PARENTHESES)

	Exposure category			U.S. white males
	0 − 2 rem	2 − 5 rem	5 + rem	
All causes	7.8 (± 0.9)	7.5 (± 1.4)	6.7 (± 1.3)	11.0
All malignant neoplasms	1.7 (± 0.4)	2.1 (± 0.8)	1.4 (± 0.6)	2.1

at the plant was a major chemical company, and many employees in the early
cohorts had previously worked in chemical plants including munitions
factories. The role of chemical exposure warrants further consideration
in view of the tentative report of an excess of deaths due to carcinoma
of the pancreas and malignant lymphoma in chemists [24].

In considering analyses of the Hanford data by other investigators,
the studies by Sanders [1-4] were directed principally to a comparison
of longevity among study and control groups, and to a possible relationship
between all cancer deaths or all deaths from other causes and mean
cumulative radiation dose. Sanders found that life span was greater for
exposed than unexposed employees and for exposed employees than their
siblings. He also concluded that, to date, his analysis of the relationship of radiation exposure to cancer or other mortality did not indicate
any adverse effect of radiation on the exposed workers. The analysis by
Sanders did not treat specific causes of death in depth.

The study by Milham in 1974 was a proportional mortality analysis
of the deaths that occurred between 1950 and 1971 among workers in
numerous occupations in the State of Washington and was supplemented by
1972 and 1973 data. His results in summary form for the individual
occupations were published in a monograph [5], which included a category
of atomic energy workers associated with the Hanford project. Milham
found that cancer of the pancreas showed a significant elevation of the
proportional mortality ratio (PMR)[4] in men 20 years of age or older
while cancer of the large intestine had an elevated PMR in men aged 20-64.
Leukemias had low PMRs and multiple myeloma only a small PMR increase
based on four deaths. The study by Milham was considered preliminary
because information on less than a fourth of the deaths was available to

---

[4] PMR refers to the ratio of the proportion of deaths due to a specified cause or set of
causes in the study population to the proportion of deaths due to that cause or set of causes
in the reference population (the population of all deaths in the State of Washington for
1950–1971 in this case).

him, and the bias introduced by the marked healthy worker effect for
causes other than cancer in this population could seriously affect his
proportional analysis.

The study by Stewart and Kneale, conducted for Mancuso in 1976,
approached the analysis in several different ways as a result of which
they reached striking conclusions [7]. They stated that at certain ages
'there is probably a cancer hazard associated with low-level radiation
which affects bone marrow cancers more than other neoplasms and cancers
of the pancreas and lung more than other solid tumors'. In addition, they
concluded that 12.2 rad would double the normal risk of dying from any
cancer, and that the doubling dose for pancreas is 7.4, for lung 6.1 and
for reticuloendothelial system or bone marrow cancers 0.8 rad. The
authors estimated that 25.8 deaths in the study population were induced
by radiation and provided a breakdown of the deaths by cancer type.

In their analyses, Mancuso et al. found a greater percentage of
exposed workers among all cancer deaths than the percentage of exposed
workers among all noncancer deaths in the total population and concluded
that this constitutes evidence of a radiation causation of cancer. As
we indicated above, the SMR for all causes other than cancer is lower
than the SMR for all cancer in the long-term, predominantly exposed
workers but not in the short-term, predominantly unexposed workers.
Therefore, diseases other than cancer are associated with a higher percentage of unexposed workers than one would expect if long- and short-term
workers had the same distribution of noncancer causes of death. Conversely,
cancer as the complement of noncancer is associated with a higher percentage of exposed workers despite similar SMRs for cancer for long-
and short-term workers. Thus, a bias in this population due to the
differential healthy worker effect in the long-term, exposed workers has
led to Mancuso's inference regarding a radiation causation of cancer.

Much of the analysis by Mancuso was concerned with a comparison
of mean cumulative radiation exposures for various disease categories.
Use of this approach ignores the severely skewed distribution of exposures
(Figure 1), which results in the undue influence of single or a few high
values when the sample size is small. Mancuso used the t test improperly
to test for statistical significance between the means of cumulative
exposures for disease categories. The skewed distribution of exposures
makes the t test inappropriate when samples are small. Their Monte
Carlo simulation of their test of significance for bone marrow neoplasms
when compared with their use of a t test increased the p value from
$p < .0001$ to $p < .06$ and for carcinoma of the pancreas from $p < .001$ to
$p < .01$. The excessive influence of isolated large values also undermines
the credibility of their calculation of doubling doses. An additional
factor that may influence the length of work and, consequently, level
of radiation exposure at various intervals before death is the
self-selection practiced by victims of chronic diseases. They are likely
to transfer into less strenuous work assignments or terminate employment
earlier than do patients suffering from diseases having a rapid clinical
course such as cancer of the lung and pancreas. This factor can bias
the mean cumulative exposures used by Mancuso to estimate the magnitude
of radiation effect.

Mancuso calculated proportional mortality ratios, which they improperly named standardized mortality ratios. However, these ratios are not
adjusted for age and calendar year of death. Furthermore, the authors

used as a basis for comparison, proportions based on U.S. vital statistics for 1960, which precedes the period when most Hanford deaths occurred. A substantial increase in mortality from cancer of the lung has occurred as well as nontrivial increases in mortality rates for pancreas and multiple myeloma between 1960 and 1974. The problem of bias due to low noncancer SMRs for this population further weakens the validity of proportional mortality ratios as discussed above.

Mancuso et al. calculated doubling doses that are hardly credible. The unorthodox grouping of myeloid leukemia and multiple myeloma into cancer of bone marrow was assigned a doubling dose of .8 rad; the doubling doses for lung and pancreas were 6.1 and 7.4 rad, respectively. The variation in natural background radiation among the states in the U.S., due to such factors as altitude and terrestrial composition, results in as much as a threefold difference in natural background exposure between populations at sea level and in mountain states [25]. With an estimated difference of 120 mrem per year in background exposure between the State of Colorado and the United States as a whole, several doubling doses for myeloid leukemia and multiple myeloma would be accumulated in Colorado during an average lifetime and at least one doubling dose for pancreas and lung. The average annual age-adjusted white male mortality rates for the period 1950-1969 for carcinoma of the pancreas were 9.23 in Colorado and 9.63 in the U.S.; for lung 28.29 in Colorado and 37.98 in the U.S.; for multiple myeloma 1.75 in Colorado and 1.76 in the U.S.; and for leukemia and aleukemia 8.59 in Colorado and 8.81 in the U.S. These comparisons indicate that at higher altitudes we do not encounter the excess mortality from these diseases that we might expect on the basis of the doubling doses reported by Mancuso.

Land has carried out a refined contingency table analysis of the relationship of radiation exposure to mortality for various causes of death [8]. His method of analysis included adjustment for age and calendar year of death. He demonstrated a statistically significant correlation of carcinoma of the pancreas and multiple myeloma with exposure.

In reviewing the various studies, the results of our population-based analysis and the lack of evidence for a correlation between all cancer deaths and radiation exposure contradict the conclusion by Mancuso et al. that radiation has increased overall cancer mortality in the employee population. Land's study and ours indicate a positive correlation between radiation exposure and mortality from cancer of the pancreas and multiple myeloma. These findings are in agreement with those of Mancuso concerning these particular diseases if one separates myeloid leukemia, for which we established no effect, from multiple myeloma in the broader category 'cancer of the bone marrow' used by Mancuso. However, the absence of increased mortality for more typically radiation related cancer types such as leukemia and carcinoma of the lung, as well as the small numbers of cases that determined statistical significance for cancer of the pancreas and multiple myeloma, led us to consider these findings promising leads rather than definitive relationships. Observation and analysis will be continued in the future to check further our current findings and monitor any new developments that might occur in this employee population.

ACKNOWLEDGEMENTS

We acknowledge the superb performance of Mrs. Clever Kirklin in collecting and organizing the data file that was used in the study and that made this and other studies of this data possible; K.R. Heid for his excellent cooperation in providing the radiation dosimetry data; Kent B. Stewart and E.L. Kelley for their valuable support in the computer programming; and W.W. Weyzen of the Department of Energy for his encouragement.

REFERENCES

[1] MANCUSO, T.F., SANDERS, B.S., BRODSKY, A., Study of the Lifetime Health and Mortality Experience of Employees of AEC Contractors, Progress Report Nos 1 – 8 (1965–1972).

[2] MANCUSO, T.F., SANDERS, B.S., Study of the Lifetime Health and Mortality Experience of Employees of AEC Contractors, Progress Report Nos 9–11 (1973–1975).

[3] MANCUSO, T.F., SANDERS, B.S., BRODSKY, A., "Study of the lifetime health and mortality experience of employees of AEC contractors, Part I: Methodology and some preliminary findings limited to mortality for Hanford employees", Proc. 6th Ann. Health Phys. Soc. Topical Symposium, 1971, AEC Publication No. C00-3428-1 (1971).

[4] SANDERS, B.S., Low level radiation and cancer deaths, Health Phys. (in press).

[5] MILHAM, S., Jr., Occupational Mortality in Washington State, 1950–1971, I, HEW Publication No. (NIOSH) 76–175–A (1976) 29.

[6] GILBERT, E.S., Methods of analyzing mortality of workers exposed to low levels of ionizing radiation, Annual Meeting of the Biometric Society, Western North American Region, Palo Alto, CA, June 1977.

[7] MANCUSO, T.F., STEWART, A., KNEALE, G., Radiation exposures of Hanford workers dying from cancer and other causes, Health Phys. 33 5 (1977) 369.

[8] LAND, C.E., Report to be published, 1978.

[9] OTT, M.G., HOLDER, B.B., LANGNER, R.R., Determinants of mortality in an industrial population, J. Occup. Med. 18 3 (1976) 171.

[10] FOX, J.P., HALL, C.E., ELVEBACK, L.R., Epidemiology, Collier-Macmillan Ltd., London (1970) 292.

[11] MONSON, R.R., Analysis of relative survival and proportional mortality, Comput. Biomed. Res. 7 (1974) 325.

[12] McMICHAEL, A.J., HAYNES, S.G., TYROLER, H.A., Observations on the evaluation of occupational mortality data, J. Occup. Med. 17 2 (1975) 128.

[13] McMICHAEL, A.J., Standardized mortality ratios and the "healthy worker effect": Scratching beneath the surface, J. Occup. Med. 18 3 (1976) 165.

[14] GAFFEY, W.R., Cause-specific mortality, J. Occup. Med. 17 2 (1975) 128.

[15] MANTEL, N., HAENSZEL, W., Statistical aspects of the analysis of data from retrospective studies of disease, J. Natl. Cancer Inst. 22 (1959) 719.

[16] MANTEL, N., Chi-square tests with one degree of freedom: Extensions of the Mantel-Haenzsel procedure, J. Am. Stat. Assoc. 58 (1963) 690.

[17] UNITED NATIONS, "Radiation carcinogenesis in man", Sources and Effects of Ionizing Radiation, UN Scientific Committee on the Effects of Ionizing Radiation, Report to the General Assembly, with Annexes, UN, New York (1977) 361.

[18] BEEBE, G.W., KATO, H., LAND, C.E., Studies of the Mortality of A-Bomb Survivors: 8. Mortality Experience of A-Bomb Survivors, 1950–74, Radiation Effects Research Foundation, RERF Technical Report 1–77 (1977).

[19] MATANOSKI, G.N., SELTSER, R., SARTWELL, P.E., et al., The current mortality rates of radiologists and other physician specialists: specific causes of death, Am. J. Epidemiol. 101 3 (1975) 199.

[20] MATANOSKI, G.N., Unpublished observations (1978).

[21] NISHIYAMA, H., ANDERSON, R.E., ISHIMARU, T., et al., The incidence of malignant lymphoma and multiple myeloma in Hiroshima and Nagasaki A-bomb survivors, 1945—1965, Cancer 32 6 (1973) 1301—1309.

[22] JABLON, S., "Environmental factors in cancer induction: Appraisal of epidemiologic evidence — leukemia, lymphoma and radiation", Excerpta Medica International Congress Series No. 351, 3, Cancer Epidemiology, Environmental Factors (Proc. XI Int. Cancer Congress, Florence, 1974) 239.

[23] COURT BROWN, W.M., DOLL, R., Mortality from cancer and other causes after radiotherapy for ankylosing spondylitis, Br. Med. J. ii (1965) 1327.

[24] LI, F.P., FRAUMENI, J.F., Jr., MANTEL, N., MILLER, R.W., Cancer mortality among chemists, J. Natl. Cancer Inst. 43 5 (1969) 1159.

[25] KLEMENT, A.W., Jr., MILLER, C.R., MINX, R.P., SHLEIEN, B., Estimates of Ionizing Radiation in the United States, 1960—2000, U.S. EPA Document ORP/CSD72—1(1972) 8.

DISCUSSION

A.M. STEWART: How do you account for the falling trend with rising dose for the 649 non-cancer deaths in your Mantel-Haenszel analysis? If the P value was indicative of a significant trend in this direction, it would suggest that you have not fully controlled for differences between survivors and non-survivors. For instance, workers from recent cohorts (which have not yet experienced many deaths) could be more at risk than workers from remote cohorts (which are biased in favour of non-survivors).

S. MARKS: Mrs. Gilbert did test for the statistical significance of the mortality due to diseases other than cancer, and found that the correlation between those deaths and the levels of exposure was not significant when testing for either positive or negative correlation.

RE-ANALYSIS OF DATA RELATING TO THE HANFORD STUDY OF THE CANCER RISKS OF RADIATION WORKERS

G.W. KNEALE, A.M. STEWART,
T.F. MANCUSO
Department of Industrial Environmental
    Health Sciences,
University of Pittsburgh Graduate School
    of Public Health,
Pittsburgh,
Pennsylvania,
United States of America

Abstract

RE-ANALYSIS OF DATA RELATING TO THE HANFORD STUDY OF THE CANCER
RISKS OF RADIATION WORKERS.
    A study of workers in the nuclear industry who had linked records of external radiation
doses and certified causes of death (1944–72 deaths of Hanford workers) was followed by
a similar analysis of a larger sample of Hanford data (1944–77 deaths). The second study
included one test which showed that, in surveys of the delayed effects of low-level radiation,
comparisons between observed and expected doses of cancer cases (CMD method) are more
informative than comparisons between observed and expected cancer deaths of exposed workers
(SMR method). A second test (which took the form of a Mantel-Haenszel analysis and included
exposure period and internal radiation among the controlling factors) showed that there were
genuine differences between the radiation doses of two groups of certified deaths (cancers and
non-cancers). Both studies produced evidence of a cancer hazard from low doses of external
radiation even when delivered at low dose rates. According to the second study, approximately
5% of the cancer deaths of Hanford workers were radiation-induced, and these extra deaths were
probably concentrated among cancers of tissues which rate high in the ICRP 14 classification
of radiosensitivity (e.g. bone marrow, pharynx and lung, pancreas and small intestine).

A recent study of men and women who were repeatedly exposed to measured
doses of low-level radiation before dying of cancers and other causes (Hanford
data) [1] has raised uncertainties about the cancer hazards of workers in the nuclear
industry by producing risk estimates of a different order of magnitude from ICRP
26 recommendations [2]. The analysis of Hanford data was designed to take full
advantage of the fact that for all badge-monitored workers there were annual
doses of external or penetrating radiation. It therefore followed unusual lines
and was open to criticism by advocates of an alternative and more familiar method.

TABLE I.   NUMBERS OF BADGE-MONITORED AND URINE-MONITORED WORKERS IN THE LARGER SAMPLE OF HANFORD DATA

Badge-monitored (external radiation)	Urine-monitored (internal radiation)	Certified deaths (1944–77)			Uncertified deaths	Survivors
		Cancers	Non-cancers	All causes		
Monitored males	Not monitored	264	1188	1452	67	4 386
	Monitored (negative)	194	782	976	28	2 739
	Monitored (positive)	285	1029	1314	34	10 884
	Total	743	2999	3742	129	17 929
Monitored females	Not monitored	33	95	128	20	2 114
	Monitored (negative)	21	50	71	8	1 155
	Monitored (positive)	35	57	92	7	2 487
	Total	89	202	291	35	5 756
All monitored workers	Not monitored	297	1283	1580	87	6 500
	Monitored (negative)	215	832	1047	36	3 894
	Monitored (positive)	320	1086	1406	41	13 371
	Total	832	3201	4033 [a]	164	23 765
Not monitored	Males	181	771	952	46	2 362
	Females	88	196	284	51	3 191
	Total	269	967	1236	97	5 553

[a]   This is the population of badge-monitored workers included in later analyses.

It was clearly important to know which was the more reliable method and to observe the effects of simultaneous control of several factors with radiation or cancer associations. Therefore we first tested the relative efficiency of the two methods, and then applied the more efficient one to a larger sample of Hanford data after applying a Mantel-Haenszel test [3] to the null hypothesis of no difference in the external radiation doses of cancers and non-cancers.

The method actually used in the earlier study compared observed with expected radiation doses, and had as cases and controls cancer and non-cancer deaths (Comparative Mean Dose or CMD Method). The alternative was to compare observed with expected cancer deaths and to have as cases and controls exposed and non-exposed workers (Standardized Mortality Ratio or SMR Method). The earlier study was based on 3520 men and 412 women who died between 1944 and 1972, and the larger sample of Hanford data included 4694 men and 575 women who died between 1944 and 1977 (Table I).

TEST OF THE RELATIVE EFFICIENCY OF THE SMR AND CMD METHODS

(1)   Let a population of size N (in man years of observation) be exposed to a radiation dose distribution of $f(x)$ with a mean dose (R) and a variance (V) such that

$$R = \int_0^\infty xf(x)\,dx \quad \text{and} \quad V = \int_0^\infty (x - R)^2 f(x)\,dx$$

(2)   Let the risk of a cancer death increase linearly with the radiation dose from level A at zero dose (normal cancer risk) according to doubling dose (D), such that the risk for dose x is $A(1 + x/D)$.

(3)   Let n be the number of cancer deaths actually observed in a study population with a mean radiation dose r.

Given these conditions the necessary size of the population for detecting a given doubling dose (at a given size and power of the test) will depend upon which approach is taken. Thus the SMR method will require a known value of A which can usually be obtained from official sources (e.g. in Great Britain, the male cancer death rate is currently in the region of 2600 per million). Under the hypothesis of no radiation effect, the number of cancer deaths actually observed (n) would have a Poisson distribution with AN as the mean value. Therefore,

TABLE II.   MEAN RADIATION DOSES OF CANCERS
AND NON-CANCERS

Sex	Certified causes of death	ICD 8th Revision	Cases	Penetrating radiation [a]	
				Total	Mean
Males	Cancers	140−209	743	150 952	203
	Cardiovascular	390−458	1988	314 636	158
	Respiratory	460−519	198	29 578	149
	Digestive	520−577	140	31 694	226
	Violence	800−999	424	55 985	132
	Other causes	Residue	249	38 804	156
	All causes	000−999	3742	621 649	166
Females	Cancers	140−209	89	7 901	89
	Cardiovascular	390−458	106	6 518	61
	Respiratory	460−519	15	808	54
	Digestive	520−577	16	912	57
	Violence	800−999	36	975	27
	Other causes	Residue	29	872	30
	All causes	000−999	291	17 986	62
All non-cancer deaths	Males		2999	470 697	157
	Females		202	10 085	50

[a]   All doses in centirads.

provided N was large enough to apply a normal approximation to the Poisson distribution, the condition for significance would be

$$n > AN + t\sqrt{AN}$$

where t is the critical normal deviate corresponding to a given significance level (or size of the test).

One now requires the power of the test, or the probability of the significance condition being satisfied under the hypothesis of some radiation effect (with D as the doubling dose). Under this hypothesis the number of cancer deaths

TABLE III. BASIC DATA FOR THE MANTEL-HAENSZEL ANALYSIS

Factors	Levels	Cases (Cancers)	Controls (Non-cancers)
Sex	Male	743	2999
	Female	89	202
Final age	Under 40 years	38	206
	40–49 years	96	396
	50–59 years	223	707
	60+ years	475	1892
Death year	1944–54	69	284
	1955–59	79	327
	1960–64	123	575
	1965–69	181	715
	1970–77	380	1300
Internal radiation	Not monitored	297	1283
	Monitored (negative)	215	832
	Monitored (positive)	320	1086
Exposure period	Under 2 years	280	1223
	Over 2 years	552	1978
External radiation	Under 8 centirads	256	1068
	8–31 centirads	131	592
	32–63 centirads	119	428
	64–127 centirads	123	448
	128–255 centirads	91	320
	256–511 centirads	48	147
	over 511 centirads	64	198

actually observed (n) would have a Poisson distribution with $AN(1 + R/D)$ as the mean value. Therefore, the required power would be

$$\Phi\left[\frac{AN + t\sqrt{AN} - AN(1 + R/D)}{\sqrt{AN(1 + R/D)}}\right]$$

where Φ is the integrated normal distribution.

TABLE IV.   RESULTS OF THE MANTEL-HAENSZEL ANALYSIS [a]

Test factors	Levels	Cancer deaths		t-values		Relative risk [b]
		Observed	Expected	O−E	Progressive component	
Sex	Male	478	496.6	−3.0*		1.00 (1.00)
	Female	81	62.4	+3.0*	—	1.57 (1.78)
Final age	Under 40 years	34	46.4	−2.3*		0.61 (0.73)
	40−49 years	92	97.3	−0.7		0.93 (0.96)
	50−59 years	220	188.8	+3.0*		1.30 (1.25)
	60+	468	481.4	−1.2	+0.8	1.00 (1.00)
Death years	1944−54	66	61.7	+0.7		0.99 (0.83)
	1955−59	78	77.9	+0.0		0.91 (0.83)
	1960−64	120	138.1	−2.0*		0.77 (0.73)
	1965−69	178	183.7	−0.6		0.88 (0.86)
	1970−77	360	340.6	+1.7	+0.9	1.00 (1.00)

Internal radiation	Not monitored	249	251.6	− 0.3		1.00 (1.00)
	Monitored − ve	201	197.8	+ 0.4		1.06 (1.12)
	Monitored + ve	273	273.6	− 0.1	+ 0.1	1.00 (1.27)
Exposure period	Under 2 years	245	250.5	− 0.8		1.00 (1.00)
	Over 2 years	229	223.5	+ 0.8	—	1.12 (1.22)
External radiation	Under 8 centirads	235	240.6	− 0.6		1.00 (1.00)
	8−31 centirads	129	146.5	− 1.9		0.86 (0.92)
	32−63 centirads	119	108.9	+ 1.2		1.15 (1.15)
	64−127 centirads	121	117.9	+ 0.4		1.14 (1.14)
	128−255 centirads	91	89.9	+ 0.2		1.10 (1.19)
	256−511 centirads	47	43.9	+ 0.6		1.08 (1.36)
	over 511 centirads	64	58.8	+ 0.9	+ 2.0*	1.26 (1.35)

* Significant at the 5% level or higher.

a The observed number of cancer deaths in the results of a Mantel-Haenszel analysis are necessarily smaller than those in the basic data because of the necessity of excluding from the fully controlled analysis non-informative cases (or cases without controls matched for every factor except the one of immediate interest). The methodology necessitating this exclusion is described in the appendix to Ref.[13].

b Uncontrolled risk estimates in brackets, see Table III.

TABLE V. ICRP CLASSIFICATIONS OF CANCERS

ICRP classification of cancers	ICD Nos (8th Rev.)	Males		Females	
		Cases	Mean R dose in centirads	Cases	Mean R dose in centirads
High sensitivity					
I. Established					
(a) Bone marrow	203	10	861	1	0
	205	15	125	–	–
(b) Thyroid	193	1 (26)	44 (405)	– (1)	– (0)
II. Apparent					
(a) Lymph nodes	200–1	33	136	2	117
Reticular tissue	202	7 (40)	29 (117)	1 (3)	1573 (602)
(b) Pharynx	146–9	10	481	–	–
Lung	162–3	215 (225)	258 (268)	10 (10)	52 (52)
(c) Pancreas	157	52	391	5	13
Stomach	151	44	240	2	109
Large intestine	153	69 (165)	132 (242)	9 (16)	80 ((63)
III. *Low sensitivity*					
Mouth and salivary	140–5	15	133	–	–
Oesophagus	150	19	43	–	–
Small intestine	152	2	32	–	–
Liver and gall bladder	155–6	18	252	2	230
Nose and larynx	160–1	14	143	–	–
Bone, C.T. and skin	170–3	18	149	6	30
Testis and penis	186–7	3	114	–	–
Kidney	189	23	178	2	44
Eye and CNS	190–2	28	170	5	35
Other endocrine	194	– (140)	– (152)	– (15)	– (60)
IV. *Unclassified*					
Rectum	154	20	101	2	30
Other digestive	158–9	2	38	1	3
Breast	174	1	0	19	120
Uterus and ovaries	180–4	–	–	11	37
Prostate	185	52	119	–	–
Bladder	188	13	87	–	–
Lymphatic leukaemia	204	3	19	3	70
Other haemopoetic	206–9	8	23	3	1
Ill-defined	195–9	48 (147)	93 (96)	5 (44)	140 (83)
All high sensitivity groups		456	253	30	111
Residual cancers		287	123	59	78

If the power of the test is given the convenient value of $1/2$ (so that one is equally likely or unlikely to detect a significant difference between actual and expected cancer deaths), the argument to Φ will become zero — or $t\sqrt{AN} = ANR/D$ — and the necessary man-years of observation will be $t^2 D^2/(AR^2)$. Therefore, assuming: (a) a doubling dose of 30 rad; (b) a mean radiation dose of 1.6 rads; (c) a normal cancer risk of 2600 per million; and (d) a 5% level of significance, the SMR method would require 540 000 man-years or a data base approximately five times larger than the Hanford one.

The corresponding calculations for the CMD method are as follows. On the hypothesis of no radiation effect the mean cancer dose (r) would have an approximately normal distribution with mean R and variance V/n. Therefore, the condition for significance would be $r > R + t\sqrt{V/n}$. On the alternative hypothesis (of some radiation effect with D as the doubling dose) the mean radiation dose (r) would have an approximately normal distribution with $[R + (R^2 + V)/D]/(1 + R/D)$ as the mean value [1] and the condition for a power of $1/2$ would be

$$t\sqrt{V/n} = \frac{R + (R^2 + V)/D}{(1 + R/D)} - R$$

By allowing the approximate mean value of n to be AN the necessary size of the base population would be $t^2(D+R)^2/(AV)$. Therefore, to detect a doubling dose of 30 rads with a mean radiation dose of 1.6 rads (and the additional information that for Hanford males $\sqrt{V} = 3.6$ rads), the CMD method would only require 145 000 man-years of observation or a data base similar in size to the current Hanford one.

Finally, the general formula for the efficiency of the CMD method (compared with the SMR method) is $D^2 V/((D+R)^2 R^2)$. Therefore, should the radiation doses have a wide scatter about the mean, as was certainly the case in Hanford data, comparisons between actual and expected radiation doses of cancer cases should be more reliable than comparisons between actual and expected cancer deaths of exposed workers.

Following this vindication of the CMD method, steps were taken to ensure that factors other than external radiation were not influencing the results.

AVOIDANCE OF SPURIOUS ASSOCIATIONS

In the original study and again in the larger sample of Hanford data the mean radiation doses were higher for cancers than non-cancers (Table II). Therefore the first question requiring a reliable answer was whether these were genuine findings or the result of accidental differences between two groups of certified deaths.

TABLE VI.   CMD ANALYSIS OF MALE CANCERS:
(i) DISTRIBUTION OF EXPOSED MALES BY PRE-DEATH YEARS

Pre-death years	Non-cancers	Cancers (ICRP classification)				All cancers
		I	II	III	IV	
29	377	3	56	11	32	102
28	513	4	72	16	39	131
27	642	4	99	23	44	170
26	767	5	119	28	49	201
25	929	8	148	39	56	251
24	1059	9	173	45	70	297
23	1200	11	196	51	79	337
22	1330	13	212	58	85	368
21	1470	14	227	66	92	399
20	1600	15	247	73	97	432
19	1735	16	260	77	100	453
18	1854	20	273	83	106	482
17	1983	20	288	87	110	505
16	2096	20	305	93	114	532
15	2198	20	327	97	118	558
14	2287	21	337	100	123	581
13	2363	22	352	103	124	600
12	2442	22	365	108	128	623
11	2509	22	372	114	130	638
10	2578	22	380	118	132	652
9	2640	22	393	122	134	671
8	2702	22	402	125	136	685
7	2762	23	408	126	138	695
6	2806	23	411	129	140	703
5	2854	26	418	131	140	715
4	2891	26	424	134	141	725
3	2927	26	426	138	141	731
2	2953	26	429	138	144	737
1	2987	26	430	138	146	740
0	2999	26	430	140	147	743

In the earlier study the radiation dose differences remained after controlling separately for five possible sources of bias, including age at death. In the repeat analysis they remained after simultaneous control of the following factors: sex, age at death, date of death, internal radiation and exposure period (Tables III and IV). The second test took the form of a Mantel-Haenszel analysis which also showed that:

(1) Relative risks for different levels of external radiation were only slightly altered in the controlled compared with the crude analysis (changing from a relative risk of 1.35 to 1.26 in the highest dose category);

(2) The progressive component for seven dose levels was suggestive of a dose-dependent effect without threshold (i.e. a stochastic effect, see ICRP 26);

(3) Controlling for internal radiation which was strongly correlated with external radiation and therefore suspected of causing most if not all of the dose difference between cancers and non-cancers [4, 5], actually strengthened the external radiation effect;

(4) Hanford females were more cancer sensitive than Hanford males; and

(5) Cancers accounted for a higher proportion of deaths between 50 and 60 years than of earlier or later deaths.

DETECTION OF CANCERS WITH DEFINITE RADIATION EFFECTS

Since the null hypothesis of no difference in the radiation doses of cancers and non-cancers was rejected by the Mantel-Haenszel test there were strong reasons for suspecting that some of the cancer deaths were radiation-induced. But the question remained: were the extra deaths evenly distributed between the different malignant diseases or concentrated in radiosensitive tissues?

Even in the larger sample of Hanford data there were insufficient numbers to treat the 59 malignant diseases listed under different ICD numbers as separate entities. In the earlier study we allowed the choice of suitable groups to be influenced by the radiation doses. In the repeat analysis the choice was determined solely by ICRP 14 [6] or the publication which included a totally independent classiciation of radiosensitive tissues under the following headings: I. High Sensitivity Established; II. High Sensitivity Apparent; III. Low Sensitivity; and IV. Not Classified (Table V).

In the larger sample of Hanford data the first and second categories included 456 males and 30 females and the third and fourth categories included 287 males and 59 females. For males the mean radiation doses (reading from I to IV) were 405, 244, 152 and 93, and for females they were 0, 115, 60 and 83.

MEAN RADIATION DOSES BY PRE-DEATH YEARS

For three quarters of all the certified deaths of badge-monitored men in Table I there were records of annual radiation doses for at least 15 years before death (Tables VI and VII). For each of these years the mean cumulative radiation dose (which was strongly correlated with the number of separate exposures) was greater by a significant amount for cancers than non-cancers (Table VIII and Fig.1), but

TABLE VII. CMD ANALYSIS OF MALE CANCERS:
(ii) OBSERVED AND EXPECTED RADIATION DOSES
FOR FOUR TYPES OF CANCERS

Pre-death years	Expected mean doses	Actual mean doses of cancer cases [a]				All cancers
		I	II	III	IV	
29	21	52	27	31	25	28
28	22	44	30	37	26	28
27	23	49	29	23	26	28
26	26	41	32	26	27	30
25	27	26	33	26	32	31
24	30	25	30	29	28	32
23	34	34	39	31	30	35
22	37	31	44	31	34	40
21	40	39	50	30	38	43
20	44	47	55	33	40	47
19	48	59	63	38	42	54
18	51	57	68	46	46	59
17	56	83	75	52	51	67
16	61	112	85	57	55	75
15	66	140	100	63	59	83
14	71	161	105	69	61	91
13	77	179	116	76	64	100
12	84	204	125	89	66	109
11	91	235	138	93	68	119
10	98	271	150	97	71	128
9	106	313	160	102	73	137
8	114	346	173	111	75	147
7	121	365	185	121	78	158
6	129	386	1987	128	80	167
5	137	374	203	137	83	175
4	143	389	214	142	86	183
3	148	403	229	143	90	190
2	152	413	234	149	92	197
1	155	414	242	153	95	202
0	157	414	244	153	96	204

[a] For cancer classifications see Table V and for expected doses see non-cancers in Table VI; all radiation doses in centirads.

TABLE VIII. CMD ANALYSIS OF MALE CANCERS:
(iii) *t*-VALUES FOR DIFFERENCES BETWEEN
OBSERVED AND EXPECTED RADIATION DOSES

Pre-death years	*t*-values for the difference between observed and expected doses [a]				All cancers
	Ca I	Ca II	Ca III	Ca IV	
29	+1.4	+1.1	+0.5	+0.3	+1.5
28	+1.0	+1.4	0.0	+0.4	+1.5
27	+1.2	+1.3	−0.2	+0.3	+1.3
26	+0.7	+1.5	−0.2	+0.1	+1.3
25	−0.1	+1.4	−0.5	+0.6	+1.2
24	−0.3	+1.1	−0.3	−0.4	+0.5
23	0.0	+1.1	−0.3	−0.7	+0.4
22	−0.3	+1.5	−0.7	−0.5	+0.5
21	−0.1	+1.7	−0.9	−0.4	+0.7
20	+0.1	+1.8	−0.8	−0.5	+0.8
19	+0.4	+2.1	−0.7	−0.6	+1.1
18	+0.2	+2.1	−0.4	−0.6	+1.3
17	+0.8	+2.3	−0.3	−0.5	+1.6
16	+1.4	+2.5	−0.3	−0.6	+1.9
15	+1.8	+2.7	−0.2	−0.7	+2.1
14	+2.0	+2.9	−0.3	−0.8	+2.2
13	+2.1	+3.1	−0.2	−0.9	+2.3
12	+2.3	+3.0	+0.1	−1.1	+2.4
11	+2.5	+3.2	−0.0	−1.3	+2.4
10	+2.8	+3.3	−0.1	−1.4	+2.5
9	+3.2	+3.3	−0.0	−1.6	+2.4
8	+3.6	+3.6	0.0	−1.9	+2.7
7	+3.7	+3.7	+0.0	−1.9	+2.8
6	+3.6	+3.7	0.0	−2.0	+2.7
5	+3.4	+3.7	+0.0	−2.1	+2.7
4	+3.5	+3.9	+0.0	−2.3	+2.8
3	+3.5	+4.1	−0.1	−2.2	+2.9
2	+3.6	+4.4	−0.1	−2.4	+3.1
1	+3.6	+4.7	−0.1	−2.4	+3.2
0	+3.5	+4.6	−0.1	−2.4	+3.1

[a] Because of the skewness of the dose distribution normal approximations to
one-sided significance levels for *t*-values only apply if the number (n) in Table VI
exceeds the given value; thus:
$n > 20$ and $t > 1.7$ means $p < 0.05$
$n > 50$ and $t > 2.3$ means $p < 0.01$
$n > 200$ and $t > 3.0$ means $p < 0.001$

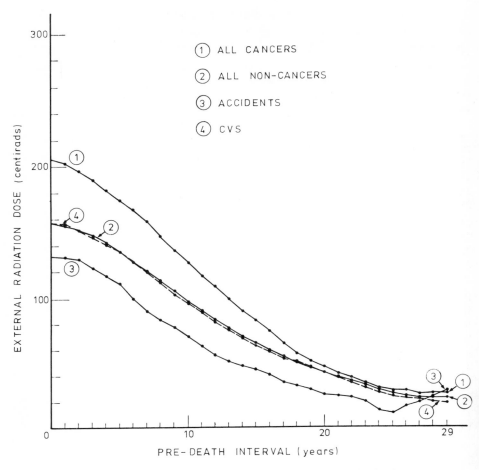

FIG.1.   Male cancer and non-cancer deaths;   CMD analysis by pre-death years.

only two of the four cancer groups (I and II) were responsible for these differences
(Table VIII and Fig.2). For females there were similar findings but owing to
the small numbers differences between cancers and non-cancers only achieved
statistical significance towards the end of the time scale (Table IX and Fig.3).

ESTIMATED DOUBLING DOSES FOR CANCERS SHOWING
DEFINITE RADIATION EFFECTS

Comparisons between the two methods had shown that, given a population
of 30 000, the CMD method would be more efficient than the SMR method.

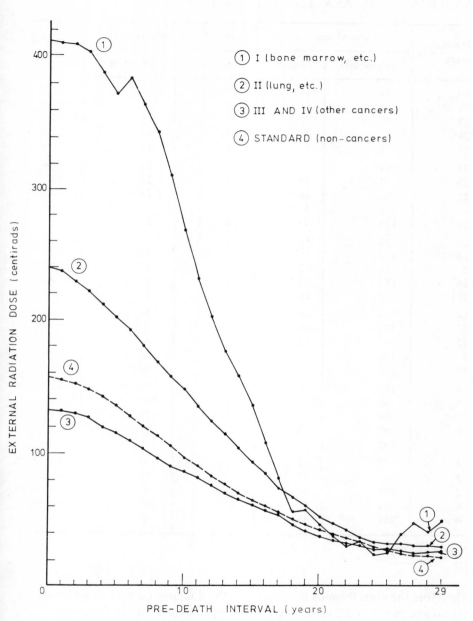

FIG.2. Male cancers by ICRP classification; CMD analysis by pre-death years.

TABLE IX.   CMD ANALYSIS OF FEMALE CANCERS

Pre-death years	Exposed females		Mean R dose for all cancers		t-Value 0−E
	Non-cancers	Cancers	Expected	Observed	
29	34	11	10	29	+1.7
28	41	19	9	18	+1.7
27	52	26	8	14	+1.0
26	63	29	9	19	+1.8
25	74	32	9	21	+1.9
24	84	37	11	21	+1.6
23	94	39	13	23	+1.7
22	103	43	16	23	+1.1
21	118	46	17	25	+1.0
20	124	49	20	24	+0.5
19	133	50	21	27	+0.7
18	139	57	23	26	+0.3
17	152	62	23	25	+0.2
16	156	64	24	27	+0.3
15	163	66	25	29	+0.5
14	166	68	37	32	+0.5
13	170	69	30	37	+0.6
12	172	72	33	44	+0.9
11	176	75	36	52	+1.1
10	179	76	39	60	+1.2
9	182	78	41	64	+1.3
8	183	79	43	69	+1.4
7	186	80	45	73	+1.5
6	190	82	46	75	+1.5
5	193	86	47	77	+1.6
4	196	87	47	81	+1.7 [a]
3	201	87	47	84	+1.9 [a]
2	201	88	49	85	+1.8 [a]
1	201	89	49	88	+1.9 [a]
0	201	89	50	88	+1.9 [a]

[a] See Table VIII.

Therefore the same formula for estimating the doubling dose was used in the repeat analysis as in the earlier study (see Appendix ii of the 1977 report).

On the first occasion only two of nine groups of malignant diseases showed definite evidence of a radiation effect (cancers of bone marrow and pancreas), but lung cancer also showed doubtful evidence of this effect. For these three groups the estimated doubling doses were 0.8, 7.4 and 6.1 rads. On the second

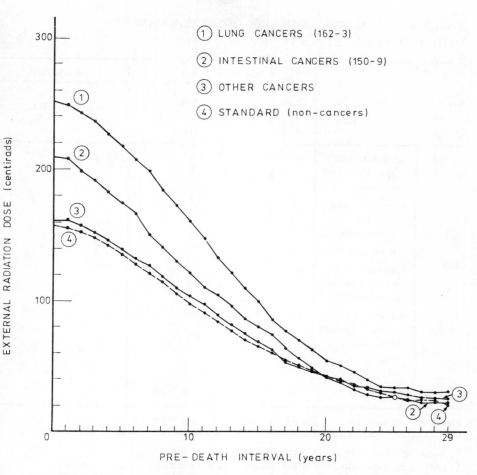

FIG.3.   Male cancers by ICD numbers;   CMD analysis by pre-death years.

occasion (Table X) there was definite evidence of a radiation effect for cancer
groups I and II and for the following subgroups: (a) myeloma and myeloid
leukaemia with a doubling dose of 3.6 rads; (b) lung cancer with a doubling dose
of 13.7 rads (Fig.4); and (c) cancers of the pancreas, stomach and large intestine
with a doubling dose of 15.6 rads. For one component of group II (lymphoma
and reticulum cell sarcoma) there was no evidence of any radiation effect among
the male cases. However, the female cases included the woman with the highest
dose (1573 centirads) and for all female cancers the estimated doubling dose was
8.6 rads.

      For all male cancers the doubling dose was higher in the repeat analysis
(33.7 rads) than in the earlier study (12.2 rads). As, however, the lowered

TABLE X.   ESTIMATED DOUBLING DOSES FOR CANCERS
WITH RADIATION EFFECTS

Sex	Cancers	Cases	Doubling dose in rads [a]			Pre-death years [b]	
			Estimate	95% Confidence limits		Exceptional ones	Maximum t-value
Males	Myeloma and myeloid leukaemia	25	3.6	1.7	10.3	15—0	*3.7**
	Lymphoma and reticulum cell sarcoma	40	—	—	—	—	0.7
	Lung cancer	215	13.7	7.3	28.7	20—0	*3.7**
	Pancreas, stomach and large intestine	165	15.6	7.3	55.0	8—0	*2.7**
	All high sensitivity groups (I and II)	456 [c]	13.9	8.4	21.2	21—0	*5.3**
	Other cancers (III and IV)	287	—	—	—	—	0.6
	All cancers	743	33.7	15.3	79.7	16—0	*3.2**
Females	All cancers	89	8.7	2.6	∞	4—0	*1.9**

[a] Assuming a linear model (see Ref.[1]).
[b] Exceptional years when the total radiation dose was significantly higher than the corresponding dose for non-cancer deaths.
[c] Including cancers of thyroid and pharynx (see Table V).
*   See Table IV.

estimate of risk still allowed 35 of the 743 male cancers to be radiation-induced (and the ICRP 26 expected number was 4.8) [2], there remained a wide gap between risk estimates based on workers in the nuclear industry and ones based on A-bomb survivors and patients with ankylosing spondylitis.

EFFECT OF AGE ON THE CANCER INDUCTION EFFECTS
OF RADIATION

On the basis of the earlier findings we concluded that sensitivity to the cancer induction effects of radiation decreased with age before 30 years and

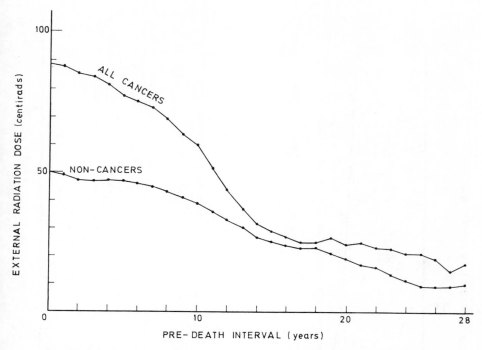

FIG.4.   *Female cancer and non-cancer deaths; CMD analysis by pre-death years.*

increased with age thereafter. On the basis of the repeat analysis (Fig.5), we concluded that more data were needed before we could be certain of age trends before 30 or after 60 years, but between these ages there was definite evidence of an increase in sensitivity (Fig.5).

CHECKING THE VALIDITY OF HANFORD BASED RISK ESTIMATES

In the earlier study we used differences between actual and expected cancer deaths (or the SMR method) to test the validity of the risk estimates derived from the CMD analysis. In the repeat analysis we compared relative risks from the Mantel-Haenszel analysis, first, with the corresponding risks in a crude analysis (Table IV) and then with the doubling dose for all male cancers (Figs 6 and 7).

The first test showed that the risk estimates were only slightly altered in the controlled compared with the crude analysis (changing from a relative risk of 1.35 to 1.26 in the highest dose group), and the second showed that seven points on the curve for relative risks at different dose levels in the controlled analysis were clustered reasonably close to the doubling dose projection line (assuming a linear model).

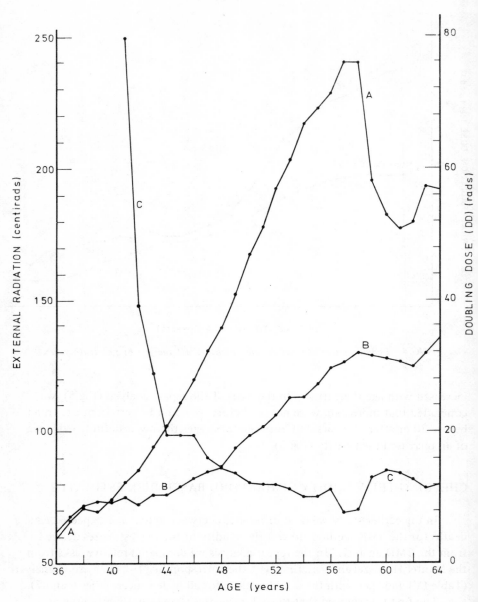

FIG.5.   *Male cancers in Groups I and II;   CMD analysis by age.*
A.   *Mean cumulative radiation doses for Cancer Groups I and II*
B.   *Ditto Non-cancers*
C.   *Doubling Dose (DD) for Cancer Groups I and II*

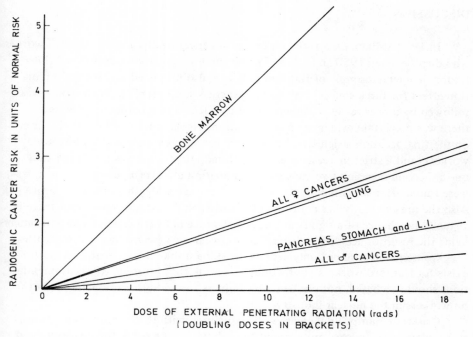

FIG.6. Projection lines for various forms of radiation-induced cancers.

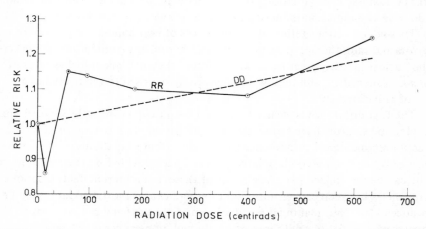

FIG.7. Male cancers; Doubling Doses (DD) and Relative Risk Estimates (RR) from the Mantel-Haenszel analysis.

DISCUSSION

In 1974 Milham discovered an excess of cancer deaths among Hanford worker
who died between 1950 and 1973 [7], and three years later we confirmed this
finding in a larger sample of Hanford data and also produced evidence of a radiation effect for three cancers (myeloma, pancreas and lung) [1]. Each report was
followed by a peer review (commissioned by ERDA) purporting to show that
there was no certain evidence of any radiation effects in Hanford data. However,
on the first occasion a significant difference between exposed and non-exposed
workers (and a strict increase of effect with radiation dose) was found [8], and
on the second occasion two cancers with radiation effects (myeloma and pancreas)
were found after adjusting for the effects of sex, age at death and date of death [4].
Also the present study has confirmed the earlier findings, and shown that there is
virtually no chance of a significant dose difference between cancers and non-cancers
being the result of accidental differences between two groups of certified deaths.

Consequently we not only agree with Milham that 'an occupational hazard
exists for Hanford workers', but would also think that future ICRP recommendations should be based, not on A-bomb survivors and radiotherapy patients, but
on workers in the nuclear industry.

Critics of Hanford data were well-acquainted with ICRP recommendations,
and evidently saw no reason to doubt the validity of the risk estimates contained
in the most recent publication [2]. Therefore they expected bone marrow to
be more sensitive to the cancer induction effects of radiation than other tissues,
and expected some effect from low-level radiation. However, they also expected
the bone marrow effect to take the form of myeloid leukaemia, and expected the
dose response curve to be highly sigmoid, thus making it unlikely that Hanford
Works (which has kept radiation doses far below ICRP maximal permissible doses)
would have any radiation-induced cancer deaths among its employees.

These expectations reflect the experiences of two populations (A-bomb
survivors and radiotherapy patients) who differ from any population of workers
in the nuclear industry in at least two respects: they had much higher rates of
non-cancer mortality, and they were only briefly exposed to relatively large
doses of radiation.

The first difference is clearly important because data from the Oxford Survey
of Childhood Cancers have shown that the pre-cancer state is associated with
lowered immunological competence to such an extent that children are in grave
danger of dying from secondary infections and accidents before the true state of
affairs can be recognized [9]. As a result of these 'latent period deaths' serious
discrepancies between cancer initiation rates and cancer mortality rates may be
introduced [10], thus making it peculiarly unsafe to base any radiation risk
estimates on populations with exceptionally high non-cancer death rates.

The second difference could be the reason why bone marrow effects have taken the form of myeloid leukaemia in three populations with brief exposures to relatively large doses of radiation (i.e. A-bomb survivors, early entrants to Hiroshima and Nagasaki after the explosions, and radiotherapy patients) and the form of myeloma in two populations with prolonged exposures to small doses (i.e. radiologists [11] and Hanford workers). It is true that we know very little about the effects of dose fractionation per se. On the other hand clinical experience suggests that the greater the insult the greater the probability of diffuse disease and the smaller the insult the greater the probability of localized disease.

Although 'cumulative radiation doses' played an important role in the CMD analysis of Hanford data, this does not imply any cumulative effects of the exposures. For Hanford workers even one exposure to a sizeable dose of radiation was a rare event. Therefore the total radiation dose of each worker was strongly correlated with the number of separate exposures, or the number of times that there was any probability of a stochastic effect.

According to ICRP 26, the mortality risk factor for radiation-induced cancers is about 10^{-2} Sv^{-1} (as an average for both sexes and all ages), and the corresponding figure for leukaemia is 2×10^{-3} Sv^{-1}. However, a recent follow-up of 'early entrants' (or persons who entered Hiroshima and Nagasaki less than four days after the explosions and therefore combined brief exposure periods with relatively low rates of non-cancer mortality), has produced a much higher figure for leukaemia, namely 18×10^{-3} Sv^{-1} [12]. Consequently the Hanford study is no longer the only one to question the validity of the risk estimates contained in ICRP 26.

Since two populations with low rates of non-cancer mortality have produced higher risk estimates than two populations with high rates, it is no longer safe to assume that the dose response curve is highly sigmoid [2]. On the contrary, since any non-stochastic effects of radiation necessarily have some effect on non-cancer mortality it is possible that linear extrapolation for high doses will slightly underestimate the risk at low doses.

Finally, an important reason for suggesting that future estimates of risk be based on Hanford data is because this population is currently the only one to provide a suitable model for studying the effects of low doses of radiation delivered at low dose rates to individuals whose non-cancer death rate is not increased.

ACKNOWLEDGEMENTS

The Hanford study was supported by the Division of Biology and Medicine, and Division of Occupational Safety of the former Atomic Energy Commission, AEC Contracts No. (AT(30-1)-3394) and No. CH-AT(11-1)-3428, and ERDA Contract No. E(11-1)-3428. The mortality data was supplied by the Social Security Administration and State Offices of Vital Statistics.

REFERENCES

[1] MANCUSO, T.F., STEWART, A., KNEALE, G., Radiation exposures of Hanford workers dying from cancer and other causes, Health Phys. **33** 5 (1977) 369.

[2] INTERNATIONAL COMMISSION ON RADIOLOGICAL PROTECTION, Publication No. 26, Recommendations of the International Commission on Radiological Protection, adopted 17 January 1977, Pergamon Press, Oxford, New York.

[3] MANTEL, N., HAENSZEL, W., Statistical aspects of the analysis of data from retrospective studies of disease, J. Natl. Cancer Inst. **22** (1959) 719.

[4] LAND, C., Analysis of Hanford proportional mortality data, adjusted for age and year of death (unpublished).

[5] JABLON, S., Comment on Ref. [1] (1978, unpublished).

[6] INTERNATIONAL COMMISSION ON RADIOLOGICAL PROTECTION, Publication No. 14, Radiosensitivity and Spatial Distribution of Dose, Pergamon Press, Oxford, New York (1969).

[7] MILHAM, S., Occupational Mortality in Washington State, 1950–1971, HEW Publication No. (NIOSH 76–175), Vols A, B & C (1976).

[8] GILBERT, E.S., BUSCHBOM, R.L., An evaluation of Milham's analysis of Hanford deaths (1975, unpublished).

[9] KNEALE, G.W., STEWART, A.M., Pre-cancers and liability to other diseases, Br. J. Cancer (in press).

[10] KNEALE, G.W., The excess sensitivity of pre-leukaemics to pneumonia: A model situation for studying the interaction of an infectious disease with cancer, Br. J. Prev. Soc. Med. **25** (1971) 152.

[11] LEWIS, E.B., Leukemia, multiple myelomatosis and aplastic anemia in American radiologists, Science **142** (1963) 1492.

[12] ROTBLAT, J., Risk factor for radiation-induced leukaemia among entrants to Hiroshima, Nature (London) (in press).

[13] KNEALE, G.W., STEWART, A.M., Mantel-Haenszel analysis of Oxford data, J. Natl. Cancer Inst. **56** (1976) 879.

DISCUSSION

G.W. DOLPHIN: In Table 10 the doubling dose for myeloma and myeloid leukaemia is shown as 3.6 (1.7 to 10.3) rads. This value is $4\frac{1}{2}$ times higher than the value, 0.8 rad, given in your paper in Health Physics (Ref. [1]). Why does the inclusion of more data in the survey cause such a large change in doubling dose? Surely the doubling dose value must contain more uncertainty than the statistical 95% limits quoted above.

G.W. KNEALE: In a very large sample the 95% limits would be very close together, whereas the point estimate from a small sample would fluctuate widely, so it is not true that the 95% limits from a large sample should include the point estimate from a small one. The converse is, however, true that the 95% limits from a small sample (not quoted in the Health Physics paper) should include the point estimate from the larger one. Even if it did not, there is an explanation, since in the Health Physics estimate we treated non-film-badge wearers as if they had zero dose.

D. BENINSON: The assessment of doubling dose in your paper is based on values of σ for the total population, the average dose in the total population and the average dose in the critical group. It seems that the assessment would depend on the inclusion of doses from natural radiation in the basic dose data. The inclusion would in turn depend on what is recorded in the case of low doses (0 or a nominal value), which are the most frequent.

G.W. KNEALE: According to our conversations with the health physicists, who know how the badges were measured, a correction was made for natural background radiation. If the data are plotted on a logarithmic scale of dose (which makes the distribution approximately symmetrical) it is noticeable that between 1 and 8 centirads there are irregularities in the distribution probably caused by some such rounding of low doses as you mention. With regard to the analysis it is only possible to take the data as we find it, noting, as we do, that the actual estimates of doubling dose depend quite critically on the assumption that any effect of such procedures is negligible. It would, of course, be desirable to have a method of estimating doubling dose that was not sensitive to such things, but such a method would necessarily be very complicated.

D.J. MEWISSEN: In Fig.1, it is seen that accidents, all non-cancers and all cancers decreasingly correlated in terms of pre-death intervals versus cumulative radiation dosage. Obviously the cumulative radiation doses are related to the age of the individuals involved, as the latter is also in some way related to the length of occupational exposure. On the pre-death interval scale, how are the various groups (non-cancer versus all cancers versus accidents cohorts) corrected for their relative age-specific peak incidences in a non-irradiated control population?

G.W. KNEALE: In Fig.1 they are not corrected for the factors you mention. However, in the controlled or Mantel-Haenszel analysis of cancers and non-cancers these factors are taken into account and we still find a dose effect, therefore the difference between cancers and non-cancers cannot be explained in this way. Since we have not done a Mantel-Haenszel analysis of accidents and non-accidents it is possible, and indeed likely, that the dose difference is accounted for by some such factor. Finally Fig.7, showing the relation between the relative risks (from the controlled analysis) and the fitted linear dose response (from the uncorrected difference in dose between cancers and non-cancers) shows that the uncorrected analysis cannot be exaggerating much.

P.G. GROER: You mentioned that the follow-up period was longer in your study than in Mr. Marks'. Did additional cancers occur during this period?

G.W. KNEALE: In the Health Physics paper (Ref.[1]) there were 670 male and 126 female cancers; in the present paper we have 924 male and 177 female cancers. The increase was particularly marked in the case of lung cancers. The estimate of radiation-induced cases was 28 in the Health Physics paper compared with 35 in the present paper.

Mr. Marks, I hope I was correct in stating that the cut-off date for deaths in the data on which your present paper is based was 1974.

S. MARKS: It is correct that we have not included deaths occurring since 1974 in our analysis. We do have death certificates available on some additional deaths, but have been reluctant to include them in our data base at this point because that could not be done systematically. We fear that haphazard additions to the data set might cause undesirable biases in the analyses.

RISK ASSOCIATED WITH OCCUPATIONAL EXPOSURE TO IONIZING RADIATION KEPT IN PERSPECTIVE

J.A. BONNELL
Nuclear Health and Safety Department

G. HARTE
Berkeley Nuclear Laboratories,
Central Electricity Generating Board,
London,
United Kingdom

Abstract

RISK ASSOCIATED WITH OCCUPATIONAL EXPOSURE TO IONIZING RADIATION KEPT IN PERSPECTIVE.

The risks associated with exposure to ionizing radiations are placed in perspective by a study of the natural incidence of those diseases in the United Kingdom that can be induced by radiation exposure. It is apparent that at ICRP recommended annual dose equivalent limits the small risks associated with exposure to ionizing radiations are acceptable, bearing in mind the obvious benefits that accrue from activities such as power production. This applies both to genetic and somatic diseases.

INTRODUCTION

In view of the widespread public debate on the acceptability of nuclear power it is necessary for those scientists and physicians who have a duty to advise governments and institutions on the health and safety implications of exposure to ionising radiations to express themselves clearly and in terms which are understood by the lay public.

In an attempt to do this we have taken the risk factors proposed by ICRP and calculated the risks of development of disease in individuals exposed to different levels of radiation.

These figures are most clearly conveyed to the public if they are compared with other chances of harm in everyday life; and to keep these risks in perspective we have chosen to compare the risks from cancer and leukaemia resulting from exposure to ionising radiation with the natural mortality risks from these diseases. The latter

413

risks have been calculated from data given in the mortality
tables published by the Registrar General in the U.K. We
have also extracted from this data the chances of death
from all causes in the U.K. at different ages.

In its latest recommendations (ICRP 26; 1977)[1]the
International Commission on Radiological Protection has
formulated its new protection philosophy. Having classified
the biological effects of radiation exposure as 'stochastic'
and 'non-stochastic', the document states that the aim of
radiation protection should be to prevent non-stochastic
effects (those such as cataract of the lens and non-
malignant skin damage for which the severity of the effect
varies with dose) and to limit the probability of stochastic
effects to an acceptable level.   The stochastic effects of
irradiation are those for which the probability of occurrence
of the effect is a function of dose. Carcinogenesis – the
chief somatic effect of irradiation at low doses – is
stochastic in nature, as is the induction of genetic damage.

In pursuance of its aims, the Commission has moved
away from the concept of limiting the dose to a critical
organ, and now recommends a protection procedure which takes
account of the total risk attributable to the exposure of all
irradiated tissues in the body.   A concomitant of a
protection system based on risk limitation is the assignment
of a risk per unit dose to the tissues of the body
susceptible to the induction of stochastic effects, and
Table I lists the risk factors put forward by the Commission.
These risk factors may be used in conjunction with postulated
exposure regimes to estimate the risk to an average member
of the working population or of the general public arising
out of the operation of nuclear power plants.

In the calculations carried out here, a rectangular
time variation of risk after exposure has been assumed,
similar to that used by Kay and Reissland (1977).[2]   For
leukaemia a latent period of 5 years is followed by 20 years
of constant risk, whilst for other cancers a latent period
of 15 years is assumed to be followed by a 30 year period of
constant risk.   The annual risk per Sievert (Sv) for
leukaemia is then 10^{-4} over the period of finite risk, and
for all other cancers is 2.7×10^{-4}.

The risk of genetic damage can be assessed by
adopting a similar approach and this is discussed in detail
at a later stage.

ICRP have proposed that the acceptability of the
level of risk from occupational exposure may be judged from
a comparison with other occupations which have a low
incidence of accidents or occupational disease. It is
difficult however to obtain accurate risk estimates from the
wide range of occupations necessary to make this assessment,
especially in the case of occupationally induced diseases,
though Pochin (1975)[3] collected data which he has expressed
as deaths per million persons employed per year for various
occupations and activities.

TABLE I. ICRP RISK FACTORS per Sv

SOMATIC EFFECTS (Mortality)

Red bone marrow	Leukaemia	2×10^{-3}
Bone	Cancer	5×10^{-4}
Lung	Cancer	2×10^{-3}
Thyroid	Cancer	5×10^{-4}
Breast	Cancer	2.5×10^{-3}
Other tissues[a]	Cancer	$<5 \times 10^{-3}$
Uniform whole body	Cancer	10^{-2}

GENETIC EFFECTS

Gonads	Hereditary disease[b]	
	In first two generations	10^{-2}
	All generations	2×10^{-2}
Uniform whole body	Hereditary disease[b]	
	In first two generations	4×10^{-3}
	All generations	8×10^{-3}

[a] The combined risk of malignancy in all other tissues is thought unlikely to exceed 5×10^{-3} Sv^{-1}, with no one tissue contributing more than one fifth this value.

[b] The average risk factor for hereditary effects is taken as $\sim 4 \times 10^{-3}$ Sv^{-1} when account is taken of the proportion of exposures that is likely to be genetically significant.

We have chosen to compare the levels of risk associated with exposure to radiation, whether in the working environment or outside it, with the natural risk of contracting one of the various forms of cancer, or of genetic damage. The UK Office of Population Censuses and Surveys (OPCS) have kept accurate records of deaths from these diseases in the U.K., and naturally occurring risks can therefore be calculated.

SOMATIC EFFECTS

Let us therefore examine some results obtained from OPCS data

(a) The probability of death within one year from all causes at different ages.

(b) The probability of death within one year from

    (i)   leukaemia   )

    (ii) all cancers) at different ages.

$1 \, mSv = 0.1 \, R$

$1 \, Sv = 100 \, R$

PROBABILITY OF DEATH WITHIN ONE YEAR

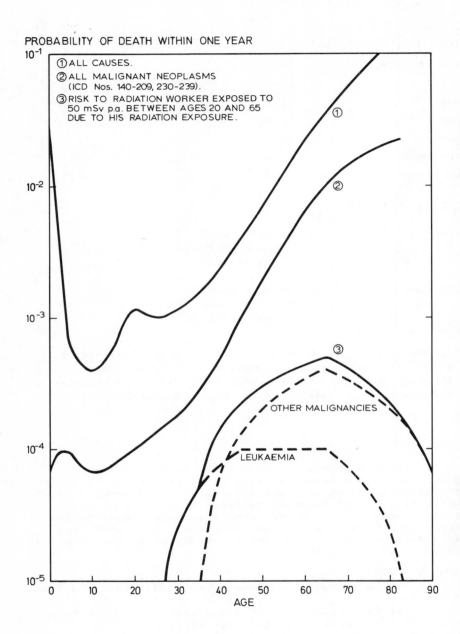

① ALL CAUSES.
② ALL MALIGNANT NEOPLASMS
(ICD Nos. 140-209, 230-239).
③ RISK TO RADIATION WORKER EXPOSED TO
50 mSv p.a. BETWEEN AGES 20 AND 65
DUE TO HIS RADIATION EXPOSURE.

OTHER MALIGNANCIES

LEUKAEMIA

AGE

FIG.1.   *Annual risk of death for males at various ages (England and Wales).*

In addition we have made an assessment of the
increased probability of developing these diseases if
individuals are exposed to different doses of ionising
radiations either through occupational exposure or as
members of the general public.

Figure 1 shows the probability of death within one
year from any cause plotted as a function of the age of the
individual.   This curve, which applies only to males in
England and Wales, is based on data obtained from the
Annual Abstract of Statistics 1976.[4]   A man aged 25 has
a probability of 1 in 1000 of dying within one year;   at
age 45 this probability is 1 in 250, and at 65 it is 1 in 27.

The principal causes of death vary from age-group to
age-group, accidents being the commonest cause for people
under 35 (OPCS, 1977)[5].

In middle age, however, cancer shares, with heart
disease, top place amongst natural causes of death.   As an
illustration the main causes of death for 1976 are shown in
Table II.   Data presented in the Registrar General's Review
(HMSO, 1969-1973)[6] have been used to estimate the annual
probability of death from cancer at different ages, and
these results are also plotted in Figure 1.   At age 25 a
man has an annual risk of death from cancer of about 1 in
7,500, at 45 this risk is 1 in 1000 and at 65 is 1 in 100.

The annual dose equivalent limit for whole body
irradiation of workers is 50mSv; and although workers are
very rarely exposed at such levels it is theoretically
possible for a particular individual to receive such a dose
every year of his working life.   This has been taken
therefore as our worst case.

The additional risks to a radiation worker exposed
from age 20 to the dose limit of 50 mSv per year proposed
by ICRP are given below.   The risks from these exposures
have been calculated using ICRP risk factors and the risk-
time relationship mentioned previously.

The time variation of the cancer risk to this worker
is shown in Figure 1 split up into components from leukaemia
and from other cancers.   It has been assumed that this
worker retires at age 65 and irradiation ceases.   The
radiation risk is about one fifth the natural risk between
ages 35 and 45 - it is at this point that it forms the
greatest fraction of the natural risk of cancer.   These
results are set out in more detail in the tables which
follow.

Table III shows the naturally occurring cancer risk
for males of various ages, together with the annual risk to
a notional radiation worker who has received a dose of
50mSv p.a. whole body from age 20, and the annual risk to a
member of the public who has received 1mSv p.a. from birth
due to operation of nuclear installations.   The average

TABLE II. CAUSES OF DEATH IN ORDER OF FREQUENCY PER MILLION TOTAL POPULATION 1976

Age	Death rates (All causes)			
1–4	552	Accidents 135 (24%)	Congenital anomalies 101 (18%)	Respiratory diseases 97 (18%)
5–14	276	Accidents 90 (33%)	Cancer 57 (21%)	Congenital anomalies 32 (12%)
15–34	703	Accidents 249 (35%)	Cancer 122 (17%)	Suicide 61 (9%)
35–44	1784	Cancer 562 (32%)	Heart disease 434 (24%)	Accidents 165 (9%)
45–54	5626	Cancer 2006 (36%)	Heart disease 1864 (33%)	Respiratory diseases 392 (7%)
55–64	14717	Heart disease 5268 (36%)	Cancer 4955 (34%)	Respiratory diseases 1382 (9%)
65–74	36750	Heart disease 13069 (36%)	Cancer 9670 (26%)	Respiratory diseases 4968 (14%)
75+	112360	Heart disease 37448 (33%)	Respiratory diseases 23490 (21%)	Cerebrovascular disease 18475 (16%)

TABLE III. RISK OF DEATH FROM RADIATION-INDUCED CANCER & CANCER FROM NATURAL CAUSES

Age	Natural risk[a]	1 mSv per annum from birth[b]	50 mSv per annum from age 20[c]
5	8.2×10^{-5} (1 in 12 000)	0	—
15	7.6×10^{-5} (1 in 13 000)	10^{-6} (1 in a million)	—
25	1.3×10^{-4} (1 in 7 700)	4.7×10^{-6} (1 in 210 000)	0
35	2.7×10^{-4} (1 in 3 700)	7.4×10^{-6} (1 in 140 000)	5.0×10^{-5} (1 in 20 000)
45	1.0×10^{-3} (1 in 1 000)	10^{-5} (1 in 100 000)	2.3×10^{-4} (1 in 4 300)
55	3.5×10^{-3} (1 in 300)	10^{-5} (1 in 100 000)	3.7×10^{-4} (1 in 2 700)
65	9.6×10^{-3} (1 in 100)	10^{-5} (1 in 100 000)	5.0×10^{-4} (1 in 2 000)

[a] Annual risk of death from malignant neoplasms (ICD Nos 140–209, 230–239) in age group centred on specified age, estimated from analysis of deaths by cause (males) in Registrar General's Review of England and Wales, 1969–1973 [5].

[b] Supposed member of a critical group receiving 1 mSv (100 millirem) per annum from birth due to operation of nuclear installations.

[c] Supposed worker receiving the maximum dose of 50 mSv (5 rem) per annum from age 20 till retirement at 65.

member of the public receives only a very small dose as a result of nuclear operations, so once again we have taken as a worst case a notional member of a critical group who receives 1 mSv (100 mrem) of radiation as a whole body dose. The risk to this notional member of a critical group attendant upon his radiation exposure is small both in absolute as well as relative terms. The radiation worker exposed at the ICRP dose limit would be exposed to an increasing annual cancer risk which in fact reaches its maximum at age 65. Should exposure at that rate continue beyond age 65, the annual risk will remain constant at one chance in 2000 of death from a radiation-induced malignancy.

It is however rare for a worker to receive the maximum dose of 50 mSv even in 1 year, let alone over all the years of his working life. An annual dose of 10mSv or less is more usual for workers in the British Nuclear power industry (UNSCEAR 1977)[7], and the annual average dose to radiation workers at CEGB power stations for 1976 was 2.6 mSv.

Therefore, abandoning the 'worst case' approach, the increase in natural risk due to a more realistic 10mSv per annum may be examined.

TABLE IVA.   INCREASE IN LEUKAEMIA RISK FOLLOWING 10 mSv p.a.
FOR MALES FROM AGE 20

Age	Naturally occurring	Radiation-induced	Total risk
25	2.0×10^{-5} (1 in 49 600)	0	2.0×10^{-5} (1 in 49 600)
35	2.3×10^{-5} (1 in 43 500)	10^{-5} (1 in 100 000)	3.3×10^{-5} (1 in 30 300)
45	4.0×10^{-5} (1 in 25 100)	2.0×10^{-5} (1 in 50 000)	6.0×10^{-5} (1 in 16 700)
55	7.4×10^{-5} (1 in 13 600)	2.0×10^{-5} (1 in 50 000)	9.4×10^{-5} (1 in 10 600)

TABLE IVB.   INCREASE IN TOTAL CANCER RISK FOLLOWING 10 mSv p.a.
FOR MALES FROM AGE 20

Age	Naturally occurring	Radiation-induced	Total risk
25	1.3×10^{-4} (1 in 7 700)	0	1.30×10^{-4} (1 in 7 700)
35	2.7×10^{-4} (1 in 3 700)	10^{-5} (1 in 100 000)	2.80×10^{-4} (1 in 3 600)
45	1.0×10^{-3} (1 in 1 000)	4.7×10^{-5} (1 in 21 000)	1.05×10^{-3} (1 in 955)
55	3.5×10^{-3} (1 in 300)	7.3×10^{-5} (1 in 14 000)	3.57×10^{-3} (1 in 280)
65	9.6×10^{-3} (1 in 100)	10^{-4} (1 in 10 000)	9.70×10^{-3} (1 in 100)

It will be seen from Table IV that at any age the
risk of death from any malignancy is increased only by a
very small amount - the natural risk is increased by 5% or
less in early middle age and by 1% at age 65.   Reduction of
the dose   reduces the risk.

When leukaemia alone is considered it is apparent
that at ages 35 - 45 the natural risk is increased by 50%.
It should, however, be noted that the total number of
leukaemia cases is low, and that the risk of developing the
disease is considerably less than the natural risk of
contracting any other malignancy or the risk of death from
all causes.

In absolute terms, therefore, the increase in the
incidence of leukaemia is small.

GENETIC EFFECTS

No discussion of the biological effects of ionising
radiation is complete without an assessment of the risk of
genetic harm.   Usually this subject is only discussed in

TABLE V. NATURAL OCCURRENCE OF GENETIC DEFECTS PER 1000 LIVE BIRTHS

Defect	Frequency of occurrence
Numerical chromosome abnormalities	5
Dominant monogenic disorders	7
Structural chromosome rearrangement	2
Total defects	14
Individual risk	1 : 70

relation to exposure of populations, and the measure of harm is expressed in statistical terms. If the facts are to be presented to radiation workers and their families or to the general public the risk to the individual must be expressed clearly.

The genetically determined diseases to be considered when estimating the risk of damage from ionising radiation are those whose frequency is closely linked to the mutation rate as estimated from the incidence in live births. These disorders, most of which are serious, include those which are listed in Table V together with their frequency of occurrence   (Ash, Vennart and Carter 1977)[8].   The total frequency is 14 per 1000 live births.

Table I gives two risk factors for hereditary disease occurring in all generations 8.10^{-3} per Sv (1 in 125 or 1 in 12,500 per rem) following irradiation of either parent, for radiation protection purposes and 2.10^{-2} per Sv (1 in 50 or 1 in 5000 per rem) where the figure is to be used for a population of pre-reproductive individuals. This is to take account of the added risk to the latter group of individuals since the whole dose will be genetically significant. In the present discussion of the risk of genetic damage the risk figure of 2.10^{-2} has been used.

It has been suggested (Ash et al.)[8] that the 'doubling dose' for chronic irradiation is 1 Sv (100 rems). This is the dose of radiation which, spread over a period of time, would give a risk of radiation-induced hereditary disease equal to the naturally occurring risk. On the basis of the ICRP proposals, a dose of 1 Sv would lead to 20 cases of serious genetic disease in the descendants of 1 000 people who receive such a dose. This is rather higher than the natural incidence of 14 per 1 000 quoted by Ash et al. (1977)[8], presumably because ICRP have added a contribution for the occurrence of disorders of multi-factorial complex inheritance yielding a rounded value of 20 per 1 000.   This means that the risk factor of 2.10^{-2} is a conservative one.

Using ICRP risk factors an individual radiation
worker exposed to 50mSv (5 rem) p.a. from age 20 will have
received a doubling dose by age 40.

A notional member of a critical group who from birth
receives a dose of 1 mSv p.a. as a result of nuclear plant
operations will have received a total dose of 25 mSv (2.5 rem)
by the age of 25.   There will be a 1 in 2000 chance
therefore for the occurrence of genetic disease in his
descendants due to this exposure.   This should be compared
with the naturally occurring risk of 1 chance in 50 (on the
basis of the figure 20 per 1000 live births implicitly
used by ICRP).

DISCUSSION

In this paper the risks of somatic and genetic
disease incurred by people exposed to ionising radiation
have been calculated using ICRP risk factors and a simple
risk-time relationship.

It can be seen that the annual risk of death due to
radiation-induced cancer, even when the person has been
exposed for a long time at the dose limit of 50mSv p.a., is
small compared with the naturally occurring cancer mortality
risk except where this natural risk is itself small.   In
general, when the radiation-induced risk is added to the
naturally occurring risk no significant difference is made
to the total risk of the individual.

Leukaemia, when considered on its own, provides an
exception to this.   In middle life (age 30 - 50) the natural
risk run by the individual is of the order of 1 in 40 000
to 1 in 20 000 annually;   if that individual had been exposed
to 50mSv p.a. his extra risk could be up to 1 in 10 000, i.e.
greater than the natural risk of contracting the disease.
However, even after such exposure, the risk in absolute
terms is small.   After the age of 20 the individual's annual
risk of death never falls below 1 in 1000 (males), and at
age 45, which is when the leukaemia mortality risk first
reaches 1 in 10 000 (its maximum), the individual's annual
chance of death is 1 in 250 and increasing.

It has been pointed out already that no occupationally
exposed person receives the annual dose limit as a regular
event, and indeed ICRP 26 specifically condemns such a
policy.   It is therefore more realistic to discuss the
significance of annual doses of the order of 10 mSv.   On
this basis an individual exposed at the rate of 10 mSv p.a.
from age 20 has incurred a risk of death from radiation-
induced leukaemia of between 1 in 100 000 and 1 in 50 000.

The risk factor proposed by ICRP for the occurrence
of serious hereditary disease in the immediate descendants
of an irradiated individual is 10^{-2} Sv^{-1}, which is the same
as the risk factor for cancer mortality.   It seems to be
commonly accepted that for chronic irradiation the doubling

dose for genetic effects is about 1 Sv.   Therefore the
individual exposed from age 20 to the annual dose limit of
50mSv will have received the doubling dose by age 40.   As
pointed out above, average annual doses received by radiation
workers are in fact of the order of 10mSv or less.

The worker who has been exposed at 10mSv per annum
from age 20 will, if he produces children at age 40, incur
an overall risk of 1 in 250 of some serious genetic disease
appearing in his descendants, the risk being 1 in 500 for his
children and grandchildren.   The natural risk over all
generations of his descendants in the absence of irradiation
is 1 in 50.

The notional member of a critical group who, as a
result of nuclear operations, has received 1 mSv per year
from birth will have a chance at age 40 of 1 in 1250 of
producing a descendant suffering from serious genetic disease
due to this exposure.

So far, no conclusions have been drawn about the
acceptability of these extra risks.   No risk can be
acceptable if it is not accompanied by substantial benefits,
and it is now part of ICRP philosophy that risk-benefit
analysis be carried out.   A very crude analysis of this type
may be carried out for the British Electricity Supply
Industry using data from various sources.   In the most
recent UNSCEAR report (1977)[7] the collective dose
commitment from nuclear power is estimated at 7 man-rads per
MW(e)-year.   This includes doses to plant personnel as well
as to the public.   The current generating capacity of the
CEGB is 56 gigawatts to supply roughly 50 million people in
England and Wales.

On this basis an 1100 MW(e) power station will give a
collective dose commitment of about 8000 man-rads as a result
of supplying one million people with their electricity needs
for a year.   One can therefore expect about one cancer death
as the price of that year's energy supply.   This death may
or may not occur in the population receiving the electricity.
The normal cancer death rate, based on cancer deaths in
England and Wales in the early 1970's, is about 2400-2500 per
million per annum.   Further, if all of the exposed population
were of reproductive age, one could, as a result of the
8000 man-rads, expect two cases of serious genetic disease
over all generations of their descendants.   The 'natural
background' of genetic diseases is 20 000 occurring in the
descendants of one million people.

It is suggested that by taking factual data concerning
disease patterns in the U.K. and presenting the probability of
contracting malignant disease at different ages, the very
small additional risk posed by radiation exposure to levels of
radiation recommended by ICRP is clearly acceptable, bearing
in mind the obvious benefit which accrues.   It should in
addition be emphasised that power generated by the nuclear
process will result in the reduction of risks which currently
exist due to power production from other processes: no
account has been taken of such benefits.

ACKNOWLEDGMENT

Table II reproduced by kind permission of the Controller, HMSO.

REFERENCES

[1]   INTERNATIONAL COMMISSION ON RADIOLOGICAL PROTECTION, Recommend-
        ations of the ICRP, ICRP Publication No. 26, Pergamon Press, Oxford, New York (1977).
[2]   KAY, P., REISSLAND, J.A., Late Effects on a Population exposed to Activity released
        into the Environment, NRPB Report R-56 (1977).
[3]   POCHIN, E.E., Br. Med. Bull. 31 (1975) 184.
[4]   HER MAJESTY'S STATIONERY OFFICE, Annual Abstract of Statistics, English Life
        Table No. 12, 1960–62, HMSO, London (1976).
[5]   U.K. OFFICE OF POPULATION CENSUSES AND SURVEYS, Deaths by Cause,
        OPCS Monitor Ref. DH2 77/3 (1977).
[6]   HER MAJESTY'S STATIONERY OFFICE, Statistical Review of England and Wales
        (for the years 1969–1973), Part 1 Tables, Medical, Registrar General, HMSO, London
        (1971–75).
[7]   UNITED NATIONS, Sources and Effects of Ionizing Radiation, United Nations
        Scientific Committee on Effects of Atomic Radiation, Report to the General Assembly,
        UN, New York (1977).
[8]   ASH, P., VENNART, J., CARTER, C.O., The incidence of hereditary disease in man,
        Lancet i (1971) 849.

DISCUSSION

I. SCHMITZ-FEUERHAKE: I feel that your paper has not so much to do with radiation protection as with justifying radiation burdens to workers in the nuclear industry. For your approach it would be best to have an extremely high 'spontaneous' cancer incidence so that you can make the number of radiation-induced cancers appear less. In your Table III a cumulative risk of 1% is shown for workers receiving the maximum permissible dose: one out of 100 workers will die from cancer as a result of his occupation. This is unacceptable. You will say that the maximum values will not be reached, but on the other hand the ICRP risk values employed are not conservative. They should be increased by a factor of 2 or 4 for several reasons, and notably in view of the breast cancer risk we heard about in Session 5. Furthermore, you neglect the non-fatal diseases. A 'cured' breast cancer means that the breast has been amputated. A non-fatal thyroid cancer means surgical intervention or radiation therapy and then for the rest of the patient's life substitution of the thyroid function by pharmaceuticals which are not always well tolerated. So the only conclusion we can draw is that the maximum permissible doses ought to be lowered.

J.A. BONNELL: In previous discussions at this symposium you have clearly not understood the philosophy of the ICRP dose limits. No person would be permitted to accumulate a dose of 5 rem (50 mSv) annually. This is the dose limit, i.e. provided it is not exceeded, the risk is not unacceptable, and further recommendations are made specifically condemning this as a regular practice. By taking this as an annual limit (as the worst case) the added risk over and above the existing cancer risk is still small. If you look at Table IVB, at the age of 55 a worker exposed to 10 mSv per annum from age 20 has increased his existing risk of 1 : 300 to 1 : 280, an increase of 0.15%. It is desirable not to make emotional comments and I do not agree with your opinions. Radiation workers accept and understand the approach made in this paper.

INDICATORS FOR LATE EFFECTS
Session 6

AN APPROACH TO EARLY EVALUATION
OF POSSIBLE LATE EFFECTS
OF RADIATION

E. RIKLIS, R. KOL
Israel Atomic Energy Commission
    Nuclear Research Center-Negev,
Beer-Sheva,
Israel

Abstract

AN APPROACH TO EARLY EVALUATION OF POSSIBLE LATE EFFECTS OF
RADIATION.
    DNA repair is a dominant factor in determining the radiosensitivity or resistance to
mutational and carcinogenic changes at the cellular or molecular level. The induction of
'error prone' repair is thought to control not only cellular radiosensitivity (cell survival),
but may also be one of the major causes of detrimental late effects. It is necessary to
develop a reliable and simple biochemical test for determining DNA repair capability
following radiation damage of high or low doses and dose rates. Lymphocytes have been
used for studying biological effects of low-level radiation. Although it is accepted that
chromosome aberrations are increased upon exposure to ionizing radiation, it is not a
reliable test of the effects of very low-level radiation which may potentially result in late
effects. Aberrations are secondary in nature to the primary events in the cell, affecting
primarily DNA, events whose outcome depends on the efficiency and accuracy of the repair
systems. Impairment of repair capability, an indicator of the cellular capacity to overcome
damage, is of greater significance to possible future harmful effects from different possible
types of damage, whereas aberrations are the somatic manifestation of an immediate unrepaired
certain type of damage. Transformation capability and repair capability via repair synthesis
of DNA and their relation to chromosome aberrations in lymphocytes are therefore being
studied. Subjects who have been exposed for a long time to very low dose radiation are
available among persons occupationally exposed to soft beta radiation from tritium during
the preparation of beta lights, or of labelled organic molecules for medical-research use.
Slight differences could be found between such persons and control subjects, in the
concentration of PHA mitogen for stimulation of optimal transformation, and in the response
to additional in-vitro gamma radiation dose as measured by uptake of tritium-labelled
thymidine into stimulated transforming lymphocytes. A dose of 40 rads, additional to the
continuous very low-level beta radiation, resulted in a decreased uptake of thymidine,
compared with control subjects. The possibility that such changes may be indicative of a
slight impairment of the potential repair capability of the cells is being currently investigated.

INTRODUCTION

The main problem that stems from the fact that no 'theoretical threshold' can be decided upon, and no 'practical threshold' can be overlooked, is in the need to perfect assay methods which will allow prediction, if no immediate damage is observed, of possible potential future damage. Immediate damage to DNA is usually dealt with, in normal healthy cells, by the various DNA repair systems [1, 2, 3 and reviews]. The cellular processes of DNA repair can re-establish the molecular integrity of the genetic material when damaged by physical (radiation) and chemical (mutagenic and carcinogenic) agents, and ultimately control the response of cells to external stimuli that alter the structure of the genetic material. DNA repair is therefore a dominant factor in determining the radiosensitivity or resistance to mutational and carcinogenic changes at the cellular level. The methods conventionally used to detect mutagenic actions, such as the study of chromosomal aberrations, or the induction of dominant lethal mutations in vivo, are actually measuring indirectly the results of a whole series of actions which may either perfectly repair a damaged cell, or lead to changes. Indeed, in the process of repair itself lies the danger of whether it is 'error free' as is the excision repair [1], or 'error prone' as are pathways such as 'SOS' repair [4]. It is therefore necessary to develop a reliable biochemical test for determining DNA repair capability as well as accuracy. Such a test might be needed to monitor special cases of radiosensitivity of persons who may be subjected to occupational or medical exposures. Attention may be drawn to the possible involvement of deficient DNA repair in syndromes of various diseases accompanied with chromosome aberrations.

A question that should be asked, in particular in relation to occupational exposures is, can the natural repair system(s) be 'weakened' by prolonged low-level assaults that force it to function constantly and continuously at a rate higher than dictated by the need to repair damage invoked by background external and internal radiations. Situations like this may exist among people of different groups: those living in very high background areas, or those involved in the preparation of beta lights or tritium-labelled organic molecules for medical and research uses, where HTO contamination is a common phenomenon as it is difficult to seal hermetically the preparation boxes and avoid breathing tritium vapours.

Several such cases have been selected and followed for some time; the level of HTO in their urine was measured frequently and showed a degree of contamination below the maximum permissible body burden, but above the natural background.

Lymphocytes have been widely used for studying biological effects of low-level radiations. Although it is acceptable that chromosome aberrations increase with radiation, a minimal dose of several rads is required to obtain a significant result.

Many karyotypes prepared from lymphocytes after an in-vitro dose of 50 rads led us to conclude that meaningful results can be obtained not by scoring individual aberrations, but rather by analysing the types of aberrations in groups and looking for a typical group pattern related to dose [5], and using this as a biological dose meter. But aberrations are the end-product of events of damage and repair, and the potentiality of a damage to end as an aberration should be determined at an earlier stage. We have previously observed the efficiency of a DNA repair-synthesis system in lymphocytes following gamma irradiation, as well as the susceptibility of the repair system to external factors, such as hyperthermia [6]. These considerations led to the decision to study some of the basic characteristics of lymphocyte function which may affect immunologic competence and be reflected in chromosomal aberrations: namely, the capability for transformation and for repair synthesis of DNA following an additional acute low radiation dose to lymphocytes previously exposed to continuous very low-level beta radiation.

MATERIALS AND METHODS

Venous blood was drawn with heparinized syringes and separated on Dextran (Rheomacrodex 10% wt/vol., Pharmacia, Sweden) as described by Fitzgerald [7]. The white cell differential count was taken in a haemocytometer, and cells were suspended in Medium 199 (Gibco, USA), supplemented with 20% foetal calf serum. Lymphocyte purity varied from 50—70%, and there was a small amount of red cell contamination. Another differential cell count was taken after suspension in Ml99, and the cultures, containing approximately 0.5×10^6 cells/ml, were grown in 2 ml volume in screw-capped plastic tubes (Nunc) at 37°C.

Cultures were irradiated at room temperature in a cobalt-60 gamma source at a dose rate of 20 rads/s. Stimulants were added after irradiation in concentration shown previously to give optimal response, as described in the following section.

Two stimulants were used: phytohaemagglutinin (PHA) (Wellcome, England, reagent grade) and pokeweed mitogen (PWM) (Barker and Farnes, Gibco, USA). The contents of the commercially available vials of PHA and PWM were dissolved in 5 ml sterile distilled water and diluted into several working solutions, 0.1 ml of which was added into each culture.

The cultures were incubated for 70 h. To each tube, 0.2 μCi ^{3}H-thymidine (Nuclear Research Center-Negev, 30 Ci/mM) was added and cultures incubated for an additional 2 h.

Harvesting was done by washing the cells with cold phosphate buffered saline (PBS) and 5% cold TCA. The precipitate was air-dried and dissolved in hyamine hydroxide 10-x (Packard) and kept overnight at 4°C; samples were transferred into vials, 10 ml toluene-based scintillation mixture added, and counting was performed in a TriCarb liquid scintillation counter. Activity, expressed in counts per minute, was corrected for each culture tube according to the exact number of lymphocytes present in the tube. Mean value of triplicate cultures was calculated and final results are expressed in counts/min $\times 10^3$ per cell, as can be seen in the figures.

RESULTS AND DISCUSSION

Lymphocytes stimulated in vitro were shown to transform into 'blast' cells, basically similar in morphology to immunoblasts characteristic of lymphoid tissue involved in the generation of immunologically activated cells. It is believed that at least two classes of lymphocytes are operative in immune reactions: thymus-derived T-cells are supposed to meet with antigen, and by interaction with bone marrow derived B-cells bring about their proliferation and differentiation to plasma cells. There is much controversy on the question of radiosensitivity of T-cells and B-cells, and the relative amounts of each are often blamed for differences in radiation sensitivity of individuals [8, 9].

The interest in in-vitro activation and transformation of lymphocytes is based on the contention that these phenomena are analogous to morphological and biological properties of lymphocytes expressed in vivo during immunological reactions. DNA synthesis is used as an indication of reactivity and responsiveness of lymphocytes to the mitogens that stimulate transformation. A marked reduction in ^{3}H-TdR incorporation into DNA of lymphocytes irradiated with high doses has been previously demonstrated by several authors [10].

Our attention was focused on the question whether lymphocytes that have been previously exposed to continuous low-level radiation from an internal emitter will show (a) a reduction in transformation capability; (b) a difference in DNA repair capability; (c) a reduction in transformation capability following an additional dose of radiation given in a high dose-rate; or (d) an effect of such additional radiation on the DNA repair synthesis.

Whenever cultures of an experimental subject were prepared, a control subject who never came in touch with radiation sources was done in parallel. Although natural variation in transformation capability is quite wide [11], definite answers could be provided for the questions (a), (b) and (c). Very slight differences, yet still significant, could be found in the ability of lymphocyte cultures of experimental and control subjects to transform, following stimulation by mitogens, as can be seen in Fig. 1. The incorporation of ^{3}H-thymidine into lymphocytes was somewhat lower both in the case of pokeweed mitogen and with PHA. In the latter case, a higher concentration of PHA was required in order to obtain maximal stimulation in lymphocytes of experimental subjects than in those of control subjects. It has been suggested [11] that impairment in the rate of thymidine uptake appears to be related to impairment in the cell's ability to repair damage to DNA. An effect of extremely low dose X-irradiation on the interaction of DNA and dye — acridine orange — has already been reported by us and suggested as a possible biological dosimetry system [12].

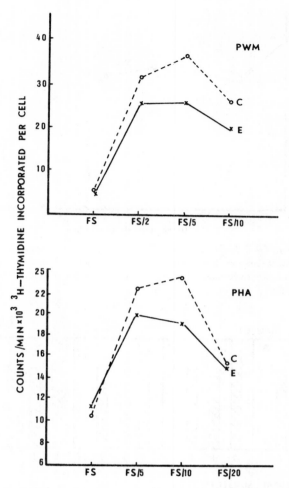

FIG.1.   Effect of mitogen concentration on optimal lymphocyte transformation; uptake of
³*H-TdR was calculated in counts/min per cell, and results as noted are multiplied by 10³.*
PWM = *pokeweed mitogen;* PHA = *phytohaemagglutinin.* o = *control subjects;*
x = *experimental subjects.*

As discussed above, the ability of the experimental subjects' lymphocytes
to transform normally following an additional acute dose of radiation was
studied. The cultures were irradiated in a gamma cell, receiving acute, but still
low doses of radiation, for very short exposure periods of one and two seconds.
When studying first a control subject, the mode of incorporation of ³H-TdR
shown in Fig. 2 was obtained, showing a decrease in incorporation after a 1 s
dose, equal to 20 rads, a slight increase after a higher dose, 40, 60 and 80 rads,
and a sharp decline following much higher doses.

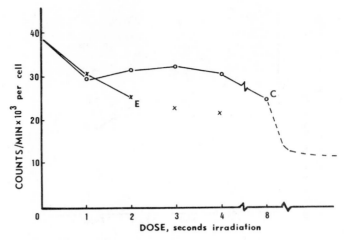

FIG.2.   Incorporation of ^{3}H-TdR into irradiated PHA-stimulated lymphocytes; PHA at 1/10th of *full strength, 0.1 ml per tube containing 1.0 × 10*^{6} *lymphocytes in 2 ml culture.* o = *control, one subject*; x = *experimental subjects. Average uptake of several experimental subjects as detailed in Fig. 3.*

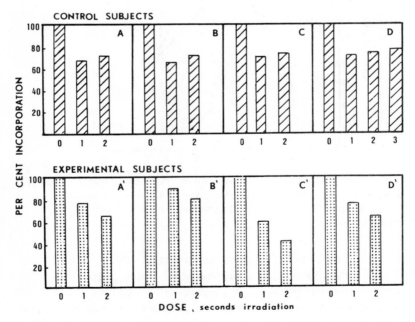

FIG.3.   *In-vitro low-dose effect on the incorporation of* ^{3}*H-TdR into transforming lymphocytes; stimulation with PHA, 1/10th full strength; control was always done in parallel with experimental subject. A B C D and* A′ B′ C′ D′ *represent individual control and experimental subjects correspondingly.*

When the same was studied in lymphocytes of an experimental subject, it was evident that the increase observed at doses of 40 to 80 rads is not apparent in this case, and a higher dose resulted in a lower incorporation. This initiated an examination of the response specifically to such a low dose, and thus four experimental subjects' lymphocytes were compared with four control subjects. Both cultures were treated and irradiated at the same time, each couple, experimental and control, done together, but the different couples done over a long period of time, so that maximum possibility for variations and errors was given. The results, nevertheless, as shown in Fig. 3, are strikingly the same: in all four cases a difference can be seen between control and experimental subjects. The incorporation of ^{3}H-TdR after a 2 s dose of gamma radiation was always higher in the controls and lower in the experimental subjects than the incorporation following a 1 s dose.

The only difference between the lymphocyte cultures of control and experimental subjects is in the fact that the experimental subjects were previously exposed to a continuous very low-level beta radiation from internal tritium burden. A conclusion must be drawn that this brings about some difference in the response to additional radiation, a response which, if dependent on the ability to repair sub-lethal damage, is somewhat resembling a reduction in the value of Dq, the term for quasithreshold dose, signifying the limit between the ability to absorb additional sub-lethal damage and the beginning of a potentially lethal damage. This indicates an impairment in the repair capability. There is, however, another possible explanation for this difference in thymidine uptake following an additional dose of radiation, namely that the basis for the difference lies in the difference in radiosensitivity between B- and T-cells [9], and that the relative number of cells of either type could be changed by the continuous low-level radiation. These points as well as DNA repair synthesis are currently being investigated.

REFERENCES

[1] SETLOW, R.B., CARRIER, W.L., The disappearance of thymine dimers from DNA: An error correcting mechanism, Proc. Natl. Acad. Sci. U.S.A. **51** (1964) 226.

[2] RIKLIS, E., Studies on the mechanism of repair of ultraviolet-irradiated viral and bacterial DNA in vivo and in vitro, Can. J. Biochem. **43** (1965) 1207.

[3] BOYCE, R.P., HOWARD-FLANDERS, P., Release of ultraviolet light induced thymine dimers from DNA of E. coli K-12, Proc. Nat. Acad. Sci. U.S.A. **51** (1964) 293.

[4] RADMAN, M., "Phenomenology of an inducible mutagenic repair pathway in E. coli: SOS repair hypothesis", Molecular and Environmental Aspects of Mutagenesis, Charles C. Thomas, Springfield (1973) 128.

[5] KOL, R., MEGED, Y., RIKLIS, E., "A computer program for characterization of radiation damage in chromosomes of lymphocytes grown in tissue culture", Israel Atomic Energy Commission Research Laboratories Report IA-1321 (1975) 217.

[6]   BEN-HUR, E., KOL, R., RIKLIS, E., "Modification of radiation response by hyper-
      thermia and its relation to DNA damage and repair", Radiobiological Research and
      Radiotherapy (Proc. Symp. Vienna, 1976) I, IAEA, Vienna (1977) 299.

[7]   FITZGERALD, M.G., The establishment of a normal human population dose-response
      curve for lymphocytes cultured with PHA, Clin. Exp. Immunol. 8 (1971) 421.

[8]   SPRENT, J., ANDERSON, R.E., MILLER, J.F.A.P., Radiosensitivity of T and B
      lymphocytes, Eur. J. Immunol. 4 (1974) 204.

[9]   VINCZE, I., CSUKA, I., FARKAS, G., STAUB, M., ANTONI, F., "DNA repair of
      human lymphocytes", DNA Repair and Late Effects (Int. Symp. IGEGM), Vienna
      (1975) 73.

[10] BARAL, E., BLOMGREN, H., Response of human lymphocytes to mitogenic stimuli
      after irradiation in vitro, Acta Radiol., Ther., Phys., Biol. 15 (1976) 149.

[11] AGARWAL, S.S., BROWN, D.Q., KATZ, E.J., LOEB, L.A., "DNA repair in human
      lymphocytes", Genetics of Human Cancer (MULVIHILL, J.J., MILLER, R.W.,
      FRAUMENI, J.F., Eds), Raven Press, New York (1977) 365.

[12] VIDER, E., YAARI, A., SHAFIR, D., RIKLIS, E., "Detection of radiation exposure
      by fluorescent microscopy of human blood cells", Proc. 1st Int. Congr. Radiation
      Protection (Rome 1966) I, (SNYDER, W.S., et al., Eds), Pergamon Press (1968) 525.

DISCUSSION

H. ALTMANN: Is the decrease in the ^{3}H-thymidine in the absence of
hydroxyurea due to a partial inhibition of semi-conservative DNA synthesis or
are membrane changes or changes in the pool of DNA precursors responsible
for this effect after low doses?

E. RIKLIS: We have shown so far a definite difference in PHA-induced
transformation, as measured by ^{3}H-TdR uptake, in the response to additional
in-vitro acute irradiation of lymphocytes previously exposed in vivo to
continuous very low-level beta radiation. Both induced transformation as well
as repair synthesis have been referred to in the literature as linked phenomena
affected by high doses of radiation (up to a certain level, above which the
remaining cells are not affected). It has been suggested that impaired transformation capability is directly related to impaired repair. We are going to look
into the questions of changes in nucleotide pool, as well as possible changes in
the relative numbers of B- and T-type lymphocytes, as part of our joint research
efforts with Mr. Castellani of Casaccia and Mr. Campagnari of ISPRA. Also, in
addition to looking for a biochemical indicator of changes in lymphocyte
response to radiation, we have begun looking into the morphological pictures in
an electron microscope, which may show membrane damage. However, we still
think that the DNA repair system or an enzymatic member of it may prove to
be the most sensitive factor determining the ultimate response of lymphocytes
to radiation.

DNA-REPAIR INVESTIGATIONS IN LYMPHOCYTES OF PERSONS LIVING IN ELEVATED NATURAL BACKGROUND RADIATION AREAS (BADGASTEIN)

H. ALTMANN, H. TUSCHL
Institute of Biology,
Seibersdorf Research Centre,
Seibersdorf,
Austria

Abstract

DNA-REPAIR INVESTIGATIONS IN LYMPHOCYTES OF PERSONS LIVING IN ELEVATED NATURAL BACKGROUND RADIATION AREAS (BADGASTEIN).

Unscheduled DNA synthesis (UDS) was studied in lymphocytes of three groups of persons living in an environment with different background radioactivity. These studies were performed by the autoradiographic and BND-cellulose technique for separation of native and single-strand breaks containing DNA. The control groups are persons living in Vienna and Innsbruck of the same age as the ^{222}Rn-exposed persons. The second group are personnel from the Badgastein spa treatment hospital working in rooms with radon content in air of 3–86 pCi/l radioactivity. The third group are working 2–4 hours daily in a ^{222}Rn atmosphere of 3 nCi/l. The first and second group were not significantly different in the DNA repair incorporation of lymphocytes, but the third group showed a highly significant increase in UDS. Semi-conservative DNA-synthesis was in this group significantly lower compared with controls. In this group a loss of supercoils of native DNA could be found by gradient centrifugation. The induction of de novo synthesis of repair enzymes induced by damage to DNA is discussed.

INTRODUCTION

DNA repair represents an important factor in the prevention of the induction of mutations and cancer [1–4]. DNA-repair deficient diseases show a close connection between the DNA repair capacity of cells and late effects. Error-free DNA repair processes therefore protect all organisms from environmental factors that can damage DNA. Under certain conditions DNA repair enzymes can be induced by damage in the DNA of the cells. These inducible enzymes are studied mainly in micro-organisms. The induction of mutations in *E. coli* after gamma irradiation seems to occur often via the operation of an inducible error-prone DNA repair system [5]. But, unlike this error-prone SOS repair system which allows increased survival at the cost of an increased mutation rate, a different set of gene products are inducible in *E. coli* after slight damage of DNA. These repair pathways seem to work error free, and the induction process can be inhibited by chloramphenicol and hence requires de novo protein synthesis [6]. The induction of malignancies is the most important effect produced at low doses in the exposed individual [7]. Tumour development is controlled by immune mechanisms of the host, and the specificity of the immune response is also dependent on good error-free DNA repair action [8]. The question is still open whether a threshold exists in man for cell-killing, mutations and cancer. Therefore epidemiological investigations have been performed in populations living in areas of different natural background radioactivity. Many publications have dealt with the hypothesis that a certain fraction of cancer mortality is possibly due to the radiation background [9—11]. But most studies have not stood the test of critical re-examination [12]. In an epidemiological study in a coastal area of Kerala in south India a high prevalence of Down's syndrome and other forms of severe mental retardation occurs [13]. Patients with Down's syndrome have DNA repair imbalances in lymphocytes [14], and the mothers of Down's syndrome children have immunological defects. But the controls were not a comparable control group, especially with respect to family size, number of females in each group and the mortality rate. Another epidemiological survey on this topic was made in the context of an 'Environmental statement project' from Argonne National Laboratory. It was interesting that an association between high backgrounds and low malignant mortalities could be found [15]. Nevertheless, this report also has been criticized.

From acute radiation exposure (Hiroshima) we know that doses between 20 and 49 rads can increase the risk of leukaemia and thyroid cancer [16, 17]. In the present study we investigated DNA repair in lymphocytes of people chronically exposed to low doses of natural radioactivity to demonstrate whether this process has something to do with the various conclusions drawn from epidemiological studies.

METHODS AND MATERIALS

Badgastein has an elevated natural background radioactivity, particularly because of the radon-222 content in air. Short-lived daughter products that take part in the radiation burden of the population are ^{218}Po, ^{214}Pb, ^{214}Bi and ^{214}Po.

Peripheral blood was obtained from people living in the Badgastein area and working in the spa treatment hospital. These personnel are continuously exposed to an alpha blood dose of 0.06—2.3 mrad per month and a gamma blood dose of 8—13 mrad monthly. The total external radiation in treatment rooms is 120—300 mrad yearly [18].

A second group of people[1] was investigated who are exposed to much higher doses for 2–4 hours daily. They work in a former gold mine that is now used as a treatment room for patients with rheumatic (mainly M. Bechterew) and vascular diseases. The treatment room is called the 'Thermal Gallery', because in addition to a mean radon activity of 3 μCi/l there are air temperatures of up to 41°C and a relative humidity of about 95%. The control group consisted of persons living in Vienna and Innsbruck of the same age as the radon-exposed group. Lymphocytes were separated from whole blood using ficoll-urografin [19]. To suppress semi-conservative DNA synthesis at a high rate, (phosphate buffered saline) cells were pre-incubated at 37°C in PBS containing 10M hydroxyurea. After 30 min pre-incubation, irradiation was performed at 254 nm with an integrated dose of 200 erg/mm^2 using a 15 W germicidal lamp.

Autoradiographs

After irradiation of lymphocytes 10 μCi/ml H^3-thymidine (specific activity 56 Ci/mmol NEN Chemicals) was added, and lymphocytes incubated at 37°C for 90 min. H^3-thymidine incorporation was stopped by addition of cold thymidine (1 mg/ml). The cells were washed with PBS and fixed in ice-cold methanol-acetic acid (3:1). Autoradiograms were prepared both by Kodak AK 10 stripping film and NTB3 liquid emulsion, and exposed at 4°C for 13 d. After development slides were stained by Giemsa. The relative reflection of silver grains per labelled cells was measured using a Zeiss PMQII photometer.

BND (benzoylated naphthoylated DEAE cellulose) method

After u.v. irradiation 10 μCi/ml thymidine was added to the lymphocyte suspension and samples incubated at 37°C in Hank's for 0, 30 and 90 min respectively. After incubation, cells were washed and re-suspended in SSC (1m) and SDS (0.2%) for lysis. Lysates were treated with RNase for 1 h and Pronase for 2 h at 37°C. After fragmentation of high molecular DNA by pressing the DNA solution through a 20 G-injection needle, lysates were layered on BND cellulose columns. Native DNA was eluted with 1M NaCl buffer (1m NaCl, 10^{-4}M EDTA, 0.01M Tris-HCl pH 7.5) and DNA containing single-stranded regions with 50% formamide-1.0m NaCl buffer according to Scudiero and co-workers [20]. For determination of the specific activity, the formamide fraction was dialysed, and aliquots taken for measurement of optical density and radioactivity.

In addition to repair investigations, semi-conservative DNA synthesis was measured by the same method, but without using hydroxyurea.

---

[1] These workers inspect the gallery; they are referred to as 'miners' in this study.

TABLE I.   UDS (AUTORADIOGRAPHS) IN LYMPHOCYTES OF MINERS
IN BADGASTEIN
^{3}H-Thymidine incorporation after u.v. irradiation (200 erg/mm^2);
standard deviation in brackets

	Number of cases	Relative reflection of silver grains	Percentage of labelled cells
Radon-exposed persons	5	39.48 (4.48)	79.76 (7.2)
Controls	3	21.57 (3.58)	57.1 (3.27)
Error probablity		0.01%	0.05%

TABLE II.   30-MIN REPAIR INCORPORATION IN DNA OF LYMPHOCYTES
OF MINERS IN BADGASTEIN
Values given as specific ^{3}H-activity of DNA;
standard deviation in brackets

	Number of cases	Double-stranded DNA	Single-strand containing DNA
Radon-exposed persons	14	123 (70)	169 (45)
Controls	7	39 (6)	52 (18)
Error probability		0.5%	0.001%

For the detection of breaks caused in nuclear DNA by very low doses of
gamma rays, the method of Cook and Brazell [20] was used with lymphocytes
of miners.

RESULTS

The autoradiograms show a significantly higher level of silver grains per cell,
and also the percentage of labelled cells within the whole lymphocyte population
was higher in the miners compared with controls (Table I).

Up to now we have investigated only a small group of people, using autoradiography, but the results are very clear and the grains/cell are nearly doubled in
the lymphocytes of personnel working in the Thermal Gallery. Non-u.v. irradiated
cells of both exposed personnel and controls did not show any incorporation of

TABLE III. 90-MIN REPAIR INCORPORATION IN DNA OF LYMPHOCYTES
OF MINERS IN BADGASTEIN
Values given as specific ³H-activity of DNA;
standard deviation in brackets

	Number of cases	Double-stranded DNA	Single-strand containing DNA
Radon-exposed persons	14	288 (77)	329 (108)
Controls	7	97 (19)	117 (56)
Error probability		0.002%	0.01%

TABLE IV. UDS IN LYMPHOCYTES OF PEOPLE LIVING IN BADGASTEIN

	Number of cases	Relative reflection of silver grains	Percentage of labelled cells
Badgastein	10	20.2 (4.5)	60.0 (3.1)
Vienna	5	19.1 (1.2)	56.0 (2.6)
Error probability		17%	0.1%

label during the investigated repair time. Thus the increased repair capacity of
lymphocytes of miners is not due to repair of lesions already produced by in-vivo
exposure to radiation. Using the very sensitive method of sedimentation of
supercoiled nuclear DNA by ultracentrifugation, loss of supercoils possibly due to
some breaks in the DNA could be detected in the mine-worker group. In Table II
the values obtained with BND-separation method after 30-min repair time are listed.

DNA repair incorporation is about three fold in radon-exposed persons
compared with controls. These data fit very well the results obtained by the
autoradiographic technique, if we take into account the two-fold increase in
average label per cell and the increase of the percentage of labelled cells. In
Table III the 90-min repair-time data are given.

Despite the higher standard deviation the difference between miners and
controls is highly significant.

The DNA repair investigations carried out on personnel working in the spa
treatment hospital showed no significant difference from controls (Table IV).

It seems of interest that only the number of labelled cells per lymphocyte
population is significantly higher compared with the control lymphocytes. Also
the 90-min repair values after BND-cellulose separation of native DNA were not
significantly different (Table V).

TABLE V.   UDS IN LYMPHOCYTES OF PEOPLE LIVING IN BADGASTEIN
Values given as specific ^{3}H-activity of DNA;
standard deviation in brackets

	Number of cases	90-min repair incorporation in native DNA
Badgastein	12	124 (54)
Vienna	6	101 (26)

The values of the semi-conservative DNA synthesis obtained after 30 and 90 min H^3-thymidine incorporation without adding hydroxyurea were not significantly different between personnel of the spa treatment hospital and controls, but were significantly lower in the lymphocytes of the miners.

DISCUSSION

The present results of our investigations on DNA repair incorporation of H^3-thymidine into DNA of peripheral blood lymphocytes from miners and controls confirm our previous findings on patients with rheumatic diseases, namely that higher background radioactivity and, in particular, treatment in the mine of Badgastein, can increase the DNA repair-capacity of cells, but decrease semi-conservative DNA synthesis [21, 22]. The reason for an increase in UDS could be a change in the lymphocyte population, because juvenile cells have a higher repair capacity than differentiated cells. The possibility of transformation of small lymphocytes to blast cells with ~ 10-fold DNA-repair capacity can be excluded by the technique used in these experiments. The fact of a lower semi-conservative DNA synthesis speaks against a shift in the lymphocyte population as well as a transformation to blast cells. The question is still unsolved whether an induction process of de novo synthesis of repair enzymes induced by damage to DNA exists also in human lymphocytes. The two inducible DNA repair pathways are described as either error-prone or error-proof in micro-organisms. The results of the chromosome-aberration-studies of Pohl-Rühling and co-workers [23] on the same radon-exposed groups in Badgastein can be correlated with an error-free pathway. In *E. coli*, the inducer of a new DNA repair system might be a DNA degradation product [24], and the induction process is connected with inhibition of semi-conservative DNA synthesis. Several genes seem to be involved in the regulation of the induction. In order to determine whether activation of preformed enzymes or induction of increased synthesis of enzymes is involved in the increased specific activity of a DNA polymerase and ATP-dependent deoxiribonuclease in *Myco-bacterium smegmatis* after DNA damage, inhibitors of protein synthesis were used [25]. The inhibitors prevented the increase in specific activity, indicating that protein synthesis is involved in the enzyme induction process. Holliday [26] suggested that this inducible repair system occurs also in eukaryotes, but up till now nothing is known of this process in human cells. The pronounced increase of DNA repair incorporation in the miner groups is possibly due to the combined effect of the fractionated radiation dose obtained in the Thermal Gallery for periods of two to four hours daily, in contrast with the more continuous exposure in the spa treatment hospital, and the temperature of about 41°C. To test the possible effect of high temperature on DNA repair capacity, we also investigated lymphocytes of persons after taking a steam bath[2] with a temperature between 90° and 100°C. Compared with repair capacity before the steam bath treatment, H^3-incorporation caused by u.v.-damage after treatment was increased. Another factor that can interfere in the results obtained in the different groups is the relation between the alpha and gamma dose applied. The proportion of these two components of radiation varies in the following mode: At low-level radiation (up to 200 mrad) the gamma fraction exceeds the alpha component by a factor of up to 100, whereas at the higher level of the Thermal Gallery this factor is inversed: the alpha fraction exceeds the gamma component by a factor of 10 [18].

The inhaled ^{222}Rn, ^{220}Rn and their daughters are very unequally distributed within the body, thereby causing different exposure of various organs and different cells to radioactivity [27]. Basal cells of bronchio-epithelium are exposed 40 fold by inhalation of RaA-RaC' compared with blood [26]. Within the normal human population there are great differences in the amount of DNA repair dependent on genetic factors. Therefore it is difficult to determine whether a threshold dose for background radiation exists that leads to an increase of the DNA repair capacity of human lymphocytes.

Further work on these lines and with animal models is necessary to explain the mechanisms of the results presented in this study.

ACKNOWLEDGEMENTS

This work was performed under IAEA Contract No.1914. We thank Mr. Sandri, Prof. R. Günther and Mr. D. Egg for selection of test persons and collection of blood for the present investigations. We thank A. Topaloglou and R. Kovacs for excellent technical assistance.

---

[2] Sauna.

REFERENCES

[1] BEERS, R.F., Jr., HERRIOTT, R.M., TILGHMAN, R.C.T. (Eds), Molecular and Cellular Repair Processes, Johns Hopkins Univ. Press, Baltimore (1972).

[2] HANAWALT, P.C., SETLOW, R.B. (Eds), Molecular Mechanisms for Repair in DNA, Plenum Press, New York/London (1975).

[3] ALTMANN, H. (Ed.), DNA-repair mechanisms, F.K. Schattauer Verlag, Stuttgart/New York (1972) 1.

[4] ALTMANN, H. (Ed.), DNA-Repair and Late Effects, Rötzer-Druck, Eisenstadt (1974, 1976).

[5] BRIDGES, B.A., Mutagenic DNA repair in Escherichia coli, Mol. Gen. Genet. 151 (1977) 115.

[6] SAMSON, L., CAIRNS, J., A new pathway for DNA repair in Escherichia coli, Nature (London) 267 (1977) 281.

[7] UNITED NATIONS, Sources and Effects of Ionizing Radiation, United Nations, New York (1977) 362.

[8] ALTMANN, H. (Ed.), DNA-Repair and Late Effects, Rötzer-Druck, Eisenstadt, in press.

[9] ADVISORY COMMITTEE ON THE BIOLOGICAL EFFECTS OF IONIZING RADIATION, The Effects on Population of Exposure to Low Levels of Ionizing Radiation, National Academy of Sciences, Washington (1972).

[10] ARGONNE NATIONAL LABORATORY, Estimation of Low Level Radiation Effects in Human Populations, Rep. ANL-7811 (1970).

[11] BAUM, J.W., Population heterogeneity hypothesis on radiation induced cancer, Health Phys. 25 (1973) 97.

[12] UNITED NATIONS, Sources and Effects of Ionizing Radiation, United Nations, New York (1977) 435.

[13] KOCHUPILLAI, N., VERMA, I.C., CREWAL, M.S., RAMALINGASWAMI, V., Down syndrome and related abnormalities in an area of high background radiation in coastal Kerala, Nature (London) 262 (1976) 60.

[14] LAMBERT, B., HANSSON, K., BUI, T.H., FUNES-CRAVIOTO, F., HOLBERG, M., STRAUSMANIS, R., DNA repair and frequency of X-ray and UV-light induced chromosome aberrations in leukocytes from patients with Down's syndrome, Ann. Hum. Genet. 39 (1976) 293.

[15] FRIGERIO, N.A., STOWE, R.S., "Carcinogenic and genetic hazard from background radiation", Biological and Environmental Effects of Low-Level Radiation (Proc. Symp. Chicago, 1975) II, IAEA, Vienna (1976) 385.

[16] ISHIMARU, T., HOSHINO, T., ICHIMARU, M., OKADA, H., TOMIYASU, T., TSUCHIMOTO, T., YAMAMOTO, T., Leukemia in atomic bomb survivors, Hiroshima and Nagasaki, 1. Oct. 1950 – 30. Sept. 1966, Radiat. Res. 45 (1971) 216.

[17] SILVERMAN, Ch., SHORE, M.L., "Low-dose ionizing radiation: carcinogenic effects in man", Biological and Environmental Effects of Low-Level Radiation (Proc. Symp. Chicago, 1975) II, IAEA, Vienna (1976) 395.

[18] POHL-RÜHLING, J., FISHER, P., "Chromosome aberrations in peripheral blood lymphocytes dependent on various dose levels of natural radioactivity", Biological and Environmental Effects of Low-Level Radiation (Proc. Symp. Chicago, 1975) II, IAEA, Vienna (1976) 320.

[19] WOTTAWA, A., KLEIN, G., ALTMANN, H., Eine Methode zur Isolierung menschlicher und tierischer Lymphozyten mit Ficoll-Urografin, Wien. Klin. Wochenschr. 86 (1974) 161.

[20] SCUDIERO, A., HENDERSON, E., NORIN, A., STRAUSS, B., The measurement of
chemically induced DNA repair synthesis in human cells by BND cellulose chromatography,
Mutat. Res. **29** (1975) 473.

[21] EGG, D., GÜNTHER, R., KLEIN, W., KOCSIS, F., ALTMANN, H., „Untersuchungen
über die DNA-Reparaturvorgänge in peripheren Lymphozyten von Arthrosepatienten
während einer Gasteiner Kur", DNA-Repair and Late Effects (ALTMANN, H., Ed.),
Rötzer-Druck, Eisenstadt (1976) 99.

[22] EGG, D., GÜNTHER, R., ALTMANN, H., KLEIN, W., KOCSIS, F., DNA-Reparatur-
untersuchungen an peripheren Lymphocyten von Rheumakranken während einer Kur in
Badgastein, Z. Angew. Bäder- Klimaheilkunde **24** 3 (1977) 223.

[23] POHL-RÜHLING, J., FISHER, P., POHL, E., "The low-level shape of dose response for
chromosome aberrations", these Proceedings **II**, IAEA-SM-224/403.

[24] GUDAS, L.J., The induction of protein X in DNA repair and cell division mutants of
E. coli, J. Mol. Biol. **104** (1976) 567.

[25] MacNAUGHTON, A.W., WINDER, F.G., Increased DNA-polymerase and ATP-dependent
DNase activities following DNA-damage in *Mycobacterium smegmatis*, Mol. Gen. Genet.
150 (1977) 301.

[26] ALTSHUBER, B., NELSON, N., KUTSCHER, M., Estimation of lung tissue dose from
the inhalation of radon and daughters, Health Phys. **10** (1964) 1137.

[27] POHL, E., POHL-RÜHLING, J., Dose calculations due to the inhalation of Re^{222}, Rn^{220}
and their daughters, Health Phys. **32** (1977) 552.

DISCUSSION

E. RIKLIS: Your observations of increased repair synthesis of DNA in
lymphocytes of people living in a high-background radiation region may indeed
indicate the appearance of induced repair enzymes. In view of our results, which
show a reduced capacity of the lymphocytes of people who have over the years
suffered continuous very low-level irradiation to absorb additional acute radiation
damage, we tend to believe that the repair systems, while functioning at an
accelerated pace, become 'tired' and perhaps show a phenomenon of 'aging'.
It will be interesting to investigate this point also on your experimental subjects.

H. ALTMANN: We found a significant increase of ^{3}H-thymidine in DNA
only in the presence of hydroxyurea, but we don't know whether it is an error-
prone or error-free repair pathway. If during aging an error-proneness develops,
an equilibrium in features in DNA could possibly be reached for a certain time
by an elevated error-free DNA repair pathway, induced by a chronically or
fractionally applied low dose of radiation.

A. ARSENAULT: In view of the positive correlation between your means
and your standard deviations in the various tables, did you make a log transformation before doing your statistical comparisons?

H. ALTMANN: Yes, this was performed by our mathematical group.

NEW APPROACHES TO THE EVALUATION
OF RESIDUAL RADIATION DAMAGE
IN THE HAEMOPOIETIC SYSTEM

J. GIDÁLI, I. FEHÉR, I. BOJTOR
National Research Institute for
    Radiobiology and Radiohygiene,
Budapest,
Hungary

Abstract

NEW APPROACHES TO THE EVALUATION OF RESIDUAL RADIATION DAMAGE IN
THE HAEMOPOIETIC SYSTEM.

In the present experiments the possible residual damage in the haemopoietic stem cell
(CFU_s) compartment was studied 1 to 5 months after low-dose irradiation. The proliferative
state of the CFU_s as well as the number of CFU_s mobilizable from the bone marrow upon
adequate stimulus were chosen as indicators to evaluate the haemopoietic state of mice at
various times after 50—64 rads acute and 16 rads daily continuous gamma irradiation. It was
observed that the number of bone marrow CFU_s reached the normal level three weeks after
64 rads accumulated dose of continuous irradiation, both the CFU_s level and the proliferative
state of CFU_s then fluctuated around the normal level. The self-maintaining capacity of the CFU_s
population was slightly lower than that of the normal 10 and 16 weeks after 64 rads continuous
irradiation. Ten weeks following continuous irradiation an increase in splenic erythropoiesis
upon the effect of serious bleeding showed no difference compared with the unirradiated group.
Induction of CFU_s mobilization into the circulation has been worked out as a sensitive tool for
evaluating relatively slight damage of the CFU_s compartment, the present results showing a
reduced mobilization rate up to 12 weeks after 50 rads acute irradiation. These findings suggest
perturbance of the haemopoietic system after the total recovery from radiation injury. An
assumed cyclic tendency in the level of the CFU_s gives rise to the idea that the basis of this
perturbance might be some alteration in the regulation of the CFU_s proliferation.

INTRODUCTION

The demonstration of a possible residual radiation damage in haemopoiesis is
a constant problem in radiobiology [1]. To find any residual damage, especially
after continuous irradiation, is not an easy task, on the one hand because of the
well-known relatively rapid restoration of injuries within the haemopoietic
system [2, 3], on the other hand because of the difficulties in finding an appropriate index for detection of the injuries [4].

447

In previous experiments we have proved that when 50 rads accumulated dose is continued for over a month no detectable changes can be found in any of the haematological indices including bone marrow stem cell count [4]. The proliferatio index of the otherwise mainly resting stem cells [5], however, significantly increased [4]. This effect has led us to suppose that the increased number of stem cells entering the S phase of the cell cycle can be used to study all types of perturbed haemopoiesis. The present experiments were intended to prove that any residual effect of low-dose irradiation can be detected by the increase in proliferation rate of stem cells. Further, in order to obtain information about the character of residual damage in haemopoiesis, these experiments were completed by investigating the self-maintaining capacity and structure of the stem cell population.

METHODS

Twelve-weeks-old $BALB/c \times CBA/F_1$ hybrid male mice were used both as donors and recipients. In each group 4 donors and 10 recipients were used. For each investigation following the irradiation, control mice derived from the same age group and kept under similar conditions were also tested.

The experimental animals and recipients were irradiated with ^{60}Co gamma rays The dose rate of acute irradiation was 96.2 rads/min and continuous irradiation was performed with a dose rate of 16 rads/22 h.

The number of colony-forming cells (CFU_s) was determined according to Till and McCulloch [6]. Bone marrow cells were obtained from the femora and transplanted into lethally (816 rads) irradiated isologous recipients. Colonies were counted 9 days after transplantation and their number was referred to the total nucleated cell count of the femur.

The proportion of CFU_s in DNA synthesis was regarded as an index for the proliferation rate and was measured according to Becker and co-workers [7].

RESULTS AND DISCUSSION

In the first experiments the regeneration and the proliferative index (number of CFU_s in S phase) of stem cells were periodically examined for 5 months after 64 rads continuous irradiation.

As the effect of 64 rads continuous irradiation, 40% reduction of stem cell count was observed which was restored 14 days after the end of the irradiation. Three weeks after irradiation even the proliferation rate of stem cells returned to normal value indicating the restoration of the normal steady state of haemopoiesis. Later, however, both the stem cell count and the number of stem cells in

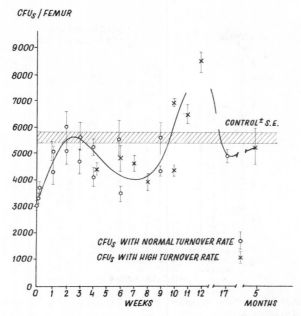

FIG.1.   *Femoral stem cell count of mice after 64 rads continuous gamma irradiation.*

TABLE I.   SELF-REPRODUCING CAPACITY OF BONE MARROW STEM CELLS 10 AND 16 WEEKS AFTER CONTINUOUS GAMMA IRRADIATION

	CFU_s/colony (mean)	Distribution of CFU_s/colony (%)				
		0	1−5	6−10	11−20	20
Control	6.12	34.7	30.2	10.4	6.3	18.8
10 weeks after irradiation	5.06	41.7	29.2	6.2	14.6	8.3
16 weeks after irradiation	5.13	47.7	20.5	13.6	11.4	6.8

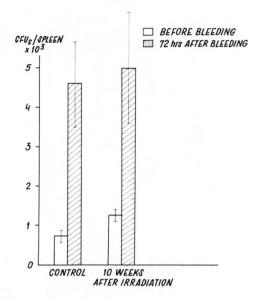

FIG.2.   The effect of 40% bleeding on splenic stem cell count of mice 10 weeks after 64 rads
continuous gamma irradiation.

the S phase seemed to show a cyclic fluctuation around the control (Fig.1).
Although no clear-cut relationship was found between the stem cell level and the
number of stem cells in the S phase, a certain correlation might be assumed
between them. Since the haemopoietic system is a strictly controlled cell renewal
system [8], this fluctuation suggests that in spite of the total regeneration measured
three weeks after irradiation, the normal steady state of haemopoiesis is still not
reached five months after the exposure. The observed unbalanced state indicates
that there was some undefined damage in the regulation of proliferation.

Since this hypothetical damage may mean either the abnormal level of regulator
agents or the abnormal reaction of stem cells to normal concentration of
regulators, it was decided to analyse this unbalanced state by studying the self-
maintaining capacity of the haemopoietic stem cells 10 and 16 weeks after 64 rads
continuous irradiation.

For maintaining normal haemopoiesis, stem cells have to keep their population size at a constant level in spite of continuous cell loss for differentiation [9].
For this purpose stem cells reproduce themselves, in other words they produce
identical daughter cells.

The self-reproducing capacity of stem cells can be characterized by the number
of newly formed stem cells in individual spleen colonies [10].

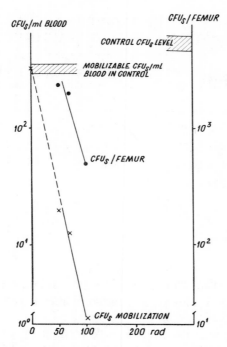

FIG.3. Stem cell level in the femur and the number of mobilizable CFU$_s$ in 50 to 100 rads irradiated mice, 24 hours after irradiation.

Table I shows the CFU$_s$ content of individual spleen colonies 10 and 16 weeks after 64 rads continuous irradiation. The mean CFU$_s$ content of the single colonies fell close to the lower limit of the control value. Distribution of CFU$_s$ among colonies is a statistical phenomenon [11] giving information about the structure of stem cell population. In irradiated groups the number of stem cells producing no new stem cells increased, and those producing a high quantity of new stem cells decreased. This finding also seemed to support the concept of the perturbance of stem cell proliferation control after irradiation.

All these results suggested some perturbance in haemopoiesis after irradiation without giving information on whether this perturbance has a profound influence on the reactivity of haemopoiesis.

As the first experimental model for studying the haemopoietic reactions a certain type of stress reaction was tested. In rodents spleen is known to be an important erythropoietic organ especially in rapid restoration of erythropoiesis when it is almost completely shunted from the bone marrow to the spleen [12]. Ten weeks after continuous irradiation 40% of total blood volume was withdrawn from the orbital sinus and the number of the stem cells in the spleen was studied 72 hours later as an indicator for the increased haemopoiesis.

TABLE II.   FEMORAL STEM CELL COUNT AND STEM CELL MOBILIZATION
AT VARIOUS TIMES AFTER 50 rads ACUTE GAMMA IRRADIATION

Time after irradiation	CFU_s/femur Mean $\pm$ S.E.	Mobilizable CFU_s/ml blood Mean $\pm$ S.E.	CFU_s mobilization % of momentary control
Control	5558 $\pm$ 188	225 $\pm$ 24.2	-
1 month	5843 $\pm$ 277	70 $\pm$ 16.2	31.1
2 months	5126 $\pm$ 339	75 $\pm$ 15.7	36.2
3 months	5637 $\pm$ 588	116 $\pm$ 8.5	88.6

The increase in splenic CFU_s level did not differ in the irradiated group from that of control (Fig.2). In this experiment no residual radiation injury could be detected.

Various inducers have the effect of making the stem cells migrate from the bone marrow to the circulation [12, 13]. In the next experiment mice were irradiated with 50 to 100 rads acute dose. Twenty-four hours afterwards 1.5 mg trypsin was injected intravenously as CFU_s mobilizer and stem cell mobilization was compared with bone marrow stem cell level. Mobilization was found to run parallel with bone marrow stem cell count, indicating a fairly good correlation between the number of bone marrow and mobilizable stem cells after relatively small damage to the population (Fig.3).

The mobilizable CFU_s fraction represents a subpopulation of bone marrow stem cells [14]. Therefore, this test can be used for evaluating the regeneration of the structure of the bone marrow stem cell population.

One, two and three months after 50 rads acute irradiation, bone marrow stem cell count was found to be normal. The mobilizable CFU_s fraction, however, did not return to normal value (Table II). This finding draws attention to some residual damage in the structure of the haemopoietic stem cell compartment.

CONCLUSIONS

The present study has been designed to find various indicators for a possible residual injury in the haemopoietic system after small doses of acute and continuous irradiation. For this purpose reliable test systems were elaborated to evaluate whether normal haemopoietic indices found some weeks after low-dose irradiations are maintained by the normal proliferation rate or only by increased proliferation, and perhaps only under physiological conditions.

The fluctuation in both the level and the proliferation rate as well as the reduced self-maintaining capacity of stem cells following the regeneration after 64 rads continuous irradiation suggested residual perturbation of proliferation control. The reduced mobilization rate of stem cells also supported the residual alteration in the compartment structure of stem cells.

The splenic stem cell reaction upon erythropoietic stress, however, seemed to be normal 10 weeks after 64 rads continuous irradiation, in contradiction to the data on residual erythropoietic injury after higher doses or shorter time periods after irradiation [15].

The applied sensitive indicators emphasize that the perfect recovery of the haemopoietic system is a slower process than was thought earlier, even after low doses.

Another problem is whether this prolonged proliferative activity of stem cells has any connection with the late effects of irradiation. The higher probability of errors in DNA replication during the increased proliferation rate is a generally accepted hypothesis. One might assume that stem cells carrying a possible latent radiation damage are better targets for 'accidents' in DNA replication, and this circumstance might affect the process of malignant transformation.

REFERENCES

[1] GONG, J.K., MacVITTIE, J., VERTALINO, J.E., Radiat. Res. 37 (1969) 467.
[2] LAMERTON, L.F., Radiat. Res. 27 (1966) 119.
[3] BLACKETT, N.M., Br.J. Haematol. 13 (1967) 915.
[4] GIDÁLI, J., BOJTOR, I., FEHÉR, I., Radiat. Res., in press.
[5] LAJTHA, L.G., J. Cell. Comp. Physiol. Suppl. 1 (1963) 143.
[6] TILL, J.E., McCULLOCH, E.A., Radiat. Res. 14 (1961) 213.
[7] BECKER, A.J., McCULLOCH, E.A., SIMINOVITCH, L., TILL, J.E., Blood 26 (1965) 296.
[8] LORD, B.I., LAJTHA, L.G., Haematologica (Pavia) 59 (1974) 259.
[9] LAJTHA, L.G., In Vitro CSSR 4 (1969) 14.
[10] VOGEL, H., NIEWISCH, H., MATIOLI, G., J. Cell. Physiol. 72 (1968) 221.
[11] FRUHMAN, G.J., in Regulation of Haemopoiesis (GORDON, A.S., Ed.), Appleton-Century-Crofts, New York (1971).
[12] VOS, O., BUURMAN, W.A., PLOEMACHER, R.E., Cell Tissue Kinet. 5 (1972) 467.
[13] MONETTE, F.C., MORSE, B.S., HOWARD, D., NISKANEN, E., STOHLMAN, F., Jr., Cell. Tissue Kinet. 5 (1972) 121.
[14] GIDÁLI, J., FEHÉR, I., ANTAL, S., Blood 43 (1974) 573.
[15] MARCHETTI, D.L., GLOMSKI, C.A., Exp. Hematol. 3 (1975) 375.

DISCUSSION

C. STREFFER: When you refer to stem cells in S-phase, do you mean proliferating cells in the bone marrow or in the spleen colonies?

I. FEHÉR: Only those in the bone marrow. The samples were taken from the bone marrow and the determination was carried out in vitro on the basis of their sensitivity to ^{3}H-thymidine of high specific activity.

POSSIBLE ROLE OF INTRAVASCULAR COAGULATION IN RADIATION NEPHRITIS*

M. KOPEĆ, T. WRONOWSKI
Department of Radiobiology and Health Protection,
Institute of Nuclear Research,
Warsaw

Z. TYRANKIEWICZ, J. MUSZKOWSKA
Department of Nephrology,
School of Medicine,
Gdańsk

J. PALESTER-CHLEBOWCZYK
Institute of Surgery,
School of Medicine,
Warsaw

K. CZEŚNIN
Department of Gynaecology,
Institute of Oncology,
Warsaw,
Poland

Abstract

POSSIBLE ROLE OF INTRAVASCULAR COAGULATION IN RADIATION NEPHRITIS.

Thrombosis contributes to pathogenic mechanisms of such late effects as organ fibrosis and premature atherosclerosis. Recently deposition of fibrin in kidney glomeruli was postulated to be of possible significance for radiation nephritis. Results of the following studies support this view. A generalized Schwartzman reaction was provoked in 24 rabbits by a single dose of 50 μg of endotoxin (*Salmonella enteritidis*, Lipopolysaccharide B, Difco) administered 24 h after whole-body exposure to 850 R of X-rays. This procedure induced similar laboratory signs of intravascular coagulation and somewhat more pronounced fibrin deposition in kidneys compared with a group (28 rabbits) treated in a classical manner, i.e. with two doses of endotoxin spaced by a 24 h interval. In about two-thirds of 29 patients with uterine carcinoma, fibrin degradation products (FDP) appeared in urine during treatment with radium and ^{60}Co. Since kidneys were exposed to only negligible doses of radiation under the applied conditions of therapy, experiments in dogs were performed aimed at elucidating the significance of direct renal exposure. Fractionated doses (19 × 400 R, 5 weeks) of X-rays were given to either the kidney or mediastinum region. Irradiation resulted in a pronounced increase in serum FDP and the appearance of FDP in the urine. The character and dynamics of changes were similar in

* This work was supported by a grant from the Polish Government Programme PR6, 1F-9s3y.

both groups regardless of whether kidneys or mediastinum were exposed. Results of other coagulation tests and histological examinations indicate that radiation induces systemic activation of blood coagulation and renal deposition of fibrin. Kidneys can be involved in this process in an indirect way.

INTRODUCTION

Disseminated thrombotic changes leading to occlusion of the capillaries and small arteries are recognized as an important intermediate mechanism of damage to major organs, especially to the kidneys [1]. Systemic or local activation of blood coagulation and multiple thrombi can occur as a consequence of various basic underlying pathological conditions, such as major surgery, complications of pregnancy, malignancies, burns or infections. Diverse as these conditions are, they all are associated with tissue damage triggering the activation of the blood clotting system. Kidney failure due to renal cortical necrosis is the most frequent direct cause of the fatal outcome of acute or sub-acute disseminated intravascular coagulation. For still unknown reasons kidney glomeruli are particularly prone to occlusion by fibrin deposits.

Disseminated thrombosis is also involved in the mechanisms of tissue damage induced by radiation. Studies on post-irradiation cardiomyopathy implicate the injury of the vascular endothelium and subsequent activation of clotting as the main pathogenic mechanism of myocardial damage and late fibrosis [2, 3]. The significance of thrombotic phenomena for radiation hepatitis has been substantiated by the protective effect of anticoagulants in this disorder [4]. Vascular changes are considered also to determine mainly early and late radiation kidney damage [5—7].

The aim of our work was to investigate the role of activation of the blood clotting system in post-irradiation kidney injury.

EXPERIMENTAL

The first step in our study was to compare whole-body exposure to 850 R of X-rays and a single injection of bacterial endotoxin as procedures preparing rabbits for the generalized Schwartzman reaction (GSR). Male and non-pregnant female albino rabbits of one strain (Popielno, Poland) were used for the experiments. GSR, which is the classical experimental model of renal cortical necrosis due to occlusion of glomerular vasculature by fibrin deposits, was induced in the conventional manner, i.e. by two intravenous injections of endotoxin appropriately spaced in time in 28 rabbits. This group was called $E_1 + E_2$. As can be seen from Fig.1, which shows the design of the experiment in another group $X + E_2$

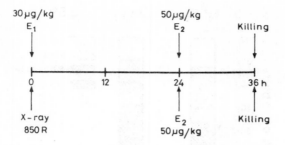

FIG.1. Design of the experiment: E = Salmonella enteritidis *endotoxin Lipopolysaccharide B*
(Difco Lab., Detroit)
E_1 = *preparative dose*
E_2 = *provocative dose*
X-ray whole body irradiation with a dose of 850 R (for conditions and dose control see Ref.[8]).

(24 rabbits), the preparatory dose of endotoxin was substituted by whole-body
exposure to X-rays. Three other groups were: X — 13 rabbits subjected only to
X-ray exposure, E_1 — 10 animals treated with a single dose of endotoxin,
C — 18 control intact rabbits.

At indicated time intervals blood samples were collected through siliconized
needles and plastic tubes by direct cardiac puncture into 0.1 vol. of 2.8 sodium
citrate containing 0.1M epsilonaminocaproic acid, an inhibitor of fibrinolytic
enzymes. The content of soluble fibrin was estimated by the protamine sulphate
test [9] in plasma obtained by blood centrifugation at 4000 × g for 15 min.
Blood was withdrawn from each animal once only to avoid additional stress and
activation of coagulation.

After bleeding rabbits were sacrificed and kidneys, lungs, spleen, liver and
thymus were removed. Organ slices were stained according to Adams [10] to
identify fibrin. Percentages of kidney glomeruli containing no (f_0), slight (f+),
moderate (f++) and abundant amounts (f+++) of fibrin were determined independently by two persons with high agreement. Three types of GSR were distinguished:
mild when percentage of f_0 plus f+ was higher than that of f++ plus f+++, moderate
when percentages of f_0, f+, f++ and f+++ were similar, and severe when f++ plus
f+++ > f_0 plus f+.

Scarce fibrin deposits in the organs, mostly in the lungs, were observed 24 h
after E_1. Histologically demonstrable deposition of fibrin in kidney glomeruli
indicating GSR occurred neither after whole-body irradiation alone nor after the
preparatory dose of endotoxin. Figure 2 shows that GSR occurred with nearly
equal frequency and was somewhat more severe in irradiated rabbits treated subsequently with endotoxin compared with the $E_1 + E_2$ group.

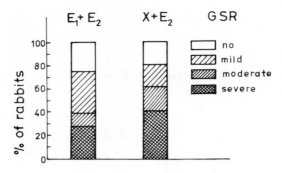

FIG.2.   Frequency and severity of GSR.

TABLE I.   FREQUENCY OF DETECTION OF SOLUBLE FIBRIN IN
PLASMA BY PROTAMINE SULPHATE GELATION TEST

	Number of rabbits examined	Protamine sulphate gelation	
		Negative	Positive
Control	18	18 (100%)	0
12 or 24 h after:			
E_1	9	4 (44%)	5 (56%)
X	13	6 (46%)	7 (54%)
3 or 12 h after:			
$E_1 + E_2$	20	1 (5%)	19 (95%)
$X + E_2$	23	1 (4%)	22 (96%)

From Table I it can be seen that the direct sign of systemic activation of
coagulation, i.e. the presence of soluble fibrin in blood plasma, was detected in
over 50% of the rabbits during 24 h after X-ray exposure as well as after the
administration of the preparatory endotoxin dose. Soluble fibrin appeared in
plasma within 12 h after the provocative injection of bacterial lipopolysaccharide
in nearly all animals of group $X + E_2$ as well as of $E_1 + E_2$.

These data indicate that whole-body irradiation with 850 R of X-rays
induces early systemic activation of the blood coagulation system and prepares
rabbits for GSR at least as efficiently as a preparatory injection of endotoxin.

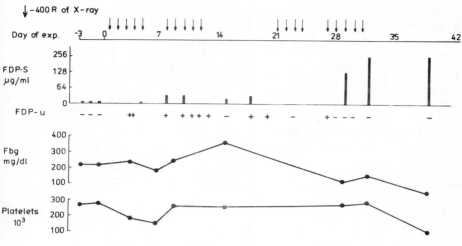

FIG.3.   Effects of local X-ray exposures of the mediastinal region in dog:
FDP-S = FDP in serum
FDP-u = FDP in urine
Fbg = fibrinogen.

The purpose of further investigation was to check whether local fractionated
doses of ionizing radiation lead to the activation of blood coagulation, and in
particular whether involvement of the kidney in this process depends on its direct
exposure.

Mongrel dogs weighing 7 to 12 kg were subjected to fractionated X-ray local
doses of 19 × 400 R applied to areas of 10 × 8 cm either in the region of the
kidneys (3 dogs) or of the mediastinum (3 dogs).

Before and at indicated time intervals during treatment platelet count,
fibrinogen concentration in plasma [11], and content of fibrin degradation
products (FDP) in serum and urine were determined. Anti-serum against dog
fibrinogen was applied for the highly sensitive immunoassay of FDP [12].

The results obtained in both groups were similar regardless of the body region
irradiated. Figure 3 presents an illustrative case of changes in the dog subjected to
mediastinal region exposure. In all animals FDP were absent in the urine before
irradiations but were detected repeatedly although not constantly during four
weeks after exposures. The content of FDP in blood serum increased gradually and
attained the highest values between the 4th and 6th week when platelet count and
fibrinogen level decreased significantly. In this period symptoms of post-radiation
syndrome were observed, such as loss of appetite and body weight, alternative
periods of diarrhoea and constipation, local skin erythema with hair loss, decreased
mobility. Similar also was the pattern of changes in dogs subjected to four

TABLE II. FDP IN URINE OF PATIENTS SUBJECTED TO
RADIOTHERAPY FOR UTERINE CERVIX CARCINOMA

Total number of patients	Age (years)	Number of cases with FDP in urine in temporal relation to radiotherapy		
		Before	2–3th week	4–8th week
29	30–74	5 (2)[a]	11 (5)[a]	21 (8)[a]
			23 (8)[a]	

[a] In brackets FDP content exceeding 10 μg/ml.

exposures of 600 R of X-rays at 2-day intervals to either the anterior (2 dogs) or posterior (2 dogs) part of the body.

FDP absent in urine before irradiation were excreted in increasing amounts, up to 10 μg/ml, in the first week after exposures. In the blood serum FDP attained the highest values during the overt post-irradiation disease when the fall of fibrinogen level and platelet count occurred.

Clinical observations were performed on 29 patients subjected to radiotherapy for uterine cervix carcinoma. Advancement of the disease was evaluated as stage I in 6, II in 11 and III in 12 cases. Radium applicators and cobalt or X-ray teletherapy was applied to most of the patients. Teletherapy alone was used in four cases. The total dose to the uterine cervix ranged from 40 to 150 Gy. The fibrinogen level [11] and the content of FDP [12] in serum and urine were determined before treatment and at weekly intervals during and after radiotherapy. It should be mentioned that in 60 control healthy people FDP in serum ranged from 0 to 4 μg/ml whereas in urine FDP were not detected in any.

Similarly to many other authors we observed that the fibrinogen level increased significantly from the initial mean of 246 ± 43 mg/dl to the mean maximum of 359 ± 66 mg/dl. Maximal values were attained most often between the 3rd to 6th week of radiotherapy. The FDP content in serum was increased (10 to 15 μg/ml) before treatment in six patients and rose to 20–40 μg in five in the 3rd week. In most cases, however, no or only minor changes in serum FDP occurred.

Table II shows that the frequency of urinary excretion of FDP increased markedly during radiotherapy. Initially FDP were detected in five out of 29 patients. Starting from the 2nd week of radiotherapy up to its termination FDP were found in the urine of 23 cases. In 14 patients the presence of FDP in urine was detected in two to six consecutive examinations at weekly intervals. In this preliminary study urinary excretion of FDP correlated neither with proteinuria, nor with advancement of the neoplastic process and any overt complications of radiotherapy.

The results presented indicate that in rabbits the whole-body exposure to ionizing radiation induces the systemic activation of blood coagulation which, when associated with endotoxaemia, can proceed to severe kidney damage, i.e. the Schwartzman reaction. If similar mechanisms operate in other species antibacterial treatment would be of benefit for protection against post-irradiation damage of renal vasculature.

The concomitant fall in platelet count, fibrinogen level and increase in FDP in the serum during the overt radiation syndrome induced in dogs by partial body exposures to heavy doses of X-rays suggest also the systemic activation of the coagulation system and fibrinolysis at this post-irradiation stage.

Excretion of FDP in urine is considered by most authors [13] to indicate intrarenal fibrin deposition followed by its proteolysis. The significance of these phenomena for pathogenic mechanism of glomerulonephritis, particularly for its proliferative forms, is now well recognized. The fact that in irradiated patients as well as in dogs the urinary excretion of FDP did not correlate with serum FDP argues against the increased passage of circulating FDP through the damaged renal filter as a probable mechanism of their appearance in urine. Local deposition of fibrin and its digestion seems more probable.

Since doses absorbed by the kidneys in the regime of radiotherapy applied for uterine cervix carcinoma were only negligible and results obtained after irradiation of the mediastinal and kidney regions in dogs did not differ, it can be concluded that renal damage leading to urinary FDP excretion can develop as an abscopal effect. This observation agrees with the results of Wachholz and Casarett [14] who found that post-irradiation nephrosclerosis in rats, although more rapid when kidneys were irradiated, occurred also after whole-body exposure but with the kidneys shielded.

The problem remains unsolved whether pharmacological prevention of thrombosis would protect the kidney against radiation injury without sacrificing any of the therapeutical effectiveness when this organ cannot be excluded from exposure during radiotherapy.

REFERENCES

[1] STEWART, G.J., Thromb. Haemostas. (Stuttg.) **38** (1977) 831.
[2] KHAN, M.Y., OKANIAN, M., Am. J. Pathol. **74** (1974) 124.
[3] FAJARDO, L.F., STEWART, J.R., Lab. Invest. **29** (1973) 244.
[4] KINZIE, J., STUDER, R., PEREZ, B., POTCHEN, E.J., Science **175** (1972) 1481.
[5] FISHER, E.R., HELLSTROM, H.R., Lab. Invest. **19** (1968) 530.

[6] KEANE, W.F., CROSSON, J.T., STANLEY, N.A., ANDERSON, W.R., SHAPIRO, F.L.,
     Am. J. Med. **60** (1976) 127.

[7] LUXTON, R.W., "Effects of irradiation on the kidney", Diseases of the Kidney II
     (STRAUSS, M.B., WELT, L.G., Eds), Little Brown and Company, Boston (1971) 1049.

[8] WĘGRZYNOWICZ, Z., WRONOWSKI, T., LATALLO, Z.S., KOPEĆ, M., Arch. Immunol.
     Ther. Exp. **22** (1974) 689.

[9] LATALLO, Z.S., WĘGRZYNOWICZ, Z., TEISSEYRE, E., KOPEĆ, M., Scand. J.
     Haematol., Suppl. **13** (1970) 387.

[10] ADAMS, C.W.M., J. Clin. Pathol. **10** (1957) 56.

[11] JACOBSON, K., Scand. J. Clin. Lab. Invest., Suppl. **7** (1955).

[12] MERSKY, C., LALEZAR, P., JOHNSON, A.J., Proc. Soc. Exp. Biol. Med. **131** (1969) 871.

[13] MICHIELSEN, P., ROELS, L., VANRENTERGHEM, Y., BOEL, A., VAN DAMME, B.,
     VERMYLEN, J., J. Urol. Nephrol. **85** (1975) 869.

[14] WACHHOLZ, B.W., CASARETT, G.W., Radiat. Res. **41** (1970) 39.

DISCUSSION

V.M. VOLODIN: What is the main cause of thrombosis of the blood vessels
in the kidney in your experiments — endotoxin or irradiation? I ask this because
endotoxin alone can cause damage to the endothelium as well as activating the
blood coagulation system. Also, what histological changes did you see in the
kidney after irradiation without administration of endotoxin?

M. KOPEĆ: Both endotoxin and X-ray exposure can induce endothelial
injury and subsequent thrombosis. However, either two doses of endotoxin
or X-ray irradiation followed by a single endotoxin dose were required to induce
fibrin deposition in the kidneys. The reverse combination, i.e. endotoxin injection
followed by irradiation, was ineffective. Neither a single dose of endotoxin nor
X-ray exposure alone provoked any definite changes in kidney histology in the
course of 48 h after administration in the preparations stained for fibrin and
with haematoxylin-eosin. We have not performed any longer-term observations
or electron microscopic studies.

IAEA-SM-224/306

EARLY DETECTION OF
RADIO-INDUCED PULMONARY CANCER

C. PĂUN, D. POPOVICI
Radiobiological Section,
Fundeni Clinical Hospital,
Bucharest

M. NICOLAE
Institute of Atomic Physics,
Bucharest,
Romania

Abstract

EARLY DETECTION OF RADIO-INDUCED PULMONARY CANCER.
An important source of information on the carcinogenic effects of radiation concerns the occurrence of lung cancer in such workers as uranium miners. A dose-time relationship for the indication of lung cancer in uranium miners is appearing between the incidence of the tumours, exposure and time. There are some difficulties in establishing with accuracy the exposure by means of length of work, radon concentration (WL), and there are considerable ambiguities regarding other physico-chemical and physiological factors. To solve these uncertainties, spit autoradiographies are being carried out to estimate the pulmonary burden with radon daughters and uranium dust. In all miners with an increased pulmonary radioactive burden after a significant period of mining cytological examination of the spit is being performed. Cytological examination shows two kinds of pathological aspects: metaplasic pavimentous forms of the cylindric opithelial cells, and metaplasic forms with a displasic character. Information obtained from a periodical cytological investigation enables some metaplasic aspects to be detected very early, which is of great importance for preventive medicine, because carcinogenic induction can be avoided, reducing exposure below the usual recommended levels.

Knowledge of the quantitative and qualitative aspects of pulmonary radio-induced carcinogenesis can only be obtained by further study.

The quantitative aspects of human carcinogenesis in uranium miners are given by the relationship between the incidence of tumours and exposure by means of the length of time spent working, and the relationship between the product of radon concentration (in so-called 'working levels') and time.

However, a simple and general statement of this quantitative relationship is now impossible because usually there are irregularities and intermittencies in the activity of the miners; also the measurement of the radioactive content of mine air was not common until recent years, and it is therefore very difficult to

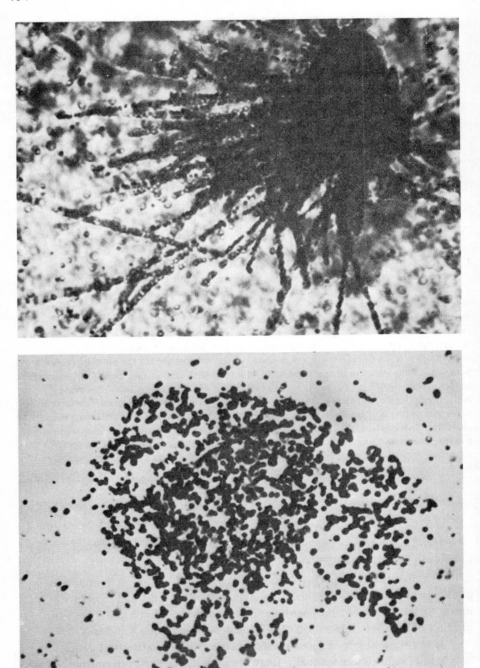

FIG.1. Alpha tracks and grains of ^{210}Pb in spit radiography.

establish the past concentration of the radioactive aerosols. Even now frequency of air sampling is inevitably low, both regarding the number of working positions examined in mines and the time interval between consecutive samples, so it is impossible to take into account the inhomogeneity of mine air.

The radioactive contamination in the mines arises from ^{222}Rn parent gas and unattached daughter products, ^{222}Rn daughter products attached to dust particles, and uranium dust of soluble and insoluble compounds.

This last-mentioned dust exhibits a low transportability, and thus the lung becomes the critical organ.

The link between air concentration and pulmonary burden depends on the content and size distribution of the particles in the inhaled radioactive aerosols.

The proportion of these various types of aerosols in the inhaled air is random, so this could explain the great variation in the radioactive, pulmonary burden which we have demonstrated by spit autoradiography.

On the spit autoradiographies there are images characteristic for accumulation at cellular level of a beta emission, and these are interpreted as the result of an agglomeration of a RaD(^{210}Pb) from radon descendants and alpha tracks easily recognized by their rectilinear appearance. Alpha-active elements contained in the spit can be identified by drawing histograms of the track length of the particles.

A quantitative appreciation of the pulmonary burden could be estimated by track density per surface unit of the measured probes, because probably the rate of the expectorated radionuclides is closely proportional to the amount of radionuclides incorporated in the lung tissue.

On the basis of our several years' experience [3] in utilizing the spit auto-radiography method in the periodic medical examinations of uranium miners, we can point out that in most of the plates autoradiography images are characteristic not only for beta emission but also at least equally for alpha tracks, as can be seen in Fig.1.

This enables us to assert that the contribution of the uranium dust incorporated in the lung tissue in the initiating dose must be by no means neglected. Finally, we require a rigorous method to estimate the dose according to different cell types within the lung and to appreciate more correctly the sensitivity of these tissues per rad. Individual variations are also most important.

The qualitative aspects of radio-induced pulmonary carcinogenesis are dependent on the variations in some individual factors.

There are many individual peculiarities of the upper respiratory tract that determine the respiration type (by nose or by mouth), or of the bronchial tree that alter the dynamics of the radioactive aerosols inhalation and retention, as well as some physiological factors of which the most important is the breathing rate.

The individual differences in some associated pathogenetic factors, which in most cases escape our investigation, should also be considered.

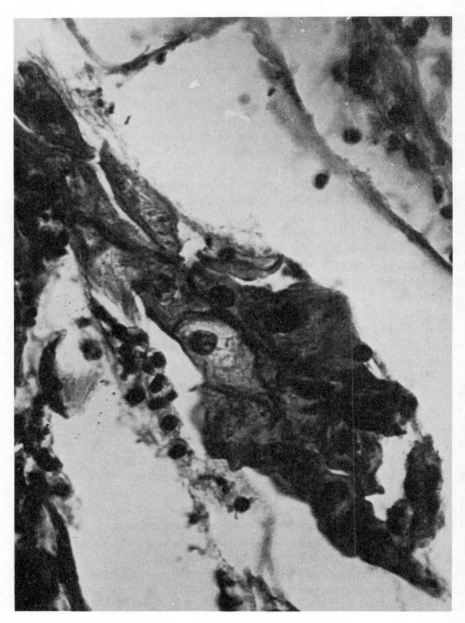

FIG. 2. *Pavimentous metaplasia, parakeratotic form.*

It is generally assumed that radio-induced cancer in man exhibits the characteristic of either a high initiating dose of short latency or a low initiating dose of long latency.

Archer and co-workers [1] and Blair [2] estimated the initiating dose to be about 400 WLM. A miner beginning exposure at 1 WL at age 20 would acquire the dose in 33 years, which would permit survival until age 76 (including the 23 years period of latency).

This is too simple to be true. As we have been trying to point out, usually in the same mine the exposure can vary from miner to miner, and it is very difficult, even impossible, to determine with accuracy the quantitative and qualitative aspects of pulmonary, radio-induced carcinogenesis.

All these individual factors do not alter the incidence of radio-induced pulmonary carcinogenesis, but surely determine both the variation in the initiating dose and the latent period, each of them varying from individual to individual independently.

In accordance with the concept of the initiating dose as a threshold dose for the individual we suggest a correlative methodology for obtaining more reliable information on the moment of the induction.

First, we assess the degree of exposure by length of work and correct monitoring of the environment so that the 'WL' would be representative as far as possible of the air breathed by the worker.

Secondly, the spit autoradiography control allows us to characterize the deposition pattern of the aerosols in the respiratory tract, taking into account any pulmonary radioactive overburden.

Thirdly, the cytological examination of the spit becomes very useful for early evaluation of radio-induced lesions. The cytological examination shows two kinds of pathological aspects: the metaplasic forms of the cylindrical epithelial cells and the metaplasic forms with a displasic character.

Among the metaplasic forms of the bronchial epithelium we are interested in the pavimentous form, which results from the complete replacement of the cylindrical epithelial cells by pavimentous ones. In the spit they appear as exfoliated cells either as isolated or small groups of cells.

The cells present the familiar cytological characteristics preserving the nucleus-cytoplasm ratio the latter being more or less eosinophilic.

The pavimentous metaplasia can be irregular, either parakeratotic (elongated cells (Fig.2), with the cytoplasm loaded with keratoeledin and picnotic nucleus) or koilocytodic (cells with excentric hyperchromatic nuclei and intracytoplasmatic vacuols).

Such metaplasia is observed in some chronic pneumopathies, lung infarcts and various cicatrized sequela but most authors consider the metaplasia as a lesion preceding the carcinogenic transformation.

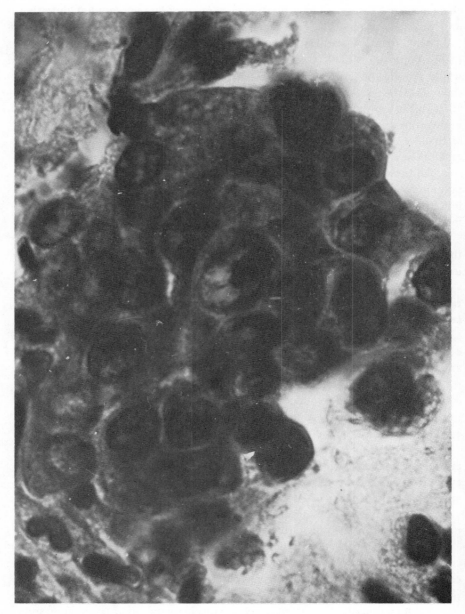

FIG.3. In the outer area, simple metaplasia; in the inner area, cells with atypical nuclei and alteration of the nucleus-cytoplasm ratio, characteristic of an advanced displasia.

Obviously, a complex clinical examination could eliminate all cases in which the metaplasia is due to a previous affection. This differentiation is very difficult only in miners with an associated silicosis.

But in cases with a long period of mining and when spit autoradiography shows a significant radioactive load, we can consider the metaplasic aspects as a warning to remove the miner from the radioactive environment.

The cytological examination of the spit can produce evidence of displasic alterations. These also have a pavimentous character (Fig.3), but the cells show loss of polarity, atypical nuclei (tachychromatic, of variable form and size) and alterations in the nucleus-cytoplasm ratio.

Displasia is no doubt a pre-cancerous state. When the exposure data and the autoradiographic spit examination allow us to incriminate the irradiation as the cause of displasia, we obtain thus an early indication of a pulmonary cancer, radio-induced by accumulation of the initiating dose.

We doubt that there is anything more which can be done to prevent such cases since the period following initiation is not altered by non-exposure, continued exposure or by increased exposure [2], thus only therapeutic measures can be taken.

Saccomanno and co-workers [4], as well as other authors, claim that the cytological spit examination offers the possibility of diagnosis and histological determination of the evolution of the bronchial epithelium metaplasia, provided a correct method of pre-lavation and processing of the spit samples is employed.

A sufficiently long time survey of a group of miners will allow us to draw the necessary conclusions to extend this correlative methodology to all the workers exposed to radioactive contamination hazards by inhalation.

REFERENCES

[1] ARCHER, V.E., et al., Lung cancer among uranium miners in the United States, Health Phys. **25** (1974) 512.
[2] BLAIR, H.A., "Dose-time relations for induction of lung cancer in uranium miners", Radiation-Induced Cancer (Proc. Symp. Athens, 1969), IAEA, Vienna (1969) 203.
[3] PĂUN, C., NICOLAE, M., Evaluation of radiation-induced pulmonary lesions by spit autoradiography, Biological and Environmental Effects of Low-Level Radiation, (Proc. Symp. Chicago, 1975) **II**, IAEA, Vienna (1976) 229.
[4] SACCOMANNO, G., et al., Lung cancer of uranium miners on the Colorado plateau, Health Phys. **12** (1964) 1195.

DISCUSSION

K.H. CHADWICK *(Chairman):* Do you notice any differences between smokers and non-smokers?

C. PĂUN: Yes, the percentage of metaplasia is higher in smokers.

A.B. DORY: In a group of over 200 Ontario uranium miners under observation for lung cancer, only in two cases out of around ten detected were early indications of carcinogenic cells discovered by sputum cytology before cancer was shown by chest X-rays. After how many years of occupational exposure do you recommend that sputum cytology be started, and at what levels of accumulated exposure to radon daughters do mortal lung cancer cases occur?

C. PĂUN: Cytological examination becomes necessary when sputum autoradiography shows a significant contamination. It is very difficult to predict for each individual the moment of the cancerous induction, so our policy is to remove a miner from the radioactive environment at the first sign of metaplasia in order to avoid dysplastic transformation.

C-TYPE RNA VIRUSES AS POSSIBLE PREDICTORS OF RADIATION-INDUCED BONE ONCOGENESIS*

V. ERFLE
Institut für Biologie der
      Gesellschaft für Strahlen- und Umweltforschung mbH München,
Neuherberg

R. HEHLMANN
Medizinische Poliklinik der Universität München,
Munich

K.-H. MARQUART, H. BÜSCHER, E. DE FRIES,
L. STRUBEL, A. LUZ
Institut für Biologie der
      Gesellschaft für Strahlen- und Umweltforschung mbH München,
Neuherberg
Federal Republic of Germany

Abstract

C-TYPE RNA VIRUSES AS POSSIBLE PREDICTORS OF RADIATION-INDUCED BONE ONCOGENESIS.
    Radium-224-induced osteosarcomas of $(C3H \times 101)F_1$ mice have been investigated for the presence of C-type RNA viruses. C-type virus particles with the typical properties of RNA tumour viruses could be detected by electron microscopic, biochemical and in-vitro studies. In a long-term experiment, the expression of C-type RNA virus particles was studied during the latency period and correlated with the appearance of osteosarcomas. The tumour incidence in this experiment was 100% with 40—50% of the tumours appearing in the 11th to 12th month after the start of the radiation. C-type RNA virus expression could be found in the 1st month and in the 11th and 12th months. These results indicate a transient virus activation shortly after starting the radiation, and a second peak of virus expression coinciding with the appearance of the osteosarcomas.

INTRODUCTION

Alpha-emitting bone-seeking radionuclides induce osteosarcomas in man and animals [1]. These and some other radiation-induced tumours, e.g. leukaemia and mammary tumours, can also be induced by RNA tumour viruses [2, 3].

---

* In association with Euratom (Contract No. 218—76—1 BIAD).

Endogenous viruses, biochemically and morphologically identical with RNA tumour viruses, are known to be present in the genome of mammalian cells [4]. These observations have led to the concept of a possible radiation-virus interaction in the development of radiation-induced tumours. The isolation of leukaemogenic C-type RNA viruses from radiation-induced leukaemias strongly supports the concept of radiation-induced tumorigenesis via activation of a tumorigenic virus [5, 6]. Recent evidence suggests that radiation-induced murine osteosarcoma may also be associated with C-type RNA viruses: (1) Radiation-induced murine osteosarcomas contain C-type particles as observed electron microscopically [7−9]; (2) Radionuclide-induced murine and canine osteosarcomas contain a 70 S RNA associated with reverse transcriptase activity [9, 10]; (3) Mice with ^{90}Sr-induced osteosarcomas develop antibodies against FBJ osteosarcoma virus [11]; (4) Cell cultures, derived from [224]Ra- and [227]Th-induced murine osteo-sarcomas, show production of C-type RNA viruses by biochemical, biological and electron microscopic methods [12]; (5) The isolation of bone tumour-inducing C-type viruses from ^{90}Sr-induced osteosarcomas of mice by Finkel and co-workers [7] suggests that some radiation-induced osteosarcomas may harbour tumorigenic viruses.

More conclusive evidence for the role of C-type RNA viruses in radiation-induced osteosarcomagenesis might be obtained from an analysis of C-type RNA virus expression in bone during the latency period before the appearance of the tumour. The high osteosarcoma yield after fractionated injection of [224]Ra in mice seems to be a suitable experimental basis for such studies (for further information see Ref.[131]). If RNA tumour viruses play an aetiological role in radiation-induced osteosarcomagenesis, their presence or at least the expression of some C-type viral information would be expected to precede the appearance of osteosarcomas. If C-type virus expression does not precede the appearance of osteosarcomas, an accidental activation of the viruses by the tumour state of the host cell would seem to be a more plausible explanation for the presence of viral particles. It is the purpose of the present study to examine radiation-induced, C-type RNA virus-induced and spontaneous murine osteosarcomas for their suitability in studies on the mechanism of tumorigenesis.

MATERIALS AND METHODS

Animals

Female (C3H X 101)F_1 mice of the Neuherberg breeding colony were used. At the beginning of the experiment the mice were 4 weeks old.

Radionuclide application

Thirty-six μCi ^{224}Ra/kg were administered as 72 ip injections of 0.5 μCi/kg with time intervals of 3.5 days, i.e. as a protracted application over 36 weeks. The radionuclide was applied as an isotonic solution. The total mean skeletal alpha-radiation dose was 1000 rads [14].

Time schedule of serial investigations

From 4 weeks (1 month) until 44 weeks (11 months) after the beginning of the injection period, animals without obvious symptoms of neoplasms were sacrificed every 4 weeks:

(a) for virological studies: 7 control animals, 7 experimental animals,

(b) for light microscopic studies of the skeleton: 2 control animals, 2 experimental animals. Electron microscopic studies were performed with lower lumbar vertebrae of selected animals of this series.

The experiment was performed with two groups of animals. The first group (A) was used for the investigations in months $1-7$. The second group (B), born 4 weeks later than the first group, was used for the investigations in months $8-11$.

Serial light microscopical studies

After X-ray examination of the animals, the total vertebral column, both humeri (proximal ends), both iliae and both knee joints were studied in H & E sections. In addition the parenchymatous organs were examined histologically.

Transplantation of normal skeleton at the end of the latency period

Thirty-six weeks after the beginning of the experiment, 5 control animals and 5 experimental animals out of the two groups with different birth dates were sacrificed. From each donor, skeletal pieces less than 1 mm^3 ($3-4$ pieces per host) were transplanted into 13 male and 13 female syngenic hosts ($2-4$ months old) according to the following schedule:

(1) intramuscularly into one thigh

(a) material from the caudal part of the lumbar vertebral column, sacrum, distal femora, proximal tibiae into 2 males and 2 females

(b)   material from the proximal humeri and the caudal part of the
       thoracic vertebral column into 1 male and 1 female
(2)   subcutaneously into the neck region
       combined material from the caudal part of the lumbar vertebral column
       into 3 males and 3 females.
       Eight weeks after transplantation, the animals were sacrificed, autopsied
and controlled by X-ray examination.

Long-term experiment

Out of the two groups with different birth dates, 40 animals of group A
(16 control and 31 experimental animals) and 77 animals of group B (50 control
and 35 experimental animals) were observed for late effects.

Out of group A, some animals with osteosarcomas, diagnosed by X-ray
picture, were used for further virological studies. In all other cases, the diagnosis
of an osteosarcoma was confirmed histologically.

Electron microscopy

Tissue specimens of bone tumours and lower lumbar vertebrae were fixed
in cacodylate-buffered 3% glutaraldehyde, postfixed in chrome-osmium,
dehydrated, and embedded in Epon 812. Thin sections were cut with a diamond
knife on a Reichert 0m U3 microtome, and stained with uranyl acetate and
lead citrate. They were examined in a TESLA BS 500 electron microscope.

Simultaneous detection test

The simultaneous detection test [15] was performed according to
Hehlmann and co-workers [16]. This test allows the simultaneous detection of
two major properties of RNA tumour viruses: a reverse transcriptase and a high
molecular weight RNA of 60—70 S size. For this test, 10 g of bone tissue
homogenates were used. The homogenates were freed from nuclei and
mitochondria by low speed centrifugation. The postmitochondrial supernatant
was density-fractionated by centrifugation through 20% sucrose on a 50% sucrose
cushion. 0.3 ml of the density-fractionated material, suspended in 0.01M Tris-HCl,
pH 8.3, 0.1M NaCl, and 0.1% Triton X-100, was used in 0.2 ml of a typical
endogenous reverse transcriptase reaction containing 25 μmole Tris-HCl,
pH 8.3, 3 μmole $MgCl_2$, 0.4 μmole each of dATP, dGTP and dCTP, 2 mCi
^{3}H-dTTP (Schwarz/Mann, 50 Ci/mmole) and 100 μg Actinomycin D per 0.5 ml
reaction volume. After a 15 min incubation at 37°C the reaction was terminated
and deproteinized with an equal volume of phenol-cresol (7:1). The resulting
aqueous phase was layered on a glycerol gradient (10—30% in TNE) and centri-
fuged for 3 h at 40 000 rev/min and 1°C (SW 41 Ti Rotor).

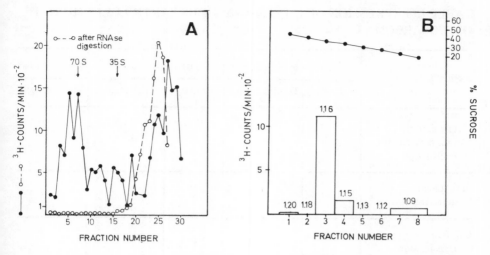

FIG.1. *Localization of 70 S RNA and reverse transcriptase activity in homogenates of a transplanted* ^{224}*Ra-induced osteosarcoma on a sucrose density gradient. (A) The sedimentation profile of a glycerol gradient from an endogenous reverse transcriptase assay, performed with density-fractionated material. (B) The* ^{3}*H-DNA counts, sedimented in the 70 S region of each glycerol gradient, were determined and plotted.*

RESULTS

C-type RNA virus particles in osteosarcomas

Electron microscopy

The electron microscopic examination of primary, transplanted and in-vitro cultured ^{224}Ra-induced osteosarcomas in $(C3H \times 101)F_1$ mice showed that typical C-type virus particles were present beside some intracisternal A-type particles. Mature C-type particles had a concentric electron-dense nucleoid, a surrounding unit membrane and an outer diameter of about 90 – 100 nm. They showed the typical morphology of mature C-type virus particles. The C-type particles were found in the extracellular space, and particles budding from cellular membranes were sometimes detected.

Simultaneous detection test

The simultaneous detection test indicated that virus particles containing a reverse transcriptase and a high molecular weight RNA are present in the osteosarcomas. The tritiated DNA-product of a reverse transcriptase reaction

TABLE I. EXPRESSION OF C-TYPE RNA VIRUS PARTICLES IN MURINE OSTEOSARCOMAS

Methods	Radiation-induced[a]		FBJ virus-induced[b]		Spontaneous[c]
	Primary	Transplanted	Primary	Transplanted	Transplanted
C-type particles found by electron microscopy	+	+	+	+	−
Simultaneous detection test	+	+	+	+	+
Cell-free transmission	−	−	+	−	−
C-type RNA virus production in cell culture	+	Not tested	+	+	+

[a] (C3H × 101)F_1 mice.
[b] C3H mice.
[c] C3H mice.

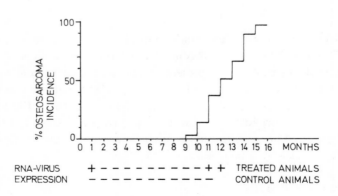

FIG.2. *Osteosarcoma incidence and RNA virus expression in the skeleton of female (C3H × 101)F_1 mice. Repeated injections of 0.5 μCi ^{224}Ra/kg with time intervals of 3.5 days during 36 weeks, i.e. total amount of injected activity 36 μCi/kg corresponding to a total mean skeletal dose of 1080 rads. The months after the start of radiation are indicated.*

with density-fractionated osteosarcomas sedimented in the $60-70$ S position
of a glycerol gradient (Fig.1A). The disappearance of the ^{3}H-DNA radioactivity
peak after RNAse treatment before sedimentation showed that the DNA was
complexed to a high molecular weight RNA. Both the primary and the transplanted osteosarcomas of $(C3H \times 101)F_1$ mice were positive in the simultaneous
detection test. The density of the particles was determined by isopycnic centrifugation of postmitochondrial supernatants from transplanted $(C3H \times 101)F_1$
osteosarcomas in $20-50\%$ sucrose gradients, and by the examination of the
gradient fractions with simultaneous detection tests. The results showed that the
virus particles banded at a density of 1.16 g/cm^3 region of the gradient which
is the typical density of RNA tumour viruses (Fig.1B). C-type RNA virus
expression was also detected in the FBJ virus-induced osteosarcomas and in a
spontaneous osteosarcoma (Dunn osteosarcoma). The results of virus particle
expression in radionuclide-induced, RNA tumour virus-induced and spontaneous
murine osteosarcomas are summarized in Table I. Only the primary FBJ virus-
induced osteosarcomas were found to harbour oncogenic viruses that induced
identical tumours by cell-free transmission in new-born C3H mice.

Tumour incidence and morphological studies

Osteosarcoma incidence

Group A: Out of 16 control animals none developed an osteosarcoma,
whereas 30 out of 31 experimental animals developed osteosarcomas $8-16$ months
after the beginning of the experiment. One animal died 3 months after the
beginning of the experiment. Since its skeleton was partly cannibalized it was
excluded from the evaluation. Group B: 2 out of 42 control animals developed
osteosarcomas 19 and 31 months after the beginning of the experiment. All
35 experimental animals developed osteosarcomas $9-17$ months after the
beginning of the experiment (see also Fig.2). More than 50% of the osteosarcomas
were located in the vertebral column, and more than 40% in the lumbar vertebral
column and in the os sacrum. Further details of the long-term experiment will
be published elsewhere.

*Light microscopic search for osteosarcomas during months $1-11$ after the
beginning of ^{224}Ra injections*

No osteosarcoma was observed in the control animals. In the experimental
animals, no osteosarcoma was observed until month 9. One of the 2 animals
sacrificed after 10 months showed an osteosarcoma of the second lumbar
vertebra. The lower half of the third lumbar vertebra of this animal was taken
for electron microscopic study. The upper half of this vertebra was obviously

free from tumour. One of the 2 animals sacrificed after 11 months had an osteosarcoma of the os sacrum. None of the control and experimental animals sacrificed in this series had leukaemia.

Transplantation experiment

None of the 260 animals with transplants of the skeleton of experimental animals and none of the 260 corresponding control animals showed outgrowth of a bone tumour.

C-type RNA virus particles in bone tissue during the latency period

Electron microscopy

During the latency period before the appearance of osteosarcomas no typical mature C-type particles could be detected in vertebral bone tissue. But extracellular virus-like particles were present in bone tissue of 4 out of 5 untreated control animals and in 9 out of 11 animals treated with ^{224}Ra. These particles resembled immature C-type virus particles. Further details will be published elsewhere.

Simultaneous detection test

The simultaneous detection test was carried out with the pooled bone tissues of seven mice monthly. All tests performed with the untreated control animals were entirely negative from months 1 − 11. In the ^{224}Ra-treated animals, the pool with the animals sacrificed 1 month after starting the treatment was positive. The bone tissue pools from months 2 − 10 did not show RNA virus particle expression. In month 11, the simultaneous detection test turned positive again in animals without macroscopically detectable tumours. Animals with osteosarcomas sacrificed in the 12th month after the beginning of treatment also showed a positive simultaneous detection test. The ribonuclease sensitive counts in the 70 S peak fraction were 105 counts/min in the 1st month, 91 counts/min in the 11th month and 115 counts/min in the 12th month. The bone tissues of osteosarcoma-bearing animals without the tumour were negative in the simultaneous detection test.

DISCUSSION

Several mechanisms have been discussed by which a normal cell is converted to a tumour cell. These mechanisms include a viral aetiology of cancer, induction by chemical and physical agents including radiation, as well as a mechanism not understood at all and merely called 'spontaneous'. Except for murine leukaemias, no defined experimental tumour model exists that allows the simultaneous study of different mechanisms. The present study introduces an experimental system for the simultaneous examination of the mechanisms causing sarcomas in the skeleton: murine osteosarcomas induced by radiation, by viruses and spontaneous osteosarcomas.

Alpha-radiation by bone-seeking nuclides induces osteosarcomas in the $(C3H \times 101)F_1$ mice, used for this study, with an incidence of 100%, whereas unirradiated mice show osteosarcomas in less than 5% during the same period. C-type particles were observed in the radiation-induced osteosarcomas by electron microscopy, and the particles were found to possess typical biochemical and physical properties of RNA tumour viruses. This observation enabled the C-type RNA virus expression to be studied and its correlation with tumorigenesis during the latency period, i.e. some time after the start of radiation and before the development of osteosarcomas.

The detection of reverse transcriptase and $60-70$ S RNA four weeks after beginning ^{224}Ra treatment is some evidence for a transient virus production as shown in radiation-induced leukaemia [17]. Which type of virus particle has been activated at this time is the subject of future investigation. The appearance of virus particles in the 11th and 12th month after the start of radiation coincides with the appearance of the tumours. Up to the 11th month, about 40% of the animals in the long-term experiment developed osteosarcomas. The animals used for the simultaneous detection test in the 11th month were macroscopically free of tumours but might have had some microscopically detectable tumours. Some of the animals used in the 12th month after ^{224}Ra treatment had macroscopically detectable tumours. It cannot be decided from these experiments whether some expression of virus particles precedes the appearance of osteosarcoma or if these virus particles appear together with the tumours.

The appearance of, or changes in expression of RNA tumour viruses or structural components of these viruses during the tumour latency time have been shown to precede the development of murine leukaemias [18, 19]. In chemically or radiation-induced leukaemias, the expression of RNA tumour viruses before overt leukaemia is strong evidence for the involvement of these viruses in leukaemogenesis [17, 20]. The appearance of complete viral particles in radiation-induced osteosarcomas argues for some role of the viruses in osteosarcomagenesis, but to decide on viral expression before tumorigenesis, the expression of viral substructures as, for example, of the structural proteins and the appearance of viral specific RNA has to be studied further.

ACKNOWLEDGEMENTS

We are indebted to M. Finkel for the provision of FBJ virus and S. Fisher for the supply of Dunn osteosarcoma.

We wish to thank U. Linzner and W.A. Müller for the dosimetry of ^{224}Ra. We also thank E. Jatho, M. Biszkup, K. Böll and S. Klemt for technical assistance.

REFERENCES

[1] VAUGHAN, J.J., The Effects of Irradiation on the Skeleton, Clarendon Press, Oxford (1973).

[2] GROSS, L., Oncogenic Viruses, Pergamon Press, Oxford (1970).

[3] BENTVELZEN, P., Host-virus interactions in murine mammary carcinogenesis, Biochem. Biophys. Acta **355** (1974) 236.

[4] AARONSON, S.A., STEPHENSON, J.R., Endogenous type-C RNA viruses of mammalian cells, Biochim. Biophys. Acta **458** (1976) 323.

[5] LIEBERMANN, M., KAPLAN, H.S., Leukemogenic activity of filtrates from radiation-induced lymphoid tumors of mice, Science **130** (1959) 387.

[6] GROSS, L., Serial cell-free passage of radiation-activated mouse leukemia agent, Proc. Soc. Exp. Biol. Med. **100** (1959) 102.

[7] FINKEL, M.P., REILLY, C.A., BISKIS, B.O., GRECO, I.L., "Bone tumor viruses", Bone – Certain Aspects of Neoplasia (PRICE, C.H.G., ROSS, F.G.M., Eds), Butterworths, London (1973) 353.

[8] LOUTIT, J.F., LLOYD, E.L., Tumours and viruses in mice injected with plutonium, Nature (London) **266** (1977) 355.

[9] ERFLE, V., MARQUART, K.-H., "Expression of type C RNA virus particles in ^{224}Ra-induced osteosarcomas", Biological Effects of ^{224}Ra: Benefit and Risk of Therapeutic Application (MÜLLER, W.A., EBERT, H.G., Eds), Martinus Nijhoff Medical Division, The Hague/Boston (1978) 158.

[10] FRAZIER, M.E., PARK, J.F., JEE, W.S.S., TAYLOR, G., "RNA-instructed DNA polymerase activity in radiation-induced osteosarcomas", The Health Effects of Plutonium and Radium (JEE, W.S.S., Ed.), The J.W. Press, Salt Lake City (1976) 707.

[11] REILLY, C.A., FINKEL, M.P., Evidence of FBJ virus antigen in ^{90}Sr-induced osteosarcomas, Radiat. Res. **47** (1971) 252.

[12] ERFLE, V.F., LUZ, A., ADLER, I.-D., MARQUART, K.-H., Attempts to recognize an oncogenic virus in ^{224}Ra-induced murine osteosarcoma, Radiat. Res. **59** (1974) 90.

[13] LUZ, A., MÜLLER, W.A., GÖSSNER, W., HUG, O., "The dependence of late effects in mice on the temporal distribution of skeletal α-doses from ^{224}Ra and ^{227}Th", Biological Effects of ^{224}Ra: Benefit and Risk of Therapeutic Application (MÜLLER, W.A., EBERT, H.G., Eds), Martinus Nijhoff Medical Division, The Hague/ Boston (1978) 135.

[14] MÜLLER, W.A., Studies on short-lived internal α-emitters in mice and rats, Part I: ^{224}Ra, Int. J. Radiat. Biol. **20** (1971) 27.

[15] SCHLOM, J., SPIEGELMAN, S., Simultaneous detection of reverse transcriptase and high molecular weight RNA unique to oncogenic RNA viruses, Science **174** (1971) 840.

[16] HEHLMANN, R., GOLDFEDER, A., SPIEGELMAN, S., RNA tumour viruses present in growing and absent in regressing mammary tumors of mice, J. Natl. Cancer Inst. **52** (1974) 49.

[17] HAAS, M., Transient virus expression during murine leukemia induction by X-irradiation, J. Natl. Cancer Inst. **58** (1977) 251.

[18] KAWASHIMA, K., IKEDA, H., HARTLEY, J.W., STOCKERT, E., ROWE, W.P.,
     OLD, L.J., Changes in expression of murine leukemia virus antigens and production of
     xenotropic virus in the late preleukemic period in AKR mice, Proc. Natl. Acad. Sci.
     U.S.A. **73** (1976) 4680.
[19] NOWINSKI, R.C., DOYLE, T., Cellular changes in the thymuses of preleukemic
     AKR mice: correlation with changes in the expression of murine leukemia viruses,
     Cell **12** (1977) 341.
[20] NEXØ, B.A., ULRICH, K., C-type virus activation during chemically induced leukemo-
     genesis in mice, Cancer Res., in press.

DISCUSSION

V. COVELLI (*Chairman*): Did you observe any biochemical differences
between your virus and the FBJ virus?

V. ERFLE: Serological investigations have shown that our virus is a
complex of an N-tropic and a xenotropic virus, whereas the FBJ virus is a
complex of an N-tropic, a B-tropic and a xenotropic virus. However, in their
biochemical properties, such as density, size of the RNA and composition of
proteins, the two viruses are identical.

J.R. MAISIN: Were the viruses or the cells cultivated in vitro able to
induce osteosarcomas in vivo in mice and, if so, what was the latency period?

V. ERFLE: The viruses did not induce osteosarcomas. Some osteomas
developed in treated animals but the statistics were not good enough to decide
whether they were really induced. The injection of $1 \times 10^6 - 5 \times 10^6$ in-vitro
cultured osteosarcoma cells induced sarcomas in new-born mice. The tumours
appeared after $7 - 10$ days with im inoculation and after 15 days with sc
inoculation.

C. STREFFER: As you certainly know, it is still a problem to demonstrate
viruses in human cancers. Have you tried to find viruses in biopsies from human
osteosarcomas, especially those which may have been radiation induced?

V. ERFLE: We have no data of our own but other groups have found
RNA specific to RNA tumour virus in spontaneous human osteosarcomas. To
my knowledge, there are no data on viruses in radiation-induced human
osteosarcomas.

ROLE OF VASCULAR DAMAGE IN THE DEVELOPMENT OF LATE RADIATION EFFECTS IN THE SKIN

J.W. HOPEWELL, J.L. FOSTER, Y. GUNN,
H.F. MOUSTAFA, T.J.S. PATTERSON,
G. WIERNIK, C.M.A. YOUNG
Churchill Hospital Research Institute,
University of Oxford,
Oxford,
United Kingdom

Abstract

ROLE OF VASCULAR DAMAGE IN THE DEVELOPMENT OF LATE RADIATION EFFECTS IN THE SKIN.

Stages in the development of late radiation atrophy have been investigated in pig skin using a number of complementary assay techniques. Evidence for vascular damage was provided 10–16 weeks after irradiation by observed changes in skin colour, a fall in skin temperature and by a dose-dependent reduction in dermal blood flow. The reduction in blood flow was transient and preceded the development of tissue atrophy; blood flow returns to normal as atrophy develops. The reduction in blood flow 12 weeks after irradiation correlated well with the degree of late damage at 6–12 months. Direct histological evidence of vascular damage in the dermis, in the form of vessels occluded by endothelial cells, coincided with the timing of the blood flow changes. Studies using fractionated radiation exposures indicated that the sensitivity of the rapidly proliferating epidermis was enhanced relative to vascular damage when the number of dose fractions was increased. These studies also showed a lack of correlation between epithelial desquamation and late damage. Many of the vascular changes observed in the dermis of the pig have also been reported in a number of other normal tissues, suggesting that it is a good model in which to investigate late effects in vascular connective tissue.

INTRODUCTION

If late radiation damage to normal tissues is to be treated or avoided, more information is required about the development of this late damage. This may lead to the development of early indicators of severe late effects. One important hypothesis to be investigated is that late damage to normal tissues is mediated through effects on the vascular system [1, 2], damage to the parenchyma being secondary to this. Alternatively late damage may develop directly in the parenchyma, the long latent period between irradiation and the expression of late damage being due to the slow turnover of the specific cell types involved in different tissues.

TABLE I.   SKIN REACTIONS AND ASSOCIATED NUMERICAL VALUES

Erythema	Pigmentation	Desquamation
Minimal ~ 1	Minimal ~ 1	Dry ~ 3
Moderate ~ 2	Light brown ~ 2	Moist $< \frac{1}{2}$ field ~ 4
Dry red ~ 3	Dark brown ~ 3	Moist $> \frac{1}{2}$ field ~ 4

		Dermal necrosis
Mauve reaction ~ 2.75		$< \frac{1}{2}$ field ~ 5.5
Dusky reaction ~ 3.5		$> \frac{1}{2}$ field ~ 6.5

The microvasculature of the dermis of the pig, which has many similarities with human skin [3], has proved to be a useful model in which to investigate vascular changes. The accessibility of the skin enables the use of a number of complementary assay methods, and the anatomical juxtaposition of the epithelium on a vascular stroma, a characteristic of a number of normal tissues, enables the separate evaluation of radiation effects on both rapid and slowly proliferating tissues.

MATERIALS AND METHODS

The flank skin of female, Large White pigs was used in all these investigations. Animals were admitted to the Institute at 16 weeks old (20 kg) and were allowed an acclimatization period of two weeks. After this time up to three 16 X 4 cm fields were tattooed on one flank and irradiated with either single or fractionated doses of 250 kV X-rays [4]. Comparable fields marked on the opposite flank acted as controls. Between 3 and 30 dose fractions were used, given either as 1, 2, 3 or 5 fractions per week. All experimental procedures were carried out under halothane/nitrous-oxide anaesthesia [4].

At regular time intervals after irradiation direct or indirect estimates of damage to the vascular system of the dermis was made using three test systems:

1. Direct visual observations (skin scoring)

For the first 16 weeks after irradiation (from mid-treatment with extended fractionation regimes), changes in the appearance of the irradiated skin were recorded weekly by up to six observers. Changes in the degree of erythema, pigmentation, desquamation and dermal necrosis were assessed separately. Numerical scores were attached according to the severity of the reaction (Table I), and numerical scores averaged over weekly time periods.

2. Skin temperature changes (thermography)

Estimates of local modifications in skin temperature, relative to adjacent areas of normal skin, were assessed using an Aga thermo-vision unit.

3. Dermal blood flow

Dermal blood flow measurements in the dermis were made using an isotope clearance technique [5]. Simultaneous measurements of clearance from irradiated and normal skin were made after the intradermal injection of 0.03 ml of technetium-99m as the pertechnetate ion.

The degree of late tissue damage to the skin was determined by measuring the length of previously delimited irradiated fields, and comparing these with comparable control fields on the other flank. The comparison 'relative linear field contraction' is a measure of late tissue atrophy [2]. Histological sections of skin were examined at selected time periods after irradiation for evidence of vascular lesions.

RESULTS AND DISCUSSION

Evaluation of skin scoring data, for areas of skin irradiated with 3 fractions/ 6 days, for example, demonstrated that two distinct waves of erythema are observed in skin in the first four months after irradiation (Fig.1). In the first wave a maximum bright red erythema can be reached after 4–6 weeks; this may be associated with dry or moist desquamation of the epidermis. The epidermal reaction heals quickly if the minimum dose required to produce this effect is not greatly exceeded. For the second wave the maximum reaction is exemplified by dusky or mauve reactions in the skin which are characteristic of ischemia. Necrosis of the dermis, which is slow to heal even in the absence of infection, results if the tolerance dose is exceeded.

Visible skin changes suggestive of ischemia were supported by the results of the thermographic and skin blood flow studies. Skin temperatures were reduced over the period 10–16 weeks, and in the case of fields irradiated with 3F/6 days the maximum reduction in skin temperature appeared to be dose-dependent. A fall in temperature of > 1 degC preceded the rapid onset of dermal necrosis.

Changes in skin temperature are often interpreted as a modification in dermal blood flow. The results of our studies, using the clearance of $^{99}\text{Tc}^{m}$ from the dermis, support this suggestion (Fig.2). For single doses of X-rays a decrease in the clearance time was first noted three weeks after irradiation; this coincides with the first wave of erythema. After 12 weeks clearance times were increased, indicating a dose-dependent reduction in blood flow, a finding that correlates well with the reduction in temperature and appearance of the skin at

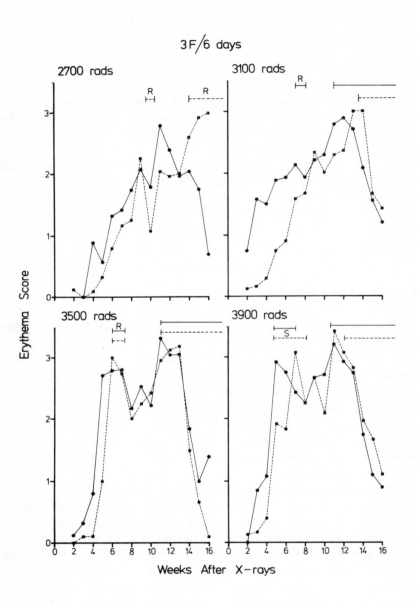

FIG.1.   Time-related changes in the intensity of the erythema reaction in individual skin fields
irradiated with varying total doses given as 3 fractions/6 days. The associated dry (⊢—R—⊣) or
moist desquamation (⊢—S—⊣) and dermal necrosis (⊢——⊣) are indicated.

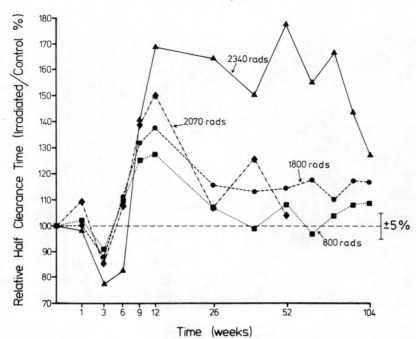

FIG.2. Time-related changes in the relative clearance of the tracer ($^{99}Tc^m$) from the dermis in areas of skin treated with single doses of X-rays. A reduction in blood flow 12 weeks after irradiation resulted in an increase in the half clearance rate and a relative clearance index of > 100%.

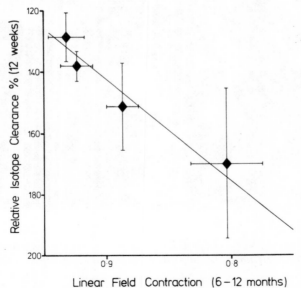

FIG.3. Correlation between the dose-dependent reduction in dermal blood flow 12 weeks after exposure to single doses of X-rays and late linear skin field contraction (correlation co-efficient, 0.94).

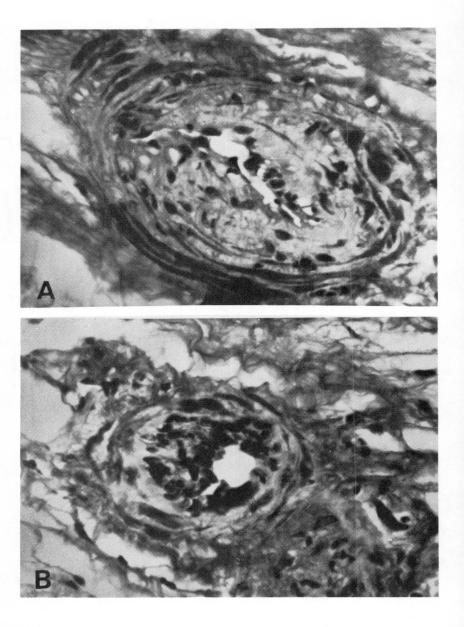

FIG.4. *Vessels in the deep dermal plexus of pig skin 11 weeks after exposure to 3500 rads
(3F/6 days). Vessels are totally (A) or partly occluded (B) by endothelial cells (Mallory × 640).*

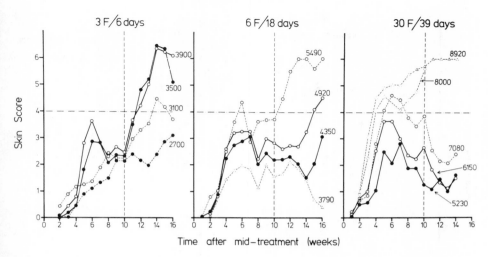

*FIG.5.   Time-related changes in the average numerical scores representing the most severe
biological reactions in areas of skin irradiated with 3, 6 or 30 fractions (○—○ = minimum dose
required to produce moist desquamation; ●—● = minimum dose required to produce dry
desquamation).*

this time. The reduction in blood flow is transient, flow returning to normal as
late tissue contraction develops. The suggestion that this reduction in blood flow
results in late tissue atrophy is supported by the excellent correlation between
reduced blood flow at 12 weeks and the degree of linear field contraction at
6–12 months (Fig.3). Linear field contraction is constant over the period
6–12 months after irradiation [2].

Evidence of a transient reduction in blood flow before the appearance of
late damage has been reported in other normal tissues including the lung [6, 7],
bone marrow [8] and the hamster cheek pouch [2].

Examination of histological sections of pig skin 10–12 weeks after irradiation
has provided direct evidence of vascular lesions. These were exemplified by the
total occlusion or partial occlusion of arterioles by endothelial cells (Fig.4). Most
of these lesions were found in the vessels of the deep dermal plexus, although
occluded vessels were found at all levels in the dermis and the underlying fat.
Similar occlusions have been reported in the vessels of the irradiated brain [9],
heart [10] and kidney [2].

Changes in dose fractionation schedules employed were found to alter the
relative importance of the first wave epithelial reaction compared with the later
vascular reaction in the dermis. A comparison of the time-related changes in the
scores for the maximum reactions observed for radiation exposures given in
3, 6 or 30 fractions illustrates this phenomenon (Fig.5). A comparison of the
minimum doses required to produce moist desquamation of the epithelium shows

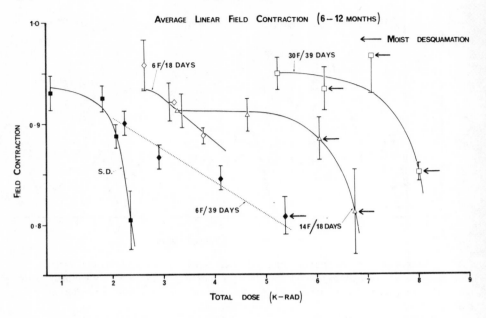

FIG.6.   Changes in relative linear field contraction (6–12 months) against total dose for
radiation given in a range of fractionation regimes.   There was no correlation between the
severity of late damage and the initial appearance of moist desquamation of the epidermis
(← irradiation doses producing an initial transient moist desquamation).

very dissimilar reactions in the vascular system of the dermis after 10–16 weeks.
For 3 fractions (3900 rads) a full thickness dermal necrosis results, for 6 fractions
(4920 rads) this was less marked, and for 30 fractions (6150 rads) no appreciable
second wave reaction was observed.   The change in relative radiosensitivity between
the epidermis and vascular dermis, presumably as a result of an increase in the
sensitivity of the epidermis, means that there is no correlation between the
severity of the first wave reaction and late damage (Fig.6).   This finding is in
disagreement with results obtained using rodents [11] where the severity of the
desquamation reaction of the epidermis did correlate with tissue deformity.   The
usual anatomical site chosen for these investigations, the hind foot, plus the high
cauterizing doses of radiation used in these studies may explain this finding.

The effects of radiation on pig skin reported here emphasize the differences
in response between the epidermis and the dermis, the relative importance of which
depends upon the radiation fractionation schedule used.   Only the radiation
response of the dermis as exemplified by the reduction in blood flow correlates
well with the late effects attested by linear field contraction.   For these reasons
pig skin is judged to provide a good model for investigating the problems pertaining
to late radiation effects in man.

REFERENCES

[1] RUBIN, P., CASARETT, G.W., Cancer 22 (1968) 767.
[2] HOPEWELL, J.W., YOUNG, C.M.A., Int. J. Radiat. Oncol. Biol. Phys. 2 Suppl. 3 (1977) 53.
[3] DONOVAN, W.E., Skin Flaps (GRABB, W.C., MYERS, M.D., Eds), Little, Brown & Co., Boston (1975) 11.
[4] BERRY, R.J., WIERNIK, G., PATTERSON, T.J.S., Br. J. Radiol. 47 (1974) 185.
[5] MOUSTAFA, H.F., HOPEWELL, J.W., Microvasc. Res. 11 (1976) 147.
[6] GLATSTEIN, E., Radiat. Res. 53 (1973) 88.
[7] MOUSTAFA, H.F., HOPEWELL, J.W., "Measurement of lung function in the pig after local X-irradiation", Radiobiological Research and Radiotherapy (Proc. Symp. Vienna, 1976) I, IAEA, Vienna (1977) 75.
[8] NIELSON, D.F., CHAFFEY, J.T., HELLMAN, S., Int. J. Radiat. Oncol. Biol. Phys. 2 (1977) 39.
[9] HOPEWELL, J.W., Br. J. Radiol. 47 (1974) 157.
[10] FAJAROO, L.F., STEWARD, J.R., Radiology 101 (1971) 429.
[11] FIELD, S.B., Radiology 92 (1969) 381.

DISCUSSION

R.A. CONARD: I should like to comment on the skin burns in 84 Marshallese people more heavily exposed to fall-out. Many of the people no doubt received thousands of rads to areas of the skin. Numerous acute lesions, so called 'beta burns', and epilation developed. However, the burns were superficial and in most cases healed in several weeks, with residual scar formation in about 15 people. Biopsies indicated only minimal persisting histological changes. No second-wave reactions, like those you have described, were noted in any of the victims, and it is noteworthy that no chronic radiation dermatitis or cancer of the skin has been found in the 23 years we have been observing these people. Perhaps the latent period for development of skin cancers is longer than for other radiation-induced malignancies.

J.L. FOSTER: Don't you think that the lack of manifestations is due to the low energy of the radiation which the Marshallese were exposed, which was not strong enough to damage the blood vessels in the dermis and thus trigger a second wave?

R.A. CONARD: Yes, the radiation was largely from low-energy beta rays with only slight penetration into the dermis. The minimal blood vessel changes we observed are no doubt related to the absence of late skin findings in the Marshallese.

Y. NISHIWAKI: I think that observations similar to those made by Mr. Conard on the radiodermatitis suffered by the Marshallese were also made in the case of some of the Japanese fishermen who were exposed to radioactive fall-out in the Bikini area in March 1954. The strongly radioactive fall-out (Bikini ash) consisted of tiny white or greyish-white particles about 0.1 − 0.3 mm (10−500 μm) in diameter. The main chemical component of the ash was calcium hydroxide derived from coral evaporated by the high temperature of the thermonuclear explosion and then condensed in particulate forms. In addition to the ordinary fission products, the neutron-induced activity ^{45}Ca, ^{237}U and some other transuranium radionuclides were detected. We measured the beta-ray energy by the ordinary absorption method, and also conducted beta spectrum analysis using a beta-ray spectrometer of the double-coil magnetic-lens type with the spectrochamber equipped with an aluminium baffle system to reduce scattered electrons. The results of these measurements showed that, although some hard components were included, the soft beta-ray components appeared to be predominant at the time we first measured the sample.

J.L. FOSTER: This confirms my opinion that the absence of a second-wave skin reaction is due to the soft beta rays being unable to reach the blood vessels in the dermis.

F.J. BURNS: Would you care to speculate on the cellular basis for the late vascular damage that you have observed in pig skin? Do the endothelial cells undergo lethal damage or in fact is there a proliferative reaction that occludes the lumen?

J.L. FOSTER: The occlusion of the blood vessel lumen is thought to be due to overcompensation by proliferating surviving endothelial cells. This overcompensation is seen in other tissues after irradiation. Occlusion by fibrin deposition is also observed. It has not been established to my knowledge whether or not this thrombus formation is independent of occlusion by proliferation of the endothelial cells.

COMPARISON OF CYTOGENETIC EFFECTS
AFTER OCCUPATIONAL EXPOSURE
TO X-RAYS WITH THOSE AFTER
FOETAL PELVIMETRIC EXPOSURE

M. KIRSCH-VOLDERS, K. POMA,
L. VERSCHAEVE, L. HENS
Laboratory of Human Genetics,
Free University of Brussels

P. VAN ELEGEM
Laboratory for Health Physics,
Free University of Brussels

C. SUSANNE
Laboratory of Human Genetics,
Free University of Brussels,
Brussels,
Belgium

Abstract

COMPARISON OF CYTOGENETIC EFFECTS AFTER OCCUPATIONAL EXPOSURE TO
X-RAYS WITH THOSE AFTER FOETAL PELVIMETRIC EXPOSURE.

In utero acute low-level exposure to X-rays (300 to 350 mrads) induces a significant
increase of band-loss in G-trypsin banded chromosomes of umbilical lymphocytes. Results,
however, have to be confirmed by dose-effect relation studies and analysis with spectro-
photometric scanning of deleted chromosomes. The same in utero exposure induces a significant
dissociation of chromosome pair 13 as revealed by centromere-centromere, angle and association
tendency analysis of chromosome distribution in comparison with a control group. Occupational
chronic low-level exposure to ionizing radiation does not modify significantly the amount of
SCE in lymphocytes of peripheral blood. However, an analysis of centromere-centromere
distances, angle values and association tendencies of the different chromosome combinations
clearly shows an association of chromosome pair 12–16 after exposure to ionizing radiation.
It is difficult to assess the exact biological importance of the observed chromosome modifications.
However, referring to the already described dissociation of human acrocentric chromosomes
after in vivo exposure to low levels of phenyl Hg acetate or inorganic Pb, the chromosome
distribution seems not to be significantly disturbed by chronic or acute low-level exposure to
ionizing radiation.

INTRODUCTION

The major problem in assessing genetic risks related to low-level radiation in humans is the insufficient sensibility of classical cytogenetic techniques.

New cytogenetic techniques might be useful: SCE counting [1] is indeed relatively sensitive but perhaps not adequate for in vivo exposure in humans, and the most sensitive for chemical mutagens [2]; studies on disappearance of chromosome bands is time consuming since they require a very large sample.

Our results with in vivo exposure in humans to chemical mutagens (phenyl-Hg acetate, anorganic Pb, depo-medroxyprogesterone acetate) showed that the chromosome distribution — and more specifically the association-pattern of human acrocentric chromosomes — is significantly modified after exposure to doses so low that they did not induce significant increase in chromosome aberrations [3]. The analyses of chromosome distribution might also be interesting for ionizing radiations since they seem to interact with the spindle apparatus [4].

To compare the three techniques (SCE, band-loss, chromosome distribution), we selected two different test populations exposed to low-level ionizing radiation; the first a population of new-born exposed in utero to acute low-level irradiation by pelvimetry, and the second a population of women exposed to chronic low-level irradiation at work.

MATERIAL AND METHODS

Material

In utero acute exposure to X-rays

Umbilical cord blood was obtained at birth from babies exposed in utero to pelvimetric irradiation either the same day or two or three days earlier.

The calculated exposure dose was about 300 to 350 mrads.

Umbilical blood for controls was obtained from babies who were not exposed in utero to medical irradiation.

Chronic occupational exposure to ionizing radiations

Blood samples were taken from nurses exposed in radiotherapic and radio-diagnostic units of the University Hospital at the Free University of Brussels. Exposure level to radioactive isotopes or to X-rays was calculated for the last 10 years according to dose meters they are obliged to wear at work.

Individuals with significant medical exposures were not analysed (Table I). Blood samples from the controls were obtained from a blood transfusion depot.

TABLE IA. DATA ON CONTROL WOMEN

Individuals	Age (years)	Amount of metaphases for SCE	SCE per metaphase	Extremes of SCE	Amount of metaphases for chromosome distribution
ABC_{33}	20	20	4.33	2—6	—
ABC_{34}	20	25	4.95	2—9	—
ABC_{68}	20	25	5.09	1—8	—
ABC_{71}	19	25	4.72	2—8	—
ABC_{95}	21	20	5.26	2—8	—
ABC_{97}	49	25	4.92	2—9	—
ABC_{101}	20	20	5.95	1—8	—
ABC_{120}	20	25	5.76	1—9	—
ABC_{202}	21	21	5.80	2—9	—
ABC_{208}	19	20	4.86	2—9	—
C_1	51	—	—	—	10
C_2	39	—	—	—	10
C_3	45.5	—	—	—	10
C_4	39.5	—	—	—	10
C_5	39.5	—	—	—	10
C_6	41.5	—	—	—	10
C_7	48.5	—	—	—	10
C_8	55	—	—	—	10
C_9	41.5	—	—	—	10
C_{10}	?	—	—	—	10

Methodology for chromosome distribution studies

Cytogenetic preparations

Within 24 hours after collection of the blood, peripheral lymphocytes were placed in culture for 48 hours and received identical colchicine, hypotonic and fixation treatment as described in detail previously [5].

A total of 91 metaphase plates were studied for the in utero exposed babies (6 ♂ and 2 ♀) as well as for the controls (5 ♂ and 3 ♀) (Table II).

TABLE IB. DATA ON OCCUPATIONALLY EXPOSED NURSES

Individuals	Age (years)	Amount of metaphases for SCE	SCE per metaphase	Extremes of SCE	Occupational dose during last 10 years (rad)	Amount of metaphases for chromosome distribution
AB_1	54	20	4.90	1–9	7.319	–
AB_2	58	19	6.15	3–10	11.661	3
AB_5	52	20	3.35	1–7	6.301	22
AB_6	53	20	7.70	4–13	12.528	–
AB_7	64	20	4.20	1–8	20.843	–
AB_8	53	20	5.15	3–11	6.426	24
AB_{10}	37	19	10.01	5–18	5.483	–
AB_{11}	51	25	8.56	5–14	7.136	–
AB_{12}	38	25	4.96	2–9	8.222	–
AB_{14}	56	–	–	–	4.800	23
AB_{15}	45	–	–	–	12.570	26

TABLE IIA. DATA ON CONTROL BABIES

Individual	Sex	Amount of metaphases for band-loss	Aneuploidy (%)	Amount of deletions /100 cells	Amount of metaphases for chromosome distribution
C_{14}	♀	25	12	28.0	12
C_{16}	♂	30	3.3	36.7	12
C_{19}	♂	24	0	16.7	12
C_{23}	♂	12	8.3	91.7	9
C_{29}	♀	15	0	33.3	12
C_{30}	♂	20	15.0	30.0	12
C_{36}	♂	15	0	0	–
C_{37}	♂	29	13.8	24.1	12
C_{39}	♀	15	13.3	26.7	10

TABLE IIB. DATA ON IN UTERO EXPOSED BABIES (300–350 mrad)

Individual	Sex	Amount of metaphases for band-loss	Aneuploidy (%)	Amount of deletions /100 cells	Amount of metaphases for chromosome distribution
S_3	♂	15	27.7	40.0	10
S_{10}	♂	4	25.0	50.0	–
S_{14}	♂	18	5.5	38.9	12
S_{16}	♂	30	10.0	30.0	12
S_{17}	♀	23	0	34.8	12
S_{18}	♂	19	5.3	52.6	12
S_{19}	♀	10	10.0	30.0	9
S_{22}	♂	19	0	42.1	12
S_{24}	♂	30	6.6	80.0	12

A total of 98 metaphase plates were studied for the occupationally exposed nurses (1 with 3 metaphases, 1 with 22 metaphases, 1 with 23 metaphases, 1 with 24 metaphases and 1 with 26 metaphases) and 100 metaphases for the controls (10 ♀ with 10 metaphases each).

Their ages ranged between 45 and 58 years (mean age: 52.8 years) for the exposed group and between 39 and 48.5 years for the controls (mean age: 44.5 years).

The individual pairs of chromosomes were identified after trypsin banding following the method of Klinger [6]. Only cells with a modal chromosome count were investigated (46 centromeres).

The mathematical aspect

A circular transformation according to Barton and co-workers [7] was performed on the co-ordinates of the 46 centromeres in order to obtain the 'generalized square distance Δ^2' (between the centromeres of two chromosomes), the 'generalized square distance d^2' (between the centromere of a chromosome and the centre of gravity of the metaphase) and the generalized angle value (angle between 2 centromeres and the gravity centre of the mitose plate). These values are dimensionless and independent of the form and the dimension of the metaphase plate. This procedure corrects the form and the width of dispersion of the centromeres in an 'ideal circular image'. Δ^2, d^2, as well as the mean angle distances for all chromosome combinations or pairs were calculated using a CDC 6400 computer (ULB-VUB mathematical centre). Mathematical details can be found in previous published papers [5,8].

In each mitosis 'generalized distances' were thus calculated between the 46 chromosomes taken in all possible combinations of pairs. For 100 metaphases, we thus obtained 103 500 values of Δ^2. These 103 500 Δ^2 values were transformed into percentage frequencies and arranged in histogram classes of equal intervals. The histogram gives a reference distribution since it represents the distribution of all possible Δ^2 values in the 100 metaphases. In an analogous way, frequency histograms were established separately for each homologous and non-homologous chromosome pair and for each possible group of four chromosomes containing two pairs of chromosomes. These histograms will be compared with the reference distribution. In order to obtain independence between the population of numbers present in the reference distribution and that of the particular histogram under study, the absolute class frequencies of the reference distribution are diminished with the absolute class frequencies of the particular histogram.

A similar methodology was used for establishing the d^2 and angle reference histograms, and histograms for d^2 or angle values of all particular chromosomes.

A χ^2 test allows us to decide in both the controls and the exposed group if the two histograms compared belong to the same population of numbers. We thus are able to decide whether the particular chromosomes or chromosome combinations do not differ from the reference distribution, or are situated more centrally or peripherally in the metaphase plate in comparison with the reference distribution. A new χ^2 test compares the position of the chromosomes of the exposed group with the corresponding chromosomes in the control group. Also we were able to decide whether two chromosomes are closer together than would be expected from the reference distribution, or, on the contrary, are more distant from each other than expected.

In order to obtain some supplementary data we attempted to study the 'tendency to be associated' as defined by Galperin [9]. Here χ^2 tests were performed considering only two classes; the first including the absolute values corresponding to the first column of the previously described histograms containing the lowest Δ^2 values, the second class containing the remainder of the absolute values. Again both cell populations (exposed and controls) were compared.

Cumulative frequencies

The cumulative frequencies of Δ^2 distances were studied for both exposed population in comparison with the corresponding control population for the following groups of chromosomes: within acrocentrics, between acrocentrics, within homologous non-acrocentrics and between homologous non-acrocentrics.

Methodology for SCE exchanges in exposed women

With the simplified technique described by Korenberg and co-workers [10], peripheral lymphocytes of 10 exposed nurses and 10 control women (Table I)

TABLE III. SIGNIFICANTLY VARYING Δ^2 DIFFERENCES BETWEEN THE IN UTERO EXPOSED GROUP AND THE CONTROLS

Chromosome pair	Δ^2 controls	Δ^2 exposed	χ^2 comparison	Degree of freedom	Probability
1– 9	4.086	3.674	20.730	10	$0.025 > P > 0.01$
2– 8	4.709	4.708	19.823	10	$0.05 > P > 0.025$
3–23	4.570	4.184	26.554	10	$P < 0.005$
4– 5	4.568	4.815	21.189	10	$0.025 > P > 0.01$
4–13	4.479	4.543	18.906	10	$0.05 > P > 0.025$
5–13	4.160	4.825	19.675	10	$0.05 > P > 0.025$
6– 7	4.519	4.012	21.185	10	$0.025 > P > 0.01$
6–19	4.077	3.515	22.866	10	$0.025 > P > 0.01$
6–21	3.896	3.884	22.724	10	$0.025 > P > 0.01$
6–23	4.618	3.938	20.960	10	$0.025 > P > 0.01$
10–21	3.665	4.044	23.905	10	$0.01 > P > 0.005$
13–13	3.397	4.692	13.047	6	$0.05 > P > 0.025$
15–16	3.712	3.320	25.998	10	$P < 0.005$
17–19	3.299	3.384	19.728	10	$0.05 > P > 0.025$
21–23	4.166	4.223	20.941	10	$0.025 > P > 0.01$

were placed for 72 hours in culture with $F_{12} Th^-$ medium supplemented with BrDu 5×10^{-5} M. After fixation, and spreading, metaphases were treated for 12 min with M NaH_2PO_2 (pH = 12), coloured with Giemsa and counted for SCE under a Zeiss III photomicroscope.

Methodology for band-loss in in utero exposed babies

Metaphases were obtained after a 48 hours culture period, and trypsin banded as described for chromosome distribution analysis.

A total of 185 metaphases from the control groups and of 168 metaphases from the exposed group were photographed, karyotyped and studied for aneuploidy and band-loss.

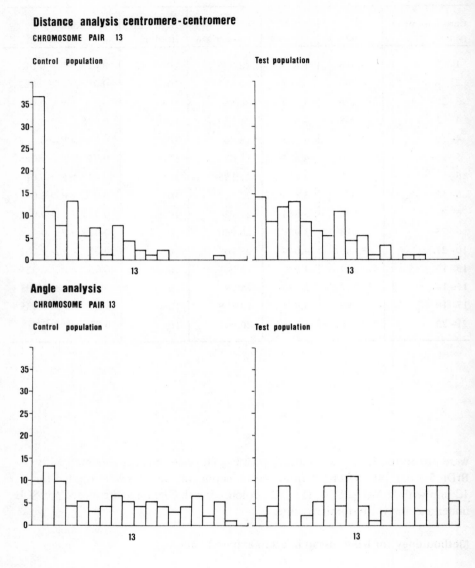

FIG.1.   Histograms of centromere-centromere analysis and angle analysis for chromosome combination 13-13.

RESULTS

In utero X-ray exposure of foetuses during pelvimetry

Analysis of aneuploidy and band-loss

Aneuploidy was of a similar level in both populations: 7.56% in the control babies and 7.73% in the exposed babies. The partial losss of G-bands, however, increased significantly ($0.05 > P > 0.025$) after irradiation: 29.72 deletions/100 cells in the controls and 45.83 deletions/100 cells in the exposed babies.

Analysis of chromosome distribution

Comparison of d^2 volumes (centromere-centre distances) between the control population and the exposed population does not show any statistically significant difference.

χ^2 tests, performed similarly on the Δ^2 values for the different chromosome combinations, point out 15 significant differences: one for the homologous chromosome combination 13-13 and 14 non-homologous chromosome combinations (Table III). The χ^2 tests, performed on angle values between the control group and the exposed group for the different chromosome combinations, confirm a statistically significant value only for the chromosome combination 13-13. Moreover, the association tendencies of combinations with significantly different Δ^2 values show a marked dissociation of chromosome combinations 13-13 ($P < 0.005$), 10-21 ($0.01 > P > 0.005$), but an association of chromosome combinations 6-19 ($P < 0.005$), 15-16 ($P < 0.0005$) after in utero exposure to X-rays.

Figure 1 illustrates that by Δ^2 analysis and by angle analysis, chromosome pair 13 clearly dissociates after exposure to X-rays.

X-ray occupationally exposed nurses

Analysis of SCE (sister chromatid exchanges)

Table I presents for the control population and for the exposed population, the age, the amount of metaphases analysed for SCE, the average SCE found per metaphase for the individual, the extreme SCE values, and the occupational dose. A Student test shows no significant difference between the average SCE in the control group ($\bar{x} = 5.164$; $s = 0.498260$) and in the exposed group ($\bar{x} = 6.10888$; $s = 4.301787$).

TABLE IV. SIGNIFICANTLY VARYING Δ^2 DIFFERENCES BETWEEN THE
OCCUPATIONALLY EXPOSED GROUP AND THE CONTROLS

Chromosome combination	Δ^2 control	Δ^2 exposed	χ^2 comparison	Degree of freedom	Probability
1−13	3.631507	3.990547	21.1157372	10	0.025 > P > 0.01
1−15	3.256694	3.149044	24.3695258	10	0.01 > P > 0.005
2−15	3.641409	3.709542	18.8555821	10	0.05 > P > 0.025
2−22	3.481801	3.841635	23.8904897	10	0.01 > P > 0.005
4−21	3.900201	3.801446	28.3709770	10	P < 0.005
6−13	4.466477	4.383697	24.8139329	10	0.01 > P > 0.005
7−14	3.927380	4.094122	18.9242531	10	0.05 > P > 0.025
7−18	5.037219	4.593777	18.5329903	10	0.05 > P > 0.025
9−16	4.364811	3.691297	20.3635117	10	0.05 > P > 0.025
9−20	4.393235	4.128925	18.5621689	10	0.05 > P > 0.025
12−16	4.788397	3.973736	34.7947840	10	P < 0.005
12−20	4.012381	4.314254	18.8087176	10	0.05 > P > 0.025
12−22	3.867691	3.854531	19.6814815	10	0.05 > P > 0.025
16−18	4.894908	3.965198	20.6847497	10	0.025 > P > 0.01
16−21	4.265129	3.874687	19.8655562	10	0.05 > P > 0.025
20−X	4.117863	3.802508	19.6270707	10	0.05 > P > 0.025

Analysis of chromosome distribution

No statistically significant differences are found between the d^2 values of
the control group and the d^2 values of the exposed group.

χ^2 tests, performed similarly on the Δ^2 values for the different chromosome
combinations, show 16 significant differences (Table IV).

Testing for association tendency the combinations with significantly
different Δ^2 values show only a significant association of chromosome combinations 9-16 (P < 0.005) and 12-16 (0.05 > P > 0.025) by exposure to X-rays.
χ^2 tests performed on the angle values between the control group and the
exposed group confirm the significant association of chromosome combination
12-16 (0.05 > P > 0.025) only.

DISCUSSION

BrDu-vizualized SCE exchanges can theoretically be used as a parameter for mutagenesis only if the mutagen studied is present during a replication cycle with BrDu. The observed mutagen-induced SCE increase is considered to be related to a parallel increase of repair [2].

However, in vivo exposure to mutagens in man excludes the possibility of the presence of BrDu in blood during exposure. Nevertheless, we thought that since SCE are repair-related, a chronic exposure to X-rays may modify some repair mechanisms resulting in a modification of SCE in cultures of peripheral blood.

Although a greater variation of SCE values was observed in the occupationally exposed group in comparison with the control group, no significant difference was found between the populations. We therefore cannot decide whether the exposure was too low or the technique inadequate.

Counting of band- loss after G-banding with trypsin seems more promising. We observed, indeed, a significant increase of partial band-loss after in utero exposure to X-rays. However, more studies are needed with photometric scanning of banding patterns in deleted chromosomes to look for dose-effect relationships.

With reference to our experience with low-level exposure to chemical mutagens, we thought that chromosome distribution analysis would be very sensitive also for exposure to ionizing radiation which might interact with the spindle. To analyse our results, we first have to make the assumption that, using a 5% significancy level in our calculations, we may logically expect to find upon the 276 performed χ^2 on Δ^2 values and upon the 23 performed χ^2 on d^2 values respectively, 14 and 1 significant values appearing not really meaningful. In the in utero exposed group we found 14 Δ^2 and no d^2 chromosome combinations significantly different from the control group; in the occupationally exposed group, we found 16 Δ^2 and no d^2 chromosome combination significantly different from the control group. We therefore will consider as biological meaningful only those chromosome combinations from which the different distribution is confirmed by angle analysis and association tendency analysis; this means a dissocation of chromosome pair 13-13 after in utero acute exposure to X-rays and an association of chromosome pair 12-16 after chronic occupational exposure to mutagens.

It seems difficult, however, to estimate the biological importance of these results. A real modification of the chromosome distribution after exposure to mutagens would be associated with a disturbance of more chromosome combinations or of a specific chromosome group as seen after in vivo exposure to phenyl-Hg-acetate or anorganic-Pb but not found after exposure to ionizing radiations (Fig.2). The analysis of chromosome distribution will therefore probably

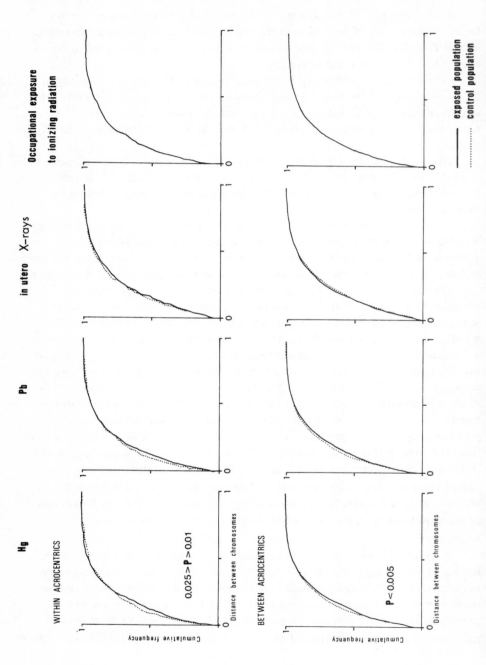

FIG. 2. A comparison of cumulative Δ^2 frequencies of acrocentric chromosomes in Hg, Pb, in utero X-rays and occupational ionizing

not be a good tool to measure low-level exposure to ionizing radiations: moreover, it seems unlikely that X-rays at low dose interact significantly with the spindle apparatus.

REFERENCES

[1]   LATT, S.A., Proc. Natl. Acad. Sci. U.S.A. 71 8 (1974) 3162.
[2]   EVANS, H.J., in Progress in Genetic Toxicology, Elsevier (1977) 57.
[3]   VERSCHAEVE, L., KIRSCH-VOLDERS, M., HENS, L., SUSANNE, C., Mutat. Res., in press.
[4]   ZAREMBA, T.G., IRWIN, R.D., Radiat. Res. 71 (1977) 300.
[5]   KIRSCH-VOLDERS, M., HENS, L., SUSANNE, C., GALPERIN-LEMAITRE, H., Cytogenet. Cell Genet. 18 (1977) 61.
[6]   KLINGER, H.P., Cytogenetics 11 (1972) 424.
[7]   BARTON, D., DAVID, F.N., MERRINGTON, M., Ann. Hum.Genet. 29 (1965) 139.
[8]   HENS, L., KIRSCH-VOLDERS, M., SUSANNE, C., GALPERIN-LEMAITRE, H., Humangenetik 28 (1975) 303.
[9]   GALPERIN-LEMAITRE, H., HENS, L., KIRSCH-VOLDERS, M., SUSANNE, C., Humangenetik 35 (1977) 261.
[10] KORENBERG, J.R., FREEDLENDER, E.F., Chromosoma 48 (1974) 355.

DISCUSSION

H. ALTMANN: Recently a paper showing direct correlation between sister chromatid exchanges and point-mutation after treatment with different mutagens was published in *Nature*. Is this direct correlation also true for X-rays?

M. KIRSCH-VOLDERS: To answer this question one would need to have more knowledge of the repair mechanisms after exposure to X-rays. Moreover, we were not looking for point mutation.

K.E. BUCKTON: Could you explain what you mean by a partial band-loss?

M. KIRSCH-VOLDERS: We compared each pair of homologous chromosomes in the karyotyped metaphases. A partial band-loss was scored when a clear difference in band length was observed. We intend to make more precise measurements of this band-loss by photometric scanning of banded chromosomes. At the moment, however, we do not regard this partial band-loss as a real deletion.

L.G. LITTLEFIELD: We have looked at SCE frequencies in human blood exposed in vitro to up to 300 R of cobalt-60 gamma radiation, and have seen no increase in SCEs. Our data thus agree with yours in that radiation exposure of human lymphocytes prior to culture does not increase SCEs.

M. KIRSCH-VOLDERS: This confirmation of our observations will probably signify that SCE-related repair at these doses is not modified by preceding radiation exposure.

SOMATIC CELL GENETICS OF URANIUM MINERS AND PLUTONIUM WORKERS
A biological dose-response indicator

W.F. BRANDOM
University of Denver,
Denver,
Colorado

A.D. BLOOM
College of Physicians and Surgeons,
Columbia University,
New York

P.G. ARCHER
University of Colorado Medical Center,
Denver,
Colorado

V.E. ARCHER
U.S. National Institute for Occupational
    Safety and Health,
Salt Lake City,
Utah

R.W. BISTLINE
Rockwell International,
Golden,
Colorado

G. SACCOMANNO
St. Mary's Hospital,
Grand Junction,
Colorado,
United States of America

Abstract

SOMATIC CELL GENETICS OF URANIUM MINERS AND PLUTONIUM WORKERS: A BIOLOGICAL DOSE-RESPONSE INDICATOR.
    Two populations of underground uranium miners and plutonium workers work in the state of Colorado, United States of America. We have explored the prevalence of structural chromosome aberrations in peripheral blood lymphocytes as a possible biological indicator of absorbed radiation late-effects in these populations. The uranium miners are divided into

four exposure groups expressed in Working Level Months (WLM), the plutonium workers
into six groups with estimated ^{239}Pu burdens expressed in nCi. Comparison of chromosome
aberration frequency data between controls, miners, and plutonium workers demonstrate:
(1) a cytogenetic response to occupational ionizing radiation at low estimated doses; and
(2) an increasing monotonic dose-response in the prevalence of complex (all exchange) or
total aberrations in all exposure groups in these populations. We also compared trends in
the prevalence of aberrations per exposure unit (WLM and nCi) in each exposure subgroup
for each population. In the uranium miners, the effects per WLM seem to decrease monotonically with increasing dose, whereas in the Pu workers the change per nCi appears abrupt,
with all exposure groups over 1.3 nCi (minimum detectable level) having essentially similar
rates. The calculations of aberrations per respective current maximum permissible dose
(120 WLM and 40 nCi) for the two populations yield $4.8 \times 10^{-2}/100$ cells for uranium
miners and $90.6 \times 10^{-2}/100$ cells for Pu workers. Factors which may have influenced this
apparent 20-fold increase in the effectiveness of plutonium in the production of complex
aberrations (9-fold increase in total aberrations) are discussed.

INTRODUCTION

    Uranium is a valuable resource for conventional nuclear power and
plutonium may figure prominently as a nuclear power source for fueling
breeder reactors in the future. The value, real or potential, of these
resources and their radiotoxicity provides challenges in radiation
protection. Retrospective epidemiological studies [1,2] provide the
primary justification for the establishment of permissible radon daughters
exposure, while permissible burdens of ^{239}Pu are based on the ^{226}Ra human
experience adjusted to reflect comparative experimental animal toxicity
findings for ^{226}Ra and ^{239}Pu [3]. Extensive animal studies have been done
on plutonium biomedical effects at high exposure levels [4-7], but little
is known about the biological effect of low doses of ionizing radiation
in humans, and no biological response related to estimated radiation doses
has been observed in non-pulmonary cells of uranium miners or in any cell
system of plutonium workers. Long-lived radon daughters are found in
uranium miner blood and vascular-rich organs, and internal plutonium is
translocated and concentrated in lymph nodes and hemapoietic tissues.
These considerations, as well as lymphocyte radiosensitivity, prompted us
to study the prevalence of structural chromosomal aberrations in the
lymphocytes of uranium miners and plutonium workers. Lymphocyte cytogenetics is a recommended method for the study of the biological effects of
radiation exposure [8], and limited populations of uranium miners [9,10]
and plutonium workers [11,12] have been studied cytogenetically, but with
mixed results. This report compares the cytogenetic data from our
present investigation of uranium miner and plutonium worker populations.

METHODS

Populations and Culture Methods

    One hundred controls and uranium miners were studied from out-patients
at St. Mary's Hospital, Grand Junction, CO., and from miners changing shifts
at mine sites in the region. Four hundred and eleven subjects from the
U.S. Department of Energy plutonium facility at Rocky Flats, Golden, CO.,
comprise the plutonium worker population. All subjects were screened by

questionnaire to elicit demographic, medical and work history data, and to
exclude those workers that showed any indications of exposure to
clastogenic agents. Microcultures were initiated with 0.3 ml whole blood
in 5 ml of Ham's F-10 medium supplemented with 15% Fetal Calf Serum
(Colorado Serum Co.), 1 000 Units/ml of pen-strep antibiotics (GIBCO) and
1% phytohaemagglutinin (PHA-M, Burroughs-Wellcome Co.). The uranium
miners' cells were cultured for 72 hr and the plutonium workers' cells
for 50 hr, the last 3 hr with 0.2 µg/ml of Colcemid (CIBA). Cells were
treated with 0.075M KCl, fixed in fresh 3:1 methanol:acetic, affixed to
cold wet slides and dried on a warming plate. The chromosomes were trypsin
G-banded using a modification of the method of Seabright [13] for karyotypic
analysis.

Cytogenetic Analyses

Approximately 100 cells were analyzed for each subject (mean = 98.5
for uranium miners and 97 for plutonium workers). Each cell was analyzed
for all structural chromosomal aberrations: symmetrical exchange
aberrations - pericentric inversions and translocations; asymmetrical
exchanges - dicentrics and rings; and, terminal and interstitial deletions.
The chromosome data are categorized for this report into: 1) complex
aberrations (dicentrics + rings + inversions + translocations); and 2) total
aberrations (complex aberrations + deletions).

Dosimetry and Analysis of the Data

The dosimetry is based on the Working Level Months (WLM) method for
the uranium miners and nCi estimated burdens for the plutonium workers.
One WLM is defined as any combination of radon and radon daughters in 1
litre of mine air which will result in the emission of 1.3×10^5 MeV of
alpha energy times 170 working hours. Systemic Pu burdens are estimated by
urine analyses [14] and lung burdens with NaI-CsI detectors, one each for
bilateral chest measurements.

The chromosomes preparation slides were decoded after cytogenetic
analysis of each of the workers and controls was completed and the subjects
assigned to estimated radiation exposure groups (TABLE I). The selection
of the exposure groups in the uranium miners was done to approximate some
of the epidemiological study groupings [1] consistent with sufficient
sample. The subgroups for the Pu workers are based on conventions used by
the Rocky Flats health physics personnel and the number of subjects in
each subgroup. Frequencies are compared using a chi-square test for two-
tailed alternate hypotheses or the chi-test (i.e. a normal approximation)
for one-tailed alternatives.

RESULTS

Dose-response in Uranium Workers and Plutonium Workers

The results for the prevalence of complex aberrations and total
aberrations are illustrated in Fig. 1. The increases in aberration
frequencies with increasing dose are monotonic and significant for both
complex and total aberrations (P<0.01).

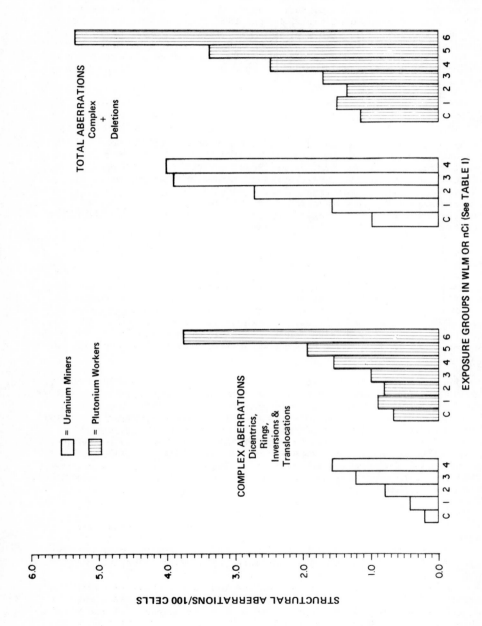

FIG.1.   Dose-response in the prevalence of complex and total aberrations in uranium miner and plutonium worker groups
(See Table I).

Comparison of Responses in the Two Populations by Dose Units and Maximum
Permissible Doses

We explored the relative frequency of aberrations per exposure unit
(either WLM or nCi) across exposure categories. The index, frequency
of aberrations/100 cells/exposure unit was calculated within each exposure
category with the results shown in Fig. 2. Since exposure units and
exposure groups were derived from quite different criteria, we also compared
the biological responses using the hypothetical working lifetime of
exposure at the current respective safety standards for two populations
(120 WLM and 40 nCi of Pu for maximum permissible systemic burden, MPSB).

The uranium miners had a total of 92 complex aberrations in the 7 926
cells examined. Adjusting for the control rate of 0.2%, about 16 of the
aberrations (0.002 x 7 926) may be attributed to factors other than
occupational radiation exposure. Dividing the remaining 76 aberrations by
the total of 189 455 WLM of estimated exposure in the miner population
yields a rate of about 4×10^{-4} complex aberrations per 100 cells per WLM
of exposure. If we use the current standard of 4 WLM/yr and assume a
working life of 30 years, we find a yield of:

$$4 \times 10^{-4} \text{ complex aberrations/100 cells/WLM} \times 4 \text{ WLM/yr} \times 30 \text{ yr} =$$
$$\underline{4.8 \times 10^{-2} \text{ aberrations/100 cells/current permissible lifetime dose.}}$$

Similar calculations for plutonium workers, after correcting for control
frequency and using the current MPSB for ^{239}Pu of 40 nCi, gives a yield
of complex aberrations for Pu workers of:

$$2.26 \times 10^{-2} \text{ aberrations/100 cells/nCi} \times 40 \text{ nCi} =$$
$$\underline{90.6 \times 10^{-2} \text{ aberrations/100 cells/MPSB.}}$$

The calculations for total aberrations yield approximately a 9-fold
increase in aberrations per maximum permissible burden in Pu workers
compared to uranium miners.

DISCUSSION

The prevalence of complex or total aberrations appears to be a valid
biological dose-response indicator of exposure to radiation in uranium
miners and plutonium workers, and the response appears to be sensitive at
low dose estimates (Groups 1 in Table I) and Fig. 1). The monotonic
increases in the frequency of aberrations with increasing dose show similar
trends in both populations, but the overall frequency of aberrations is
greater in cells of the plutonium workers (Fig. 1). The latter observation
could be attributed to several factors including the different criteria for
the selection of exposure groups, differences in the mode of burdens and
the different culture times for the two populations.

The similarity in dose-response in these populations prompted us to
explore other possible methods of comparison. The aberration frequencies
per α blood dose in each population would be the best dose response measure,
but this is not practical. Although estimates of α blood doses in rem/yr
were done by extensive measurements and calculations on subjects exposed
to radon daughters in Badgastein, Austria [15], data of comparable accuracy
are not possible for U.S. uranium miners who work at numerous mines located
over a large area. Additionally, it would be premature to generate α blood
dose estimates to lymphocytes of Pu-burdened subjects because of differences

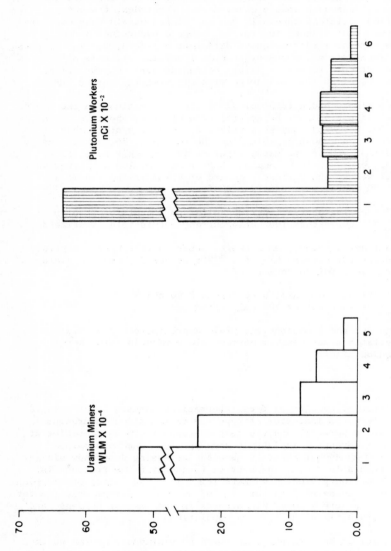

EXPOSURE GROUPS IN WLM OR nCi (See TABLE I)

COMPLEX ABERRATIONS/100 CELLS/EXPOSURE UNIT

FIG. 2.   Complex aberrations per exposure unit adjusted for control frequencies.   Uranium miner Group 4 in Table I is sub-divided into Group 4 and Group 5 (> 3000 WLM).

TABLE I. URANIUM MINER AND PLUTONIUM WORKER EXPOSURE
GROUPS BY ESTIMATED WLM AND nCi OF INTERNAL PLUTONIUM

Uranium miner groups	Estimated WLM	No. Subjects	No. Cells
C	Controls	20	1950
1	<100	5	500
2	100–470	26	2684
3	770–1725	15	1453
4	>1740	34	3263
Plutonium worker groups	Estimated nCi	No. Subjects	No. Cells
C	Controls	68	7 406
1	0.1–1.2	30	3 478
2	1.3–4.4	140	13 555
3	4.5–10.4	103	10 925
4	10.5–20.0	46	6 744
5	20.1–40.0	15	2 551
6	>40.0	9	2 504

between individuals in the site of entry, chemical and physical form of
plutonium, and different distributional patterns. In the absence of
accurate α blood dose estimates, and since the exposure groups in each
population are not divided in equal increments (Table I), we decided to
compare the dose responses in each group by aberrations per exposure unit,
though we recognize that there are disparities between the WLM and nCi
units.

In the uranium miners, the effect per WLM seems to decrease
monotonically with increasing dose (Fig. 2). In the plutonium workers,
the number of aberrations per nCi decreases abruptly after Group 1, thereafter the Pu exposure groups have essentially similar rates. The standard
deviations for WLM exposure estimates become much larger with increasing
WLM [1] and, if the WLM estimates were increasingly overestimated from
Groups 2 to 5, the uranium miner histograms could look very much like the
plutonium workers graph. Confidence in the accuracy of plutonium worker
dose estimates from urine bioassay data above $\sim$2 nCi burdens is greater
than for WLM estimates for the miners. Therefore, the trend in the
plutonium worker dose-response per exposure unit (above Group 1), is
probably more true than is the case for the uranium miners.

The value for the number of aberrations/nCi in plutonium worker Group 1 is probably an artifact. The values at these very low dose estimates (<1.3 nCi) are below minimum detectable levels for the urine bioassay method and are very variable. The very small dose estimate numbers are then used in the denominator of our aberrations/nCi calculations and the derived value expectedly is greatly exaggerated. We include these data for Group 1 for scientific completeness, while calling attention to the factors affecting the value. In absolute numbers, however, the increased prevalence of aberrations/100 cells in Group 1, compared to control frequency (Fig. 1), approaches significance for complex aberrations (P = 0.07; one-tailed test), and the difference is significant at the 5% level for total aberrations (P = 0.04; one-tailed test).

The current permissible lifetime safety standards for the two populations provide a common reference point for comparison of the biological dose response. Although permissible occupational exposures in the two populations were established from different criteria, the lifetime values of 120 WLM and 40 nCi are probably better for comparative effects than unit values of WLM and nCi. The calculation of complex aberrations/ 100 cells/working lifetime standards yields 4.8×10^{-2} for uranium miners and 90.6×10^{-2} for Pu workers. From these gross figures, it would appear that plutonium may be as much as ~ 20 times more effective (~ 9-fold for total aberrations) in the production of complex aberrations in lymphocytes at maximum acceptable levels of exposure compared to radon daughters. The calculations are, however, very rough, and random fluctuation has not been taken into account. Furthermore, the result is somewhat misleading, since it represents an average, weighted by the essentially arbitrary numbers of persons within each exposure group. The comparative effects could also be influenced by the longer culture time for the uranium miners' cells, resulting in more in vitro cell divisions and the loss of some asymmetrical aberrations [8]. Nevertheless, although it is questionable whether a precise value can be assigned, plutonium does appear to be more effective than radon daughters in generating complex aberrations. Both populations receive chronic exposures, but in many instances the plutonium workers receive a more acute initial burden than do the uranium miners, whose burdens tend to accumulate in smaller doses over time.

These findings demonstrate that, if all kinds of aberrations are analyzed, the prevalence of somatic cell chromosome aberrations may be used as a dose-response indicator of in vivo late biological effects in U.S. uranium workers and plutonium workers. We agree with the observation of other cytogeneticists that reliance solely on the prevalence of dicentrics and rings may result in an inadequate assessment of clastogen damage [11,16,17]. In the plutonium worker population, the apparent sensitivity of this test at levels below the detection capabilities of the urine assay method may prove useful as a biological monitor in the lowest exposure group. These biological findings can supplement demographic, epidemiological and medical data on these two populations.

ACKNOWLEDGEMENTS

The authors wish to thank numerous scientists and administrators on the staffs of St. Mary's Hospital, Grand Junction, CO., the Colorado State Department of Health and the Rocky Flats facility of Rockwell International for professional assistance in these studies. Special thanks is extended to the nuclear worker volunteers who have acted as subjects. The technical skills of Loris McGavran, David Braman, Ilse Brandom, Lynn Meltesen, David Lee, Janet Wilson, Laurie Quinn, Lola Brennan and Bonnie Stenger are gratefully acknowledged. These investigations were supported by the USPHS, FDA, Bureau of Radiological Health grant R01 FD 00644-03, and by the USERDA and USDOE, Division of Biomedical and Environmental Research contracts E(29-2)-3639 and EY-76-S-04-3639.

REFERENCES

[1] LUNDIN, F.E., WAGONER, J.K., ARCHER, V.E., Radon Daughter and Respiratory Cancer: Quantitative and Temporal Aspects, NIOSH and NIEHS Joint Monograph No.1, National Tech. Inform. Service, Springfield, VA (1971) 176.

[2] ŠEVC, J. KUNZ, E., PLAČEK, V., Lung cancer in uranium miners and long-term exposure to radon daughter products, Health Phys. 30 6 (1976) 433.

[3] RICHMOND, C.R., "Biomedical effects of plutonium in humans", Plutonium and Other Transuranium Elements, USAEC Rep. WASH-1359 (1974) 327.

[4] STOVER, B.J., JEE, W.S.S., Radiobiology of Plutonium, J.W. Press, Salt Lake City (1972) 552.

[5] BAIR, W.J., THOMPSON, R.C., Plutonium: biomedical research, Science 183 6 (1974) 715.

[6] BROOKS, A.L., Chromosome damage in liver cells from low dose rate alpha, beta, and gamma irradiation: derivation of RBE, Science 190 10 (1975) 1090.

[7] JEE, W.S.S., The Health Effects of Plutonium and Radium, J.W. Press, Salt Lake City (1976) 802.

[8] UNITED NATIONS, Report of the Scientific Committee on the Effects of Atomic Radiation (General Assembly Official Records: 24th Session, Suppl. No.13, A/7613, Annex C), UN, New York (1969) 165.

[9] KILIBARDA, M., MARKOVIĆ, B., PANOV, D., Etude des aberrations chromosomiques chez les personnes chroniquement exposées aux radiations ionisantes X, Ra 226, Rn 222, Stud. Biophys. 6 3 (1968) 179.

[10] BRANDOM, W.F., SACCOMANNO, G., ARCHER, V.E., ARCHER, P.G., COORS, M.E., Chromosome aberrations in uranium miners occupationally exposed to ^{222}Radon, Radiat. Res. 52 1 (1972) 204.

[11] DOLPHIN, G.W., LLOYD, D.C., PURROTT, R.J., Chromosome aberrations analysis as a dosimetric technique in radiological protection, Health Phys. 25 1 (1973) 7.

[12] HEMPELMANN, L.H., LANGHAM, W.H., RICHMOND, C.R., VOELZ, G.L., Manhattan project plutonium workers: a twenty-seven year follow-up study of selected cases, Health Phys. 25 5 (1973) 461.

[13] SEABRIGHT, M., A rapid banding technique for human chromosomes, Lancet ii 7731 (1971) 971.

[14] LANGHAM, W.H., Determination of internally deposited radioactive isotopes for excretion analyses, Am. Ind. Hyg. Assoc. Quart. 17 3 (1965) 305.

[15] POHL-RÜLING, J., FISCHER, P., POHL, E., "Chromosome aberrations in peripheral blood lymphocytes dependent on various dose levels of natural radioactivity", Biological and Environmental Effects of Low-Level Radiation (Proc. Symp. Chicago, 1975) II, IAEA, Vienna (1976) 317.

[16] CARRANO, A.V., MINKLER, J., PILUSO, D., On the fate of stable chromosomal aberrations, Mutat. Res. 30 1 (1975) 153.

[17] LUCHNIK, N.V., SEVANKAEV, A.V., Radiation-induced chromosomal aberrations in human lymphocytes, Mutat. Res. 36 (1976) 363.

DISCUSSION

G.W. DOLPHIN: I don't understand why you expect that the yield of chromosome aberrations should increase with estimated plutonium body content. In terms of radiation dose from incorporated Pu the essential parameters to be considered are the metabolic products of Pu content and their retention time in the body. The life span of a lymphocyte with an aberration must also be considered.

In my opinion the yield of aberrations in lymphocytes depends on where the plutonium is located in the body. The distribution of plutonium depends on the route of intake into the body and the chemical compound involved. Hence I would not expect a correlation between yield and estimated plutonium body content.

W.F. BRANDOM: I did not 'expect' that the yield of chromosome aberrations should or would increase with estimated plutonium body content in plutonium workers. Basing ourselves on earlier cytogenetic uranium miner studies, we did a small pilot study on plutonium workers with no preconceived or 'expected' results. The marked increase in aberrations in that study led to a more extensive investigation, but if the results had been negative we would have accepted the findings and not proceeded with the study. At the present stage of the study we have arbitrarily compared aberration yields with the estimated plutonium burdens at the date of culture. We shall also analyse the data, including the product of estimated exposure and duration of exposure. However, the results of the latter analysis would also be influenced by the life span of lymphocytes, and if you have recent information from haematology, immunology or radiation biology which gives an accurate estimate of lymphocyte life span (in sub-populations of T or B cell lymphocytes responding to phytohaemagglutinin) I should welcome such information. Certainly some lymphocytes must be long lived when one considers immunological and atom bomb survivor cytogenetics.

It is well known that the biological effects of plutonium are influenced by many factors: original site of entry, pathology or metabolism at site of entry, subsequent distribution, quantity, excretion (G.W. Dolphin, Health Phys. 20 6 (1971) 549), individual differences in response (genotype and phenotype) and so forth. We shall explore the data which are available in subsequent analyses, individual by individual. To cite only one complication, we have 117 individuals among the 411 workers who have measurable estimated lung and systemic (body) burdens. A biological response is observed in this group whether we use as our primary criterion estimated lung burden or systemic burden. With, as yet, very limited autopsy data on the distribution of plutonium in man, we cannot be more specific as to where the plutonium may be located on an individual basis. In saying that you do not expect a correlation between aberration yield and estimated plutonium body content, you are entitled to your opinion. For our part, we would not have found a correlation in our findings if we had analysed only for the prevalence of dicentric chromosomes, as you report you did in the case of eight British plutonium workers.

This report was an initial exploration of the comparison of two populations occupationally exposed to alpha-emitting radionuclides. The comparison is by rough calculations of the possible relationship between very dissimilar estimates (estimated dose in uranium miners — WLM; estimated burdens on Pu workers — nCi) and is influenced by the different relative impreciseness of the estimates. But that a relationship exists between estimated plutonium burden and the prevalence of peripheral blood lymphocyte chromosomes, I have no doubt.

Z.M. BEEKMAN: The origin of the control group for the uranium miners is stated in the paper, but not that of the control group for plutonium workers. Evidently the two control groups do not belong to the same population. Can you please indicate the origin of the plutonium worker control group? Also, how do you explain the fact that the number of complex aberrations is about a factor of two higher in the plutonium worker control group than in the uranium miner control group, whereas there is little difference in the total number of aberrations in the control groups?

W.F. BRANDOM: The plutonium worker control group consists of approximately 50 workers at the plutonium facility who have not worked in a radiation area, and the remaining controls are volunteers from the staff of the University of Denver. The similar frequency of 'total' aberrations in the controls of the two populations, compared with the prevalence of 'complex' aberrations in the respective control groups, reflects a greater increase in deletions in the uranium miner control cells compared with the plutonium worker controls. Conversely, this implies less increase in the frequency of deletions in the plutonium worker controls, perhaps due to a shorter cell culture time.

L.G. LITTLEFIELD: I should like to know whether you noted any unusual distribution of lesions in your damaged cells. Did you find disproportionate numbers of cells with multiple lesions?

W.F. BRANDOM: Except in a very few individuals, the cells do not show multiple exchange aberrations in the same cell.

D. BENINSON: External exposure to gamma radiation can be quite significant in uranium mines. Could you comment on the possible contribution of this external irradiation to the effects seen?

W.F. BRANDOM: A recent estimate of external gamma radiation in uranium mines throughout the world (UNSCEAR, 1977) is a mean dose of 1.6 rem/a. Although we cannot rule out some contribution to lymphocyte dose effect from external radiation, one advantage of lymphocyte radiation cytogenetics is that the effects of mixed radiations are integrated.

Y. NISHIWAKI; You state in your paper that the internal plutonium is translocated and concentrated in lymph nodes and haematopoietic tissues.

What chemical form of plutonium were the workers exposed to — soluble or insoluble? Plutonium may exist in many valency states, but the tetravalent form would be most important from the biological point of view. Plutonium tends to form complexes and, depending on the chemical form, the relative toxicity may vary. Monomeric plutonium is taken up preferentially by the skeleton, and polymeric plutonium by the liver. However, it is reported that in the skeleton plutonium concentrates characteristically on the endosteal surfaces, and it may also be found in the marrow especially when administered in polymeric form. Different isotopes of plutonium are known to exist: ^{239}Pu (2400 a), ^{240}Pu (6600 a), ^{238}Pu (14 a), etc. Plutonium-241 is mainly a beta-emitter and decays to the alpha-emitter ^{241}Am (430 a). Plutonium-239 and ^{240}Pu are usually mixed and difficult to distinguish from each other by alpha measurement. This mixture is usually referred to as ^{239}Pu. According to some measurements of environmental plutonium, approximately 60% of the activity would be ^{239}Pu. What was the isotopic composition of the plutonium the workers were exposed to in your mines, and could the isotopic ratio be assumed to be about the same in all the cases you studied?

W.F. BRANDOM: It is my understanding from the health physics personnel that the plutonium that the workers were exposed to was mostly ^{239}Pu in the tetravalent form. I do not know what the isotopic ratio was, but would conjecture that it was predominantly ^{239}Pu and similar in most, but not all, of the worker exposures. Also, in most cases the plutonium exposure was to the insoluble form. Where the data are available these questions will be considered in subsequent analyses of the population and for individuals.

Y. NISHIWAKI: What would be the magnitude of the accumulated dose from medical exposure of the workers you examined? Is there any possibility of the workers being exposed to other potential carcinogenic or mutagenic agents in their working environment?

W.F. BRANDOM: The magnitude of the accumulated medical exposure of the workers is nil compared with the control levels. No worker in this report has had therapeutic or recent diagnostic irradiation. We have also screened by questionnaire for possible exposure to other potential mutagenic agents or toxic substances in the working environment. We have, in fact, excluded many workers in the study on whom we have performed chromosome analyses when there was any indication of exposure to clastogenic agents other than their occupational radiation exposure.

BIOCHEMICAL LATE EFFECTS IN RAT LUNG EXPOSED TO DIFFERENT DOSES OF X-RAYS

A.M. DANCEWICZ
Department of Radiobiology and
    Health Protection,
Institute of Nuclear Research,
Warsaw,
Poland

G.B. GERBER
Department of Radiobiology,
Centre d'Etude de l'Energie Nucléaire,
Mol,
Belgium

Abstract

BIOCHEMICAL LATE EFFECTS IN RAT LUNG EXPOSED TO DIFFERENT
DOSES OF X-RAYS.
    Fibrosis represents an important late somatic effect of radiation. It can lead to the
impairment of functional capacity of the lung. The mechanisms of radiation-induced lung
fibrosis are still uncertain. Fibrosis could arise as a result of stimulation of fibrotic elements
in tissue, disturbance of collagen metabolism, impairment of blood circulation or loss of
mesenchyma cells. The biochemical study of radiation fibrosis in lung was approached by
assessing changes in several indicators at various time intervals up to 1 year after exposure of
the rat lung to 10 or 30 Gy doses of X-rays. It was found that the changes observed after each
of these doses are qualitatively similar. Quantitatively the changes observed in the 10-Gy group
of animals were less pronounced. During the whole observation period the following changes
relevant to fibrosis were noted: a decrease in fibrinolytic activity and blood flow, and an
increase in biogenic amines content. A statistically significant increase in collagen content was
observed during the gross fibrosis, i.e. several months after exposure. The role of collagen in
the development of radiation-induced fibrosis is now being investigated.

INTRODUCTION

    Lung fibrosis often develops as a late effect of exposure to ionizing
radiation [1]. Fibrosis occurs also as a sequel of exposure to other environmental agents [2]. The fibrotic alteration of lung impairs its ventilatory and

diffusion capacity. Hence, the recognition of the mechanisms and factors involved in the development of this pathological state is of importance. Because of the complexity of structural organization of the lung the relation of its biochemistry to function is not well known at present [3]. Thus, the estimation of the possible significance of alteration of a given biochemical parameter for the functional changes observed in irradiated lung is rather a matter for systematic investigation than for checking the established links between structure, biochemistry and function.

In this study we record changes in some biochemical parameters which reflect the status of connective tissue, of cellularity and of lysosomal enzymes in rat lung at different times after exposure to X-rays.

EXPERIMENTAL

Experiments were performed on Wistar male rats weighing 150—180 g at the time of irradiation. In general, for irradiation the EULEP recommendations were followed [4]. Two groups of rats were subjected to hemithoracic irradiation with a 10 Gy and a 30 Gy dose of X-rays respectively, and a third group (WB) had the whole body irradiated with a 6.5 Gy dose of X-rays. After exposure, the animals were maintained for various periods up to one year. They were sacrificed either by cutting the vena cava under ether anaesthesia or by cutting the spinal cord. The lungs were removed, washed briefly and homogenized in ice-cold water using an Ultra-Turrax homogenizer.

The following methods were used for assays: protein was determined by the Biuret method, collagen by determining hydroxyproline [5] in (a) hydrolysed in 6N HCl for 18 h at 110°C and then neutralized trichloroacetic acid extract of DNA-protein sediment precipitated from homogenate by perchloric acid, or in (b) water extract (4 h at 135°C) of powdered tissue [6]. The latter method was used in whole-body irradiated animals [7]. The activity of cathepsin D was assayed by fluorometric determination of naphtylamine liberated from Na-benzoyl-dl-arginine-betanaphtylamide after incubation for 18 h with homogenate sample [8]. The activity of beta-glucuronidase and acid phosphatase was assayed by measuring the amount of phenolphtalein released from the respective substrate incubated with the homogenate sample for 2 h [9]. Fibrinolytic activity was estimated by measuring the area of fibrin film lysed by a known amount of a homogenate supernatant [10]. Preformed peroxides were determined in homogenates using the thiobarbituric acid reaction [11]. To measure the peroxidation capacity the thiobarbituric acid reaction was repeated after a 2-h incubation of homogenate in the presence of Fe^{+2} ions. The biogenic amines, histamine and serotonin, were extracted with n-butanol from neutralized and salt-saturated perchloric acid supernatant [12], and then assayed fluorometrically by the relevant o-phtalaldehyde procedure [13, 14]. The blood flow ratio between the right (irradiated)

TABLE I. LATE EFFECT OF RADIATION ON PROTEIN AND COLLAGEN
CONTENT IN LUNG OF RATS EXPOSED TO DIFFERENT DOSES OF X-RAYS
Mean values ± S.D. are given as percentage of control values; irradiation groups:
HT-1, hemithoracic — 10 Gy; HT-3, hemithoracic — 30 Gy; WB, whole
body — 6.5 Gy

Component	Irrad. group	Time after exposure (months)					
		0.25	1	3	6	9	11
Protein	HT-1	81.4 ± 16.7	94.0 ± 2.8	91.0 ± 2.0	110.8 ± 7.8	100.0 ± 6.8	100.6 ± 5.3
	HT-3	106.3 ± 6.9	99.7 ± 16.3	100.0 ± 19.7	99.0 ± 20.7	121.7 ± 12.8	—
	WB	83.1 ± 8.0	83.1 ± 6.4	78.2 ± 5.6	74.6 ± 5.9	81.3 ± 10.9	80.8 ± 17.0
Collagen	HT-1	75.0 ± 14.7	78.7 ± 3.8	68.9 ± 15.4	—	—	155.9 ± 10.6
	HT-3	86.8 ± 28.3	85.8 ± 27.5	116.7 ± 31.7	161.4 ± 43.8	208.7 ± 33.6	—
	WB	—	110.8 ± 19.5	103.5 ± 2.5	112.7 ± 12.3	104.5 ± 8.3	114.2 ± 10.8

and left (non-irradiated) lung was estimated by measuring the retention of
^{144}Ce-labelled microspheres injected intravenously 5 min before killing the
animals. The radioactivity of the homogenate was determined by gamma
spectrometry. Lipids were extracted with a chloroform : methanol mixture
(2 : 1). The extract was assayed for phosphorus, and the composition of the
phospholipids was determined by thin-layer chromatography of the lipid
extracts [15] after saponification and methylation with boron trifluoride, using
a Hewlett Packard 5700 A gas chromatograph and a 3380 A integrator.

RESULTS AND DISCUSSION

A summary of the data obtained is presented in Tables I—III. To compare
the different experimental groups, the values of the determined parameters are
expressed as a percentage of the control values. The latter were obtained from
non-irradiated lungs in animals subjected to irradiation of the hemithorax
(HT-1 and HT-3 groups) or from the sham irradiated animals for the WB group.

TABLE II. LATE EFFECT OF RADIATION ON ENZYMIC SYSTEMS OF RAT LUNG EXPOSED TO DIFFERENT DOSES OF X-RAYS

Mean values ±S.D. are given as percentage of control values; irradiation groups: HT-1, hemithoracic — 10 Gy; HT-3, hemithoracic — 30 Gy; WB, whole body — 6.5 Gy

Enzymic system	Irrad. group	Time after exposure (months)					
		0.25	1	3	6	9	11
Acid phosphatase	HT-1	102.4 ± 11.4	109.4 ± 6.4	103.3 ± 7.3	91.5 ± 8.8	78.2 ± 7.8	86.0 ± 7.1
	HT-3	105.8 ± 50.3	95.5 ± 31.9	97.2 ± 27.3	88.2 ± 26.6	104.5 ± 36.2	—
	WB	41.2 ± 15.1	117.0 ± 6.2	90.0 ± 29.9	68.7 ± 15.6	—	65.8 ± 33.5
Beta glucuronidase	HT-1	95.4 ± 6.4	101.8 ± 5.9	72.9 ± 9.6	98.6 ± 7.5	95.4 ± 9.5	109.3 ± 6.4
	HT-3	106.1 ± 26.9	105.5 ± 34.5	104.9 ± 20.2	135.2 ± 40.7	186.8 ± 42.6	—
	WB	68.9 ± 26.2	112.4 ± 12.2	102.8 ± 20.3	101.7 ± 11.0	—	118.7 ± 21.1

Enzymic system	Irrad. group	Time after exposure (months)					
		0.25	1	3	6	9	11
Cathepsin D	HT-1	68.0 ± 6.0	58.2 ± 4.8	63.9 ± 9.3	93.6 ± 12.5	101.5 ± 20.9	105.9 ± 7.4
	HT-3	140.0 ± 26.0	111.3 ± 28.3	175.5 ± 31.9	314.3 ± 28.5	164.5 ± 14.8	–
	WB	122.9 ± 30.7	147.2 ± 12.4	129.3 ± 23.0	170.2 ± 20.2	–	122.9 ± 30.1
Fibrinolysis	HT-1	62.4 ± 7.1	69.6 ± 4.4	60.8 ± 7.2	69.6 ± 4.9	92.3 ± 6.1	86.2 ± 10.5
	HT-3	86.6 ± 31.3	71.3 ± 10.6	55.2 ± 30.6	117.6 ± 13.3	28.9 ± 10.4	–
	WB	134.5 ± 25.7	169.9 ± 15.9	129.2 ± 17.9	120.1 ± 13.7	–	130.5 ± 17.2

TABLE III. LATE EFFECT OF RADIATION ON VARIOUS BIOCHEMICAL PARAMETERS OF RAT LUNG EXPOSED TO DIFFERENT DOSES OF X-RAYS

Mean values ±S.D. are given as percentage of the control value; irradiation groups: HT-1, hemithoracic — 10 Gy; HT-3, hemithoracic — 30 Gy

Biochemical parameter	Irrad. group	Time after exposure (months)					
		0.25	1	3	6	9	11
DNA	HT-1	104.7 ±7.0	96.5 ±6.5	87.0 ±8.9	79.3 ±11.0	97.0 ±5.0	73.3 ±4.1
	HT-3	98.3 ±35.2	86.4 ±22.2	110.6 ±21.3	92.2 ±27.3	150.3 ±24.2	—
Peroxides	HT-1	67.9 ±7.0	68.4 ±21.4	89.3 ±8.8	109.7 ±19.1	74.9 ±8.4	100.5 ±12.0
	HT-3	92.6 ±27.5	59.6 ±20.8	104.7 ±43.0	135.0 ±35.7	206.9 ±38.0	—
Peroxidative capacity	HT-1	93.2 ±23.9	81.7 ±7.9	43.2 ±7.2	156.6 ±16.8	149.3 ±20.9	103.3 ±18.2
	HT-3	99.3 ±19.9	85.8 ±27.3	85.5 ±20.4	112.7 ±37.5	165.5 ±16.1	—

Biochemical parameter	Irrad. group	Time after exposure (months)					
		0.25	1	3	6	9	11
Retention of microspheres	HT-1	80.8 ±14.6	89.5 ±3.8	90.0 ±9.0	72.9 ±14.4	77.9 ±8.9	76.9 ±18.9
Phospholipids	HT-1	70.3 ±16.7	67.9 ±8.6	79.4 ±8.1	–	–	78.5 ±6.2
Serotonin	HT-3	93.6 ±62.8	153.6 ±44.9	160.7 ±52.6	310.1 ±19.8	–	–
Histamine	HT-3	115.0 ±23.5	124.7 ±32.9	187.3 ±37.8	184.3 ±19.5	–	–

Absorbed lung fibrosis becomes manifest from the 4th month after exposure onwards [16], according to the radiation dose. Morphologically this process is characterized by a thickening of the alveolar septa, a deposition of collagen and a loss of parenchymal tissue [17, 18]. The biochemical alterations underlying fibrotic changes are not clear. Our data (Table I) confirmed that the amount of collagen in the irradiated lung began to increase half a year after exposure of the hemithorax. This effect was more significant in rats irradiated with the 30 Gy dose. An increase in lung collagen occurred also in mice irradiated with 10 Gy or more [19]. In rats surviving a 6.5 Gy dose of whole-body irradiation, the content of collagen in the lung was not significantly different from the control. However, because the protein content in these animals was lowered, one can expect the occurrence of changes in the relative composition of lung proteins. Accumulation of collagen can result from earlier changes in collagen biosynthesis [20], but may also reflect radiation-induced changes in collagen properties [21]. Certainly the properties defining the uniqueness of lung collagen merit more detailed studies if the correlation between the fibrotic process and the accumulation of collagen is to be found.

Abnormal reaction of connective tissue is not considered the only, or even the main, cause of lung fibrosis [22]. In fact, more probably, the fibrotic process begins with damage of blood vessels brought about by radiation. Vascular changes are observed in irradiated lung quite early after exposure [17]. They manifest themselves in changed permeability, deposition of fibrin-rich exudates in the intra-alveolar septa and the alveolar lumina, and in the formation of microthrombi. Impaired circulation may also give rise to atrophy of parenchymal tissue and its replacement by connective tissue at later stages.

Our experiments indicated (Table III) that the irradiated lung captured fewer microspheres than the non-irradiated one, indicating that impairment of circulation manifests itself as early as the second week after exposure and lasts during the whole observation period. Reduced circulation coincides with reduced perfusion and ventilation of irradiated lungs reported by Dunjic [23] and Keyeux and co-workers [24]. These effects favour the formation of microthrombi and the deposition of fibrin. A decrease in fibrinolytic activity of irradiated lung (Table II) also favours the growth of fibrin deposits. A similar effect has been found by others [25] also after local irradiation. The reverse effect, an increase in fibrinolytic activity, was noted in the lungs of rats exposed to irradiation of the whole body (Table II). An increase in fibrinolytic activity could result from antiplasmin inhibition or from an increase in plasminogen activator. Both effects have been observed at an early stage of radiation disease [25] but no information is available for later stages.

The activity of lysosomal enzymes, reflecting cellular integrity, differs from that of the control values even at very long periods after exposure. This was especially manifest in the activity of cathepsin D (Table II). This was

increased both in rats irradiated locally with a 30 Gy dose and in rats exposed
to whole-body irradiation. No changes were noted at later periods in rats
irradiated with a dose of 10 Gy of X-rays. The activity of beta-glucuronidase
and acid phosphatase was not significantly changed during the post-acute period
of radiation disease. Thus, the observed changes in the activity of lysomal
enzymes do not form any consistent pattern in the dynamics of cellular alterations
accompanying lung fibrosis. More information to this effect is to be had from
ultrastructural studies of late effects in irradiated lung. These studies show that
there is a marked sloughing of endothelial cells from blood vessels [17, 18], an
increase in the number of mast cells and also the damage and death of alveolar
pneumocytes. The late increases in biogenic amines in irradiated lung (Table III)
could be associated with the infiltration of the lung with mast cells [18], whereas
the damage to pneumocytes and disturbances in their replacement in irradiated
lung probably impairs the formation of surfactant causing subsequent functional
disability of the organ. Such changes in the activity of the surfactant of irradiated
lungs have been reported by Rüfer and co-workers [26] and Forsberg and
co-workers [27]. Our preliminary results confirm that radiation causes changes
in saturation of fatty acids of phospholipids extracted from lung surfactant.
During the fibrotic phase there was an increase in saturation whereas at earlier
stages desaturation was observed. However, no change was seen in fatty acid
composition or phospholipid content of the whole lung (Table III). This result
is probably correct if one takes into account the fact that type II pneumocytes,
directly responsible for the production of lung surfactant, represent less than
10% of the cell population in lungs [3].

From the results presented no definite conclusion can be drawn regarding
the mechanism(s) of radiation-induced fibrosis. Comparison of several biochemical
monitors of lung structure and function makes it possible to estimate the
threshold dose level of fibrosis, and indicates that many changes persist for a
long time in irradiated lung. The origin of these changes and their participation
in the development of late structural and functional injury of the lung still
remain to be investigated.

ACKNOWLEDGEMENTS

The authors acknowledge with pleasure the participation of A. Mazanowska,
M. Jeleńska, T. Kubicka, E. Przygoda, G. Casale and B. Bessemans in performing
research reported here. This project was carried out as part of the co-operation
programme of the European Late Effects Project Group (EULEP), and was
partly supported by the Commission of the European Communities (Euratom),
Brussels, Belgium, under Contract 092-72-1 BIOC, and represents publication
No. 1523 of the Euratom Biology Division.

REFERENCES

[1] BUBLITZ, G., Morphological and Biochemical Investigations into the Behaviour of
     Fibrous Tissue in Radioinduced Pulmonary Fibrosis, G. Thieme Verlag, Stuttgart (1973).
[2] ENGELBRECHT, F.M., THIART, B.F., CLASSENS, A., Ann. Occup. Hyg. 2 (1960) 257.
[3] FULMER, J.D., CRYSTAL, R.G., "The biochemical basis of pulmonary function",
     The Biochemical Basis of Pulmonary Function (CRYSTAL, R.G., Ed.), Marcel Dekker Inc.,
     New York and Basel (1976) 419.
[4] PUITE, K.J., et al., Phys. Med. Biol. 17 (1972) 390.
[5] STEGEMANN, H., STALDER, K., Clin. Chim. Acta 18 (1967) 267.
[6] GELFON, I.A., Gig. Tr. Prof. Zabol. 13 10 (1969) 56.
[7] DANCEWICZ, A.M., KUBICKA, T., Nukleonika 21 (1976) 1029.
[8] ROTH, M., Clin. Chim. Acta 8 (1962) 574.
[9] BERGMEYER, H.U.(Ed.), Methoden der Enzymatischen Analyse, Verlag Chemie,
     Weinheim (1970).
[10] PETERSON, H.I., PETRUSSON, B., KORSAN-BENGTSEN, K., Thromb. Diath.
     Haemorrh. 30 (1973) 133.
[11] BLOOM, R.J., WESTERFELD, W.W., Arch. Biochem. Biophys. 145 (1971) 669.
[12] GILES, K.W., MYERS, A., Nature (London) 106 (1965) 93.
[13] MAICKEL, R.P., et al., Ing. J. Neuropharmacol. 7 (1968) 275.
[14] LORENTZ, W., et al., Z. Anal. Chem. 252 (1970) 94.
[15] COLOWICK, S.P., KAPLAN, N.O., LOWENSTEIN, J.M. (Eds), Methods in Enzymology
     XIV: Lipids, Academic Press, New York (1969).
[16] ADAMSON, I.R., BOWDEN, D.H., WYATT, J.P., Am. J. Pathol. 58 (1970) 481.
[17] MAISIN, J.R., Radiat. Res. 44 (1970) 545.
[18] PHILLIPS, T.L., Radiology 87 (1966) 49.
[19] LAW, M.P., HORNSEY, S., FIELD, S.B., Radiat. Res. 65 (1976) 60.
[20] PICKRELL, J.A., et al., Radiat. Res. 62 (1975) 133.
[21] DANCEWICZ, A.M., Nukleonika 20 (1975) 867.
[22] DANCEWICZ, A.M., MAZANOWSKA, A., GERBER, G.B., Radiat. Res. 67 (1976) 482.
[23] DUNJIC, A., Radiat. Res. Quart. 10 (1974) 109.
[24] KEYEUX, A., et al., Int. J. Radiat. Biol. Relat. Stud. Phys., Chem. Med. 20 (1971) 7.
[25] FLEMING, W.H., SZAKACZS, J.E., KING, E.R., J. Nucl. Med. 3 (1962) 341.
[26] RÜFER, R., MERKER, H.J., BUBLITZ, G., Strahlentherapie 145 (1973) 55.
[27] FORSBERG, S.A., JOHANSSON, J.M., LINSKONG, B., Life Sci. 9 (1970) 793.

DISCUSSION

C. STREFFER: With respect to the increase of collagen in the irradiated
lungs, I should like to ask whether you measured hydroxyproline excretion under
your conditions in order to get an idea of the collagen turnover.

A.M. DANCEWICZ: The excretion of hydroxyproline metabolite in urine
was not measured in this experiment. It is known from earlier studies by Gerber
and Altmann that the amount of collagen degradation products in urine increases
in the course of the radiation syndrome. However, we have no data about

collagen turnover at the later stages after partial or whole-body exposure when lung fibrosis develops.

C. STREFFER: I was very interested in your finding that the content of 5-hydroxytryptamine and histamine was considerably greater in the irradiated lungs. You assumed that mast cells were migrating into the tissue. Were you able to demonstrate this? Also, did you measure other parameters of the amine metabolism, as for instance excretion of 5-hydroxyindoleacetic acid?

A.M. DANCEWICZ: Morphological changes were not checked in this study, so we have no direct evidence for the migration of mast cells into lung tissue. It is known from the literature that macrophages invade lung tissue during the third week after exposure. Excretion of 5-hydroxyindoleacetic acid was measured along with other biochemical indicators of radiation injury in a group of animals that survived for one year whole-body exposure to 650 rads of X-rays. Preliminary results of this experiment indicate that the levels of some metabolites excreted in the urine are elevated even such a long time after exposure; 5HlAA is among them.

HAEMOPATHOLOGICAL CONSEQUENCES OF PROTRACTED GAMMA IRRADIATION IN THE BEAGLE
Pre-clinical phases of leukaemia induction*

T.M. SEED, D.V. TOLLE, T.E. FRITZ,
S.M. CULLEN, L.V. KASPAR, C.M. POOLE
Division of Biological and Medical Research,
Argonne National Laboratory,
Argonne, Illinois,
United States of America

Abstract

HAEMOPATHOLOGICAL CONSEQUENCES OF PROTRACTED GAMMA IRRADIATION
IN THE BEAGLE: PRE-CLINICAL PHASES OF LEUKAEMIA INDUCTION.
    Myelogenous leukaemia is the most important late effect in beagles given continuous
^{60}Co-gamma irradiation beginning at one year of age. At the optimal leukaemogenic exposure
rate of 10 R daily, the incidence is $\sim$ 50%. We recognize four distinct pre-clinical phases in
leukaemia development: (I) progressive development of severe leukopenia and thrombocytopenia;
(II) partial haemopoietic recovery after 2000 R of accumulated exposure; (III) an equilibration
of subnormal haemopoietic function; and (IV) a classical preleukaemic phase. Overt leukaemia
is the fifth and last phase of the sequences that ends in a terminal anaemia. We are characterizing
these phases haematologically and ultrastructurally through serial blood and bone marrow
sampling, and also by endotoxin-stress assays and in vitro stem cell cloning experiments. Entry
into phase II, partial haemopoietic recovery, appears to be a deciding factor for leukaemic
induction. Dogs failing to enter this phase ($\sim$ 50%) are recognized early by (a) development
of a progressive pancytopenia, and (b) morphological and functional changes in supportive
structures and cellular reserves of the bone marrow; they later die of aplastic anaemia. Dogs
eventually developing leukaemia, however, partially recover the haemopoietic functions lost
in phase I. Restoration becomes evident after 200–300 days of irradiation as an increase in
peripheral blood platelets and leukocytes. This is later accompanied by renewed marrow
function, specifically observed as a progressive increase in marrow cellularity, with partial
restoration of the granulocyte reserves and progenitor-cell compartments. Serum collected
in phase I appears to have an enhanced stimulatory effect on normal granulopoiesis, in vitro,
but this subsequently declines as marrow cellularity increases late in phase III. The preleukaemic
phase (phase IV) is most notably characterized by a greatly exaggerated oscillation in blood
platelet values, and by circulating immature granulocytes and erythrocytes with various
morphologic abnormalities. We hypothesize that human leukaemias, whether 'spontaneous',
or induced by radiation or chemicals, have preleukaemic sequences and events that are
similar to those of canine leukaemias.

---

* Work supported by the U.S. Department of Energy.

531

INTRODUCTION

The induction of either aplastic anemia or leukemia following exposure to protracted low dose irradiation has been documented both in man [1] and in a number of lower animal species [2-4]. Precise dose, dose-rate relation ships for the induction of these pathologies remain to be defined for man, but in the dog, these factors and their interrelationships are becoming understood [5-7]. In our previous studies using the beagle, continuous gamma irradiation at 5-35 R/day was shown to produce three separate, dose-rate dependent causes of death, septicemia, aplastic anemia, and myelo-proliferative disorders (MPD) [5-7]. At a given dose rate there was considerable variation in the individual response to the stress of daily irradiation. At the dose rate of 10 R/day, the incidences of aplasia and MPD (representing the two extremes of the hemopathological spectrum) both approached 50%. The most radiosensitive animals died relatively early of aplastic anemia. Dogs developing the late arising MPD passed through and reversed an early phase of deteriorating hemopoiesis which resembled progressive aplasia [3-8]. Similar types of preclinical sequences in leukemia induction have been observed with chemical leukemogens [9], as well as with the 'spontaneously' developing leukemias [10].

This paper assesses certain aspects of altered hematological function during defined phases that procede the onset of leukemia, and speculates on the role they play in the genesis of the disease and on their prognostic value.

MATERIALS AND METHODS

Animals: Twenty-three anatomically normal and healthy outbred beagles of both sexes, approximately 400 days of age, were selected from the closed Argonne National Laboratory colony [11]. Eighteen were assigned to experimental groups and the remainder served as controls. In addition, some 53 animals in other long-range gamma radiation toxicity studies [7] contributed to this investigation. All dogs were given physical examinations, which included baseline hematologic studies. Control dogs were handled in an identical fashion, except they were caged in an anteroom adjoining the radiation facility. The animals had water *ad libitum* and were given standard dog food once a day.

Irradiation: Dogs were irradiated for 22 hr/day for duration of life within a specially designed ^{60}Co gamma irradiation facility capable of delivering doses of 5-35 R/day. They received a dose of 10 R/day by arranging the two-tiered fiberglass cages (28" x 28" x 24" high) at appropriate distances from the source [5,6].

Hematology: Hemograms were performed every 14 days from blood samples collected via jugular venipuncture. Erythrocyte, leukocyte and platelet concentrations were determined, and differential white blood cell counts were made by direct microscopic examination of stained thin films.

When irradiated animals became acutely ill, or control tissues were needed from nonirradiated beagles, the animals were sacrificed by exsanguination while under sodium thiamydol anesthesia (Surital, Parke Davis). Gross pathologic changes were recorded, and tissue samples were taken for light and electron microscopic examination.

Collection of Marrow Samples: Marrow samples were collected from
irradiated and nonirradiated animals approximately every 30 days, using
alternately two types of sampling methods, namely surgical rib biopsy and
the iliac crest aspiration methods. Both techniques were performed under
general anesthesia using standard surgical procedures, and the dogs were
maintained prophylactically on a penicillin-streptomycin regimen for the
following 3 days. The iliac crest cells were withdrawn with pediatric
spinal needles into heparinized syringes (200 U preservative-free heparin).
The rib biopsy method provided pieces of intact marrow for morphological-
ultrastructural analysis, whereas the aspiration method proved more useful
for the collection of marrow cells for cell culture experiments.

Electron Microscopy: Small pieces of necropsied or biopsied tissue
were quickly excised and placed in pools of chilled glutaraldehyde-
formaldehyde. Rib sections ($\sim$ 1-2 cm) were split longitudinally and cut
into small sections with a razor blade. Sections were processed for both
scanning and transmission electron microscopy by standard methods.

Hemopoietic Stem Cell Analysis: The relative numbers of granulocytic-
monocytic progenitor cells (GM-CFUa) in sequentially aspirated marrow
samples from irradiated and control animals were assessed by the soft agar
cloning technique [12]. Mononuclear enriched cell fractions were obtained
from iliac marrow by a single ficol-hypaque-gradient centrifugation step.
Cell viability was visually assessed by trypan blue dye exclusion. Marrow
cells were placed out in concentrations of 2-6 x 10^5 nucleated cells/ml
in 1 ml of complete cloning medium (20% fetal calf serum in a supplemented
TC 199 media with 0.3% agar [12,13] with 0.2 ml of added feeder serum (normal, pooled, heated-inactivated canine serum). Cultures were incubated in
a 5% CO_2 atmosphere at 100% humidity at 37° for 7-10 days. Following the
incubation, the plates were examined for colony growth (colony $\geqq$ 50 cells)
using an inverted microscope at 15X.

To assess the colony-stimulating activity (CSA) of serum samples,
marrow aspirates from healthy stock dogs were collected, prepared as
described above, and plated out at 4 x 10^5 nucleated marrow cells/ml.
A 0.2 aliquot of the serum to be tested was added to triplicate plates of
the control marrow. Following incubation, the numbers of colonies on the
test plates were compared to those on control plates to which pooled control
serum had been added.

Granulocyte Reserve and Mobilization Assays: Dogs were subjected to
the granulocyte reserve assay (GRA) prior to being irradiated and approximately every 100 days (i.e. $\cong$ 1000 R) thereafter. On the day of the assay
the dogs were removed from the irradiation facility and bled. Subsequently,
the animals received by intravenous injection 50 ng/kg of body weight of
bacterial endotoxin (*Salmonella typhimurium*, Sigma Chemical Co.). Dogs
were subsequently bled at 1, 2, 4, 6, 8, 10, 12, 14, and 24 h after endotoxin
injection. For each blood sample collected, blood smears were made, stained,
and differential white cell counts performed. Erythrocyte and leukocyte
concentrations were determined by standard methods.

RESULTS AND DISCUSSION

Of the 18 irradiated beagles receiving 10 R per day in this longitudinal leukemogenic study, 6 dogs exhibited hematological profiles
characteristic of preclinical phases of developing MPD (e.g. leukemia).

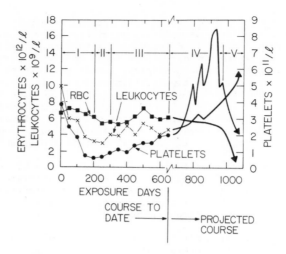

FIG.1.   Phase changes in peripheral blood values of continuously irradiated (10 R gamma/day)
pre-MPD beagles.   The values of 650 days are the means for a current experimental group of
6 dogs in suspected preclinical phases of MPD.   The projected course following 650 days is
based on data from previous studies [3, 8, 14].

Six other irradiated dogs died of aplastic anemia following a mean exposure
time of 245 days and an accumulated gamma radiation dose of ∿ 2450 R.   The
remaining 6 irradiated animals are still alive, having entered the experiment
at a later time, and have not yet reached the point of early hemopoietic
crisis (i.e.   200 days, 2000 R).

Figure 1 illustrates both the actual and the projected change in
peripheral blood cell values of the 6 irradiated dogs presently in
suspected, preclinical phases of developing MPD (e.g.   leukemia).   The
overall profile of the figure has been well documented and is typical of
the hematological sequences of some 21 previous cases of irradiation-
induced MPD in canines [3,8,14,15].   Four distinct hematological phases
precede the onset of patent disease (Fig. 1).   These are: (I) the initial
radiotoxic phase; (II) partial hemopoietic recovery; (III) subnormal
hemopoietic equilibration; and (IV) 'preleukemia'.   The fifth and final
phase in the sequence is the development of patent leukemia or other
myeloproliferative disorders.

Phase I.   The initial radiotoxic phase covers the first 150 to 200 days
of irradiation (i.e.   1500-2000 R accumulated dose at 10 R/day), and is
characterized by a rapid, severe depression of hemopoiesis.   The severe
leukopenia and thrombocytopenia (Fig. 1) corresponds in time with altered
structure-function relationships of the bone marrow.   Structural-topograph-
ical analysis of serially biopsied marrow by scanning electron microscopy
revealed reduced cellularity, with slight increases in fat deposition as
early as 100 days or 1000 R of irradiation.   In contrast to topography of
preirradiation marrow (e.g.   Fig. 2a), specimens from irradiated animals
exhibit a progressively prominent reticulum-like network (Fig. 2b).   The
latter is accounted for, most likely, by the reduced cellularity of the
marrow which enhances the visibility of underlying supportive structures.

The relative changes in size and mobility of granulocyte reserves were serially assessed, by the endotoxin-stress assay, over 500 days, representing an accumulated dose of approximately 5000 R in irradiated dogs (Fig. 3). The slope of the curve (in the linear region of the curve, i.e. 2-10 h), as well as the height of the granulocytic response, are approximate functional measures of both the mobility and the size of existing granulocyte reserves [16-18]. Progressive reduction in granulocyte reserves and their mobilization following 100 and 200 days in the radiation field (i.e. 1000 and 2000 R) is shown in Figure 3a.

In addition to the diminishing granulocyte reserves, the committed stem cell compartment which ultimately generates these reserves is similarly affected. The relative decrease in numbers of marrow GM-CFUa is shown in Figure 4. In a reciprocal fashion, the colony-stimulating activity (CSA) of sera collected during this phase is greatly enhanced (Fig. 5).

Phase II. The second phase is characterized by a partial hemopoietic recovery; blood leukocyte and platelet concentrations reach their nadir, level off, and subsequently show marginal increases (Fig. 1). Hemopoietic restoration first becomes evident, after 200 to 300 days in the field, as an increase in peripheral blood platelets and later in leukocytes (Fig. 1). These early recuperative changes are difficult to detect morphologically; biopsied marrow specimens still appear hypocellular with supportive elements prominent (Fig. 2c). Subsequently, however, we find local areas of increased cellular proliferation, particularly in the erythroid series. Many of these immature erythroid and granulocytic cells exhibit aberrant megaloblastic and monocytoid features, respectively. A slight expansion of the GM-committed stem cell compartment is suggested by the increase in clonogenic activity of culture marrow cells (i.e. GM-CFUa) obtained in mid phase II (Fig. 4).

Dogs failing to show such increases invariably die of aplastic anemia; they are recognized early, i.e. in mid phase I, by a development of a progressive pancytopenia, as well as by pronounced morphological (Fig. 2d) and functional changes in supportive structures and cellular reserves of the marrow.

During this phase of partial recovery, where a number of assayed hematological parameters show signs of improvement, granulocyte reserves and their mobilizing capacity continue to be depleted (Fig. 3a,b). The rate of granulocyte mobilization following endotoxin stress declines up to 300 days of irradiation ($\sim$ 3000 R), with increased rates noted thereafter (i.e. at 400 and 500 days) (Fig. 3b). Similarly, the peak of the granulocytic response, a rough indicator of the functional size of the reserve pool, is continually reduced up to 300 days or 3000 R. The circulating granulocyte pool (estimated from preendotoxin injection blood samples), in contrast, is slightly increased at 300 days (3000 R) (Fig. 3b) after reaching a nadir at 200 days (2000 R) (Fig. 3a). This suggests that restoration of the granulocyte storage pool lags behind the partial recovery noted in the peripheral blood values.

The recovery sequence first in peripheral blood values and subsequently in recovery of cellular reserves might well represent an adaptive process with real survival value. By increasing circulating blood cells at the expense of stored reserves during phase II, a period of hemopoietic crisis, deaths might be averted by maintaining a necessary critical level for basally required physiological functions. However, for long-term benefit to the

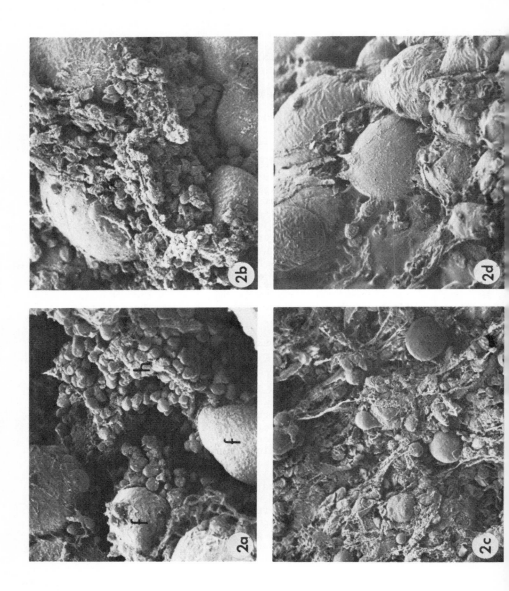

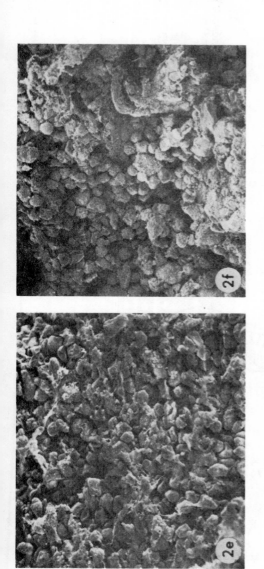

FIG.2a-f. Scanning electron micrographs of biopsied rib marrow specimens, ~300X. (a) Preirradiation specimen. Rich cellular areas exhibiting free hemopoietic cells (h) embedded in marrow matrix along with fat cells (f). (b) Phase I marrow specimen at approximately 100 days of irradiation. Note the increased reticular network and general change in cell shape. (c) Late Phase I-Early Phase II. A generalized hypocellular condition of the marrow following approximately 200 days of irradiation. Reticulum of the marrow is prominent. (d) Late Phase I. Aplastic marrow showing large fat deposits with few or no associated free hemopoietic cells. (e) Phase III. Marrow with greatly increased cellularity, with little or no fat deposits. (f) Phase V. Leukemic marrow.

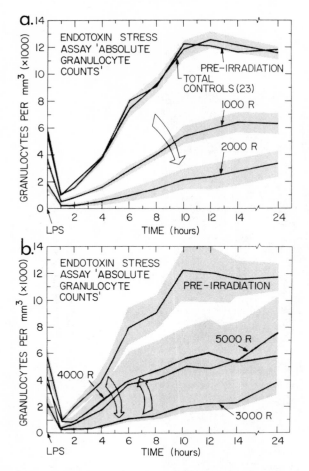

FIG. 3a, b. *Granulocyte reserve and mobilization as measured by endotoxin stress assay.*
Granulocytes per mm³ of blood are plotted versus the time after injection of 50 nm/kg body
weight liposaccharide (LPS) in groups of 12, 9, 7, 6, and 3 dogs with cumulative radiation doses
ranging from 1000 to 5000 R respectively. Twenty-three unirradiated dogs were utilized as
controls, of which 7 formed the preirradiation group. The shaded area represents the standard
deviation of the means.

animal, an increased proliferative activity within the progenitor compartments is required during this period to provide gradual cell renewal within
the depleted storage compartments. Evidence gathered to date on GM-CFUa content of marrow and our morphological observations supports this idea.

We feel it is highly likely that the critical events involved in the
partial hemopoietic recovery phase II are causally linked to the appearance
of late developing leukemia. The hemopoietic system changes, during this
relatively short interval, from a predominantly hypoplastic condition with

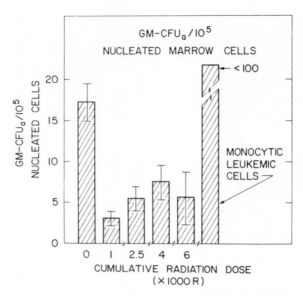

FIG.4. In vitro assessment of granulocyte-monocyte progenitors (i.e. GM-CFUa) within bone
marrow samples from 11 preirradiated beagles and groups of 6, 5, 5, and 5 beagles which
accumulated ~1000, 2500, 4000, and 6000 R at 10 R/day, respectively. Error bars indicate
the standard deviation. For comparison, the clonogenic activity of monocytic leukemic
(marrow) cells is shown.

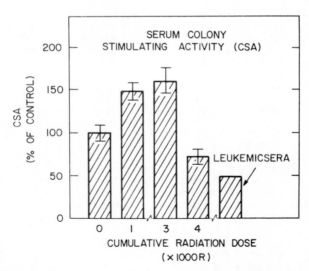

FIG.5. Colony-stimulating activity (CSA) of sera from 9 unirradiated control dogs, and
groups of 12, 6, and 6 beagles which accumulated ~1000, 3000, and 4000 R at 10 R/day,
respectively. Error bars indicate the standard deviation. For comparison serum CSA of a
dog with monocytic leukemia is shown.

marked radiosensitivity to a progressively hyperplastic condition in the face of continuous irradiation. The neoplastic involvement of a single cell line in the majority of the canine leukemias (e.g. granulocytic type), suggests that the radiation-induced neoplastic lesion occurs at the level of the committed stem cell. Altered stem cell function is suggested by the preliminary data indicating increased numbers and/or clonogenic activity of GM-progenitors (i.e. GM-CFUa) within the marrow aspirates. We hypothesize that these newly arising granulocyte-monocytic clones have altered physiological (e.g. reduced radiosensitivity) and cytological-ultrastructural properties that will relate to pre-neoplastic events.

Phase III. This period is characterized by an equilibration of subnormal hemopoietic function. Based on peripheral blood profiles this phase is gradually entered following approximately 300 days of radiation exposure and extends for several hundred days until a 'preleukemic' condition is identified (Fig. 1). Circulating blood leukocyte values tend to fluctuate at about one half their pre-irradiation levels. Concentrations of red cells show some improvement at mid phase, while blood platelet values gradually increase (Fig. 1). In contrast to the depressed blood leukocyte and platelet concentrations, the marrow becomes increasingly hypercellular (Fig. 2e). The change in marrow cellularity between phase II and III is dramatically evident by comparative scanning of intact biopsied marrow samples (Fig. 2c, e). Late phase III marrow samples generally contain scanty fat deposits, less prominent supportive elements, and highly cellular areas. Increased mitoses, especially within erythrocytic series, immature erythroid and granulocytic cells with abnormal cytoplasmic and nuclear ultrastructure are readily observed.

A corresponding expansion of the granulocyte reserves and their mobilizing capacity is noted at 400-500 days (i.e. 4000-5000 R), but still remain substantially below control levels (Fig. 3b). This increase in stored granulocytes corresponds, in time, with an apparent increase in the size of the stem cell pool committed to myeloid differentiation. The latter, presumably, provides input at an amplification stage which primes the granulopoietic system [18]. The numbers of GM-CFUa/10^5 nucleated marrow cells plated are increased in phase III ($\sim$ 7.6 CFUa/10^5 compared to 3.1/10^5 during phase II), but remain reduced in number, relative to average pre-radiation values of 17.3 CFUa/10^5.

In contrast to earlier phases when colony-stimulating activity (CSA) of sera is elevated, late in phase III, serum CSA falls below control values (Fig. 5). This decline in humoral activity appears to occur during a phase of increasing marrow plasticity.

Phase IV. 'Preleukemia' is a distinct preclinical phase of radiation-induced MPD in dogs. It is of variable duration, but most commonly extends for several hundred days prior to onset of patent leukemia. Prognostic descriptors of this phase were developed retrospectively from observations gathered from 21 cases of canine leukemia [3,8,14,15]. The most notable characteristic is the very exaggerated oscillations in blood platelet values (Fig. 1). Initially the magnitude of the oscillations are relatively small ($\pm$ 1 x 10^{11}/1) and of short duration, but gradually increase with peak blood concentrations approaching 10 x 10^{11}/1 and lasting for several months [8]. Circulating immature granulocytes, monocytes, and erythrocytes with various morphologic abnormalities are also characteristic [8,14,15].

Phase V.   Overt <u>radiation-induced canine leukemia</u> in its various forms
(i.e.   granulocytic, monocytic, and erythrocytic) has been previously
described, hematologically, pathologically, and ultrastructurally [3,5-8,14,
15,19]; and in every instance closely resembles the spontaneous disease(s)
in humans [8].   This includes the lack of any evidence suggesting oncogenic
viral involvement in the induction of this disease complex [8,19-21].   With
entry into the patent phase of disease V, the peripheral blood picture changes
dramatically (Fig. 1).   Immature granulocytes (monocytes), with severe
maturational defects, circulate in great numbers [8,15].   In a case of
monocytic leukemia, we observed a striking increase, relative to healthy
control animals, in the number of clonable circulating stem cells committed
to monocytic differentiation (i.e. GM-CFUa).   Similar high cloning rates
were found for marrow samples taken at necropsy (Fig. 4).   Serum from this
leukemic dog had a suppressive effect on normal GM-CFUa cloning (Fig. 5).

CONCLUSIONS

Results presented here indicate that four distinct preclinical phases
precede the onset of the radiation-induced leukemia in the beagle dog.   These
phases are readily recognized and reflect changing patterns of hemopoiesis.
The sum of measurable variables used to characterize these phases appear
prognostic for either the early developing aplastic anemias or the late
arising leukemias.   An early period of deteriorating hemopoiesis, followed
by partial restoration (phase II) and equilibration of subnormal hemopoietic
function (phase III) appear to be an obligatory sequence of events in leukemia
induction.

Prolonged periods of marked myelosuppression are a pathological hall-
mark of intoxication with currently recognized leukemogens, such as benzene
[9] and ionizing radiations [1].   As postulated by several workers [8,22,23],
a protracted course of myelosuppression probably functions as a strong
selective pressure for new aberrant clones of hemopoietic cells with altered
cellular properties that allow for repopulation of depleted marrow in the
face of continued intoxication.   Certainly our data showing the dramatic
reversal in marrow plasticity, especially at the level of the committed stem
cell, in these preclinical periods are consistent with the possibility that
clonal selection of aberrant cell populations is responsible for leukemia
induction by protracted low-dose irradiation.   In this regard, we are presently
attempting to evaluate the cytological and ultrastructural properties of
granulocytic-monocytic cell clones that arise in increasing numbers during
the restoration (II) and accommodation phases (III).   Evidence of aberrancy
(physical, biochemical, metabolic, morphological, etc.) would give us strong
evidence that subpatent disease exists during these very early periods, and
would therefore give us still stronger prognostic indicator(s) of impending
disease.

In summary, it is hypothesized that preleukemic sequences and events
similar to those observed in these studies exist for the radiation, chemical,
and 'spontaneous' leukemias of man.   Careful analysis of these preclinical
syndromes in the dog should be useful in understanding basic leukemogenic
mechanisms in man and for the development of prognostic indications of impending disease.

ACKNOWLEDGEMENTS

The excellent technical assistance of D. Doyle, W. Keenan, N. Kretz, J. Angerman, P. Polk, L. Bell, T. Chubb, B. Wright, and M. Sanderson is gratefully acknowledged, as the work of the Animal Care Specialists. We would like to thank Marcia Rosenthal and Jay Best for their editorial work and Lynn Purdy for her typing.

REFERENCES

[1]   MODAN, B., LUBIN, E., Radiation induced leukemia in man, Ser. Haematol. (Copenhagen) 7 (1974) 192.

[2]   DUNGWORTH, D.L., GOLDMAN, M., SWITZER, J.W., MCKELVIE, D.H., Development of a myeloproliferative disorder in beagles exposed continuously to Sr-90, Blood 34 (1969) 610.

[3]   FRITZ, T.E., NORRIS, W.P., TOLLE, D.V., Myelogenous leukemia and related myeloproliferative disorders in beagles continuously exposed to Co-60 gamma-radiation, Bibl. Haematol. 39 (1973) 170.

[4]   GRAHN, D., FRY, R.J.M., LEA, R.A., "Analysis of survival and cause of death statistics for mice under single and duration-of-life gamma irradiation", Life Sciences and Space Research X, Akademie-Verlag, Berlin (1972) 175.

[5]   NORRIS, W.P., FRITZ, T.E., "Interactions of total dose and dose-rate in determining tissue responses to ionizing radiations", Radiobiology of Plutonium (STOVER, J., JEE, S.W.W., Eds), J.W. Press, Salt Lake City, (1972) 243.

[6]   NORRIS, W.P., TYLER, S.A., SACHER, G.A., "An interspecies comparison of responses of mice and dogs to continuous ^{60}Co gamma irradiation", Biological and Environmental Effects of Low-Level Radiation (Proc. Symp. Chicago, 1975) I, IAEA, Vienna (1976) 147.

[7]   FRITZ, T.E., NORRIS, W.P., TOLLE, D.V., SEED, T.M., POOLE, C.M., LOMBARD, L.S., DOYLE, D., "Relationship of dose rate and total dose to responses of continuously irradiated beagles", these Proceedings II, IAEA-SM-224/206.

[8]   SEED, T.M., TOLLE, D.V., FRITZ, T.E., DEVINE, R., POOLE, C.M., NORRIS, W.P., Irradiation-induced erythroleukemia and myelogenous leukemia in the beagle dog: Hematology and ultrastructure, Blood 50 (1977) 1061.

[9]   FORNI, A., VIGLIANI, E.C., Chemical leukemogenesis in man, Ser. Haematol. (Copenhagen) 7 (1974) 221.

[10] LINMAN, J.W., BAGBY, G.C., The pre-leukemic syndrome: Clinical laboratory features, national course, and management, Blood Cells 2 (1976) 11.

[11] NORRIS, W.P., FRITZ, T.E., REHFELD, C.E., POOLE, C.M., The response of the beagle dog to cobalt-60 gamma radiation: Determination of the LD50(30) and description of associated changes, Radiat. Res. 35 (1968) 681.

[12] MARSH, J.C., LEVITT, M., KATZENSTEIN, A., The growth of leukocyte colonies in vitro from dog bone marrow, J. Lab. Clin. Med. 79 (1972) 1041.

[13] DEBELAK-FEHIR, K.M., CATCHATOWRIAN, R., EPSTEIN, R.B., Hemopoietic colony forming units in fresh and cryopreserved peripheral blood cells of canines and man, Exp. Hematol. (Copenhagen) 3 (1975) 109.

[14] TOLLE, D.V., FRITZ, T.E., NORRIS, W.P., Radiation-induced erythroleukemia in the beagle dog, Am. J. Pathol. 87 (1977) 499.

[15] TOLLE, D.V., SEED, T.M., FRITZ, T.E., LOMBARD, L.S., POOLE, C.M., NORRIS, W.P.,
Acute monocytic leukemia in an irradiated beagle dog (unpublished).

[16] MAGLIULO, E., GALLINA, M., SCEVOLA, D., CONCIA, E., Defect of bone marrow
granulocyte reserve in viral hepatitis, Acta Haematol. 54 (1975) 27.

[17] MARSH, J.C., PERRY, S., The granulocyte response to endotoxin in patients with
hematologic disorders, Blood 23 (1964) 581.

[18] CRONKITE, E.P., BURLINGTON, H., CHANANA, A.D., JOLL, D.D., REINCKE, U.,
STEVENS, J., "Concepts and observations on the regulation of granulocyte production",
Experimental Hematology Today (BAUM, S.J., LEDNEY, G.D., Eds), Springer-Verlag,
Berlin (1977) 41.

[19] FRITZ, T.E., NORRIS, W.P., REHFELD, C.E., POOLE, C.M., "Myeloproliferative
disease in beagle dogs given protracted whole body irradiation or single doses of Ce-144",
Proc. Symp. Myeloproliferative Disorders of Animals and Man (CLARKE, W.T.,
HOWARD, E.G., HACKETT, P.L., Eds), Oak Ridge, U.S. Atomic Energy Commission
(1970) 219.

[20] SHIFRINE, M., ZEE, Y.C., WOLF, H.G., "Attempts at transmission of the radiation-
induced canine myeloproliferative syndrome to dogs and Marmosa mitis", Annual
Report, 1969, Radiobiology Laboratory, University of California (1969) 87.

[21] HUFF, S., SCIBIENSKI, E., GALLIGAN, S.J., TAYLOR, N.J., "DNA-Polymerases from
canine tumors — Purification and properties in comparison with DNA-polymerases from
viruses and virus induced tumors", Annual Report, 1972, Radiobiology Laboratory,
University of California, Davis, (1972) 53.

[22] CRONKITE, E.P., Evidence for radiation and chemicals as leukemogenic agents, Arch.
Environ. Health 3 (1961) 297.

[23] DAMESHEK, W., Riddle: What do aplastic anemia, paroxysmal nocturnal hemogloburia
(PNA) and "hypoplastic" leukemia have in common?, Blood 30 (1967) 251.

DISCUSSION

V. ERFLE: Have you seen virus particles in your electronmicrographs?

T.M. SEED: No, and this includes all pre-clinical marrow samples as well
as tissues taken during patent leukaemia. I might add that we have extended our
search for viral particles to placental tissues, supposedly a privileged site of
c-type viral expression in many species. However, we have so far failed to observe
any c-type particles electron-microscopically.

T. OHKITA: What is the proportion of the various types of leukaemia?

T.M. SEED: At the dose rates of 5, 10 and 17 R daily of gamma irradiation,
the incidence of leukaemia is approximately 50, 50 and 15% respectively. The
cases occurring at the higher dose rates were predominantly granulocytic. There
was one case each of monocytic leukaemia and lymphocytic leukaemia. At the
lower dose rate of 5 R daily half the leukaemias were of the erythrocytic type.
Spontaneous myeloproliferative disease, i.e. myeloid leukaemia, is extremely
rare. We have not had a single case.

T. OHKITA: What are the indicators of pre-leukaemia? In human cases
we have found persisting anaemia and/or leukopenia, morphologically abnormal
(but not leukaemic) cells such as binuclear granulocytes, agranural granulocytes,

small-sized megakaryocytes, etc., and chromosomal aberrations in their pre-leukaemic period.

T.M. SEED: In the 'pre-leukaemic' phase, i.e. phase IV, there is an exaggerated oscillation in blood platelet values as well as increased numbers of circulating immature granulocytes, monocytes and red cells exhibiting various types of morphological abnormalities. Before phase IV, i.e. phase III, there is a combination of altered haematological functions, including a granulopenic thrombocytopenic blood picture, increasing marrow cellularity, specifically associated with repaired granulopoietic functions, i.e. granulocyte reserves and granulocyte-monocyte progenitors. Also during this time there is an apparent reduction in the serum activity which stimulates GM-progenitor growth in vitro.

T. OHKITA: Have you done any chromosomal studies in connection with canine leukaemia?

T.M. SEED: No, but we would certainly like to extend our longitudinal studies to include karyotyping the granulocytic elements that repopulate the marrow after phase I, i.e. phases II—V.

H.H. VOGEL: You mentioned septicaemia as one cause of radiation lethality in the dogs. I recall that neutron-irradiated mice often showed a radiation bacteriaemia when 3—8 days after exposure normal bacterial flora of the small intestine were cultured in the heart's blood and spleen of irradiated mice. E. coli was prominent. Is the dog septicaemia also from the intestinal flora?

T.M. SEED: At the daily gamma irradiation dose rates of either 35 or 17 R daily septicaemia is the primary cause of death. From typing of the micro-organisms responsible for the syndrome it appears that the agents do not derive from the intestinal tract but rather from the nasal-oral cavity. This would suggest that natural/immunological barriers, associated with the bronchial-pulmonary system, are impaired at these continuous dose rates.

F.J. BURNS: It is perhaps not surprising that the high doses employed in your experiment might cause hypoplasia as a result of cell lethality. Could you cite evidence, especially at lower doses or in controls, to support your contention that marrow hypoplasia is a necessary precursor condition for the development of leukaemia?

T.M. SEED: In the various species where 'pre-leukaemia' has been well described, some degree of myelosuppression is a common feature, and is associated with either a pancytopenic state or other cell line specific cytopenias. This appears to be the case, regardless of aetiology. We believe that the degree and time course of myelosuppression induced by protracted gamma irradiation greatly influence the incidence, and to a lesser extent the latency, of myeloid leukaemia in the dog. We have just begun to irradiate dogs at dose rates lower than 5 R daily (i.e. 0.4, 1.0 and 2.5 R daily) and, until the causes of deaths in these groups are tabulated, we shall not be able to say anything about the incidence of leukaemia. However, we feel that the incidence will rapidly fall, because of the lack of the haemosuppression assumed to be necessary for clonal selection of malignant cells.

V. COVELLI (*Chairman*): Is the myelosuppressive phase associated with a large amount of haemorrhage?

T.M. SEED: No.

R.A. CONARD: With regard to pre-leukaemic changes I would like to comment on a case of acute myelogenous leukaemia that developed in a Marshallese man 19 years after exposure to about 175 rads of gamma radiation from fall-out at one year of age. Although no pre-leukaemic bone marrow studies were performed, we were able to examine haemograms dating back to the time of exposure. Compared with cohorts of exposed and unexposed boys of the same age range, there was a consistent greater depression of the granulocyte counts over the years compared with other blood elements. This indicated reduced myelocytic reserve which might result in greater haemopoietic stimulus, possibly increasing the potential for development of a malignant clone. In view of the development of the myelogenous form of leukaemia the granulopenia would appear to be of pre-leukaemic significance.

CHAIRMEN OF SESSIONS

Session 1	L.B. SZTANYIK	Hungary
	H. KATO	Japan
Session 2	R.L. ULLRICH	United States of America
	C.F.H. PASQUIER	France
Session 3	M. COLMAN	United States of America
	R.G. GREGORIO	Philippines
Session 4	J.F. DUPLAN	France
	T. SADO	Japan
Session 5	M. COLMAN	United States of America
(Part 1)	M. KALISNIK	Yugoslavia
(Part 2)	J.L. WEEKS	Canada
	J.A. BONNEL	United Kingdom
Session 6	K.H. CHADWICK	Netherlands
	V. COVELLI	Italy
Session 7	J.L. WEEKS	Canada
	J.A. BONNEL	United Kingdom
Session 8	F.J. BURNS	United States of America
	H. ALTMANN	Austria
Session 9	R.C. von BORSTEL	Canada
	C. STREFFER	Federal Republic of Germany
Session 10	A.S. McLEAN	United Kingdom
	K. NEUMEISTER	German Democratic Republic

SECRETARIAT

Scientific Secretary:	S. KOBAYASHI	Division of Life Sciences, IAEA
Administrative Secretary:	G. SEILER	Division of External Relations, IAEA
Editor:	S.M. FREEMAN	Division of Publications, IAEA
Records Officer:	P.B. SMITH	Division of Languages, IAEA

FACTORS FOR CONVERTING SOME OT THE MORE COMMON UNITS TO INTERNATIONAL SYSTEM OF UNITS (SI) EQUIVALENTS

NOTES:

(1) SI base units are the metre (m), kilogram (kg), second (s), ampere (A), kelvin (K), candela (cd) and mole (mol).

(2) ▶ indicates SI derived units and those accepted for use with SI;

    ▷ indicates additional units accepted for use with SI for a limited time.

    [*For further information see The International System of Units (SI), 1977 ed., published in English by HMSO, London, and National Bureau of Standards, Washington, DC, and International Standards ISO-1000 and the several parts of ISO-31 published by ISO, Geneva.*]

(3) The correct abbreviation for the unit in column 1 is given in column 2.

(4) ✳ indicates conversion factors given exactly; other factors are given rounded, mostly to 4 significant figures.

    ≡ indicates a definition of an SI derived unit: [ ] in column 3+4 enclose factors given for the sake of completeness.

Column 1 Multiply data given in:	Column 2	Column 3 by:		Column 4 to obtain data in:
Radiation units				
▶ becquerel	1 Bq	(has dimensions of s^{-1})		
disintegrations per second (= dis/s)	$1\ s^{-1}$	$\equiv 1.00 \times 10^0$	Bq	✳
▷ curie	1 Ci	$= 3.70 \times 10^{10}$	Bq	✳
▷ roentgen	1 R	$[= 2.58 \times 10^{-4}$	C/kg]	✳
▶ gray	1 Gy	$[\equiv 1.00 \times 10^0$	J/kg]	
▷ rad	1 rad	$= 1.00 \times 10^{-2}$	Gy	✳
sievert *(radiation protection only)*	1 Sv	$[= 1.00 \times 10^0$	J/kg]	✳
rem *(radiation protection only)*	1 rem	$[= 1.00 \times 10^{-2}$	J/kg]	✳
Mass				
▶ unified atomic mass unit ($\frac{1}{12}$ of the mass of ^{12}C)	1 u	$[= 1.660\ 57 \times 10^{-27}$	kg, approx.]	
▶ tonne (= metric ton)	1 t	$[= 1.00 \times 10^3$	kg]	✳
pound mass (avoirdupois)	1 lbm	$= 4.536 \times 10^{-1}$	kg	
ounce mass (avoirdupois)	1 ozm	$= 2.835 \times 10^1$	g	
ton (long) (= 2240 lbm)	1 ton	$= 1.016 \times 10^3$	kg	
ton (short) (= 2000 lbm)	1 short ton	$= 9.072 \times 10^2$	kg	
Length				
statute mile	1 mile	$= 1.609 \times 10^0$	km	
nautical mile (international)	1 n mile	$= 1.852 \times 10^0$	km	✳
yard	1 yd	$= 9.144 \times 10^{-1}$	m	✳
foot	1 ft	$= 3.048 \times 10^{-1}$	m	✳
inch	1 in	$= 2.54 \times 10^1$	mm	✳
mil (= 10^{-3} in)	1 mil	$= 2.54 \times 10^{-2}$	mm	✳
Area				
▷ hectare	1 ha	$[= 1.00 \times 10^4$	m^2]	✳
▷ barn *(effective cross-section, nuclear physics)*	1 b	$[= 1.00 \times 10^{-28}$	m^2]	✳
square mile, (statute mile)^2	1 mile^2	$= 2.590 \times 10^0$	km^2	
acre	1 acre	$= 4.047 \times 10^3$	m^2	
square yard	1 yd^2	$= 8.361 \times 10^{-1}$	m^2	
square foot	1 ft^2	$= 9.290 \times 10^{-2}$	m^2	
square inch	1 in^2	$= 6.452 \times 10^2$	mm^2	
Volume				
▶ litre	1 l *or* 1 ltr	$[= 1.00 \times 10^{-3}$	m^3]	✳
cubic yard	1 yd^3	$= 7.646 \times 10^{-1}$	m^3	
cubic foot	1 ft^3	$= 2.832 \times 10^{-2}$	m^3	
cubic inch	1 in^3	$= 1.639 \times 10^4$	mm^3	
gallon (imperial)	1 gal (UK)	$= 4.546 \times 10^{-3}$	m^3	
gallon (US liquid)	1 gal (US)	$= 3.785 \times 10^{-3}$	m^3	
Velocity, acceleration				
foot per second (= fps)	1 ft/s	$= 3.048 \times 10^{-1}$	m/s	✳
foot per minute	1 ft/min	$= 5.08 \times 10^{-3}$	m/s	✳
mile per hour (= mph)	1 mile/h	$=\begin{cases} 4.470 \times 10^{-1} \\ 1.609 \times 10^0 \end{cases}$	m/s km/h	
▷ knot (international)	1 knot	$= 1.852 \times 10^0$	km/h	✳
free fall, standard, g		$= 9.807 \times 10^0$	m/s^2	
foot per second squared	1 ft/s^2	$= 3.048 \times 10^{-1}$	m/s^2	✳

Column 1 *Multiply data given in:*	Column 2	Column 3 *by:*	Column 4 *to obtain data in:*
Density, volumetric rate			
pound mass per cubic inch	1 lbm/in^3	= 2.768 $\times$ 10^4	kg/m^3
pound mass per cubic foot	1 lbm/ft^3	= 1.602 $\times$ 10^1	kg/m^3
cubic feet per second	1 ft^3/s	= 2.832 $\times$ 10^{-2}	m^3/s
cubic feet per minute	1 ft^3/min	= 4.719 $\times$ 10^{-4}	m^3/s
Force			
▶ newton	1 N	[$\equiv$ 1.00 $\times$ 10^0	m·kg·s^{-2}]✳
dyne	1 dyn	= 1.00 $\times$ 10^{-5}	N ✳
kilogram force (= kilopond (kp))	1 kgf	= 9.807 $\times$ 10^0	N
poundal	1 pdl	= 1.383 $\times$ 10^{-1}	N
pound force (avoirdupois)	1 lbf	= 4.448 $\times$ 10^0	N
ounce force (avoirdupois)	1 ozf	= 2.780 $\times$ 10^{-1}	N
Pressure, stress			
▶ pascal	1 Pa	[$\equiv$ 1.00 $\times$ 10^0	N/m^2] ✳
▷ atmosphere^a, standard	1 atm	= 1.013 25 $\times$ 10^5	Pa ✳
▷ bar	1 bar	= 1.00 $\times$ 10^5	Pa ✳
centimetres of mercury (0°C)	1 cmHg	= 1.333 $\times$ 10^3	Pa
dyne per square centimetre	1 dyn/cm^2	= 1.00 $\times$ 10^{-1}	Pa ✳
feet of water (4°C)	1 ftH$_2$O	= 2.989 $\times$ 10^3	Pa
inches of mercury (0°C)	1 inHg	= 3.386 $\times$ 10^3	Pa
inches of water (4°C)	1 inH$_2$O	= 2.491 $\times$ 10^2	Pa
kilogram force per square centimetre	1 kgf/cm^2	= 9.807 $\times$ 10^4	Pa
pound force per square foot	1 lbf/ft^2	= 4.788 $\times$ 10^1	Pa
pound force per square inch (= psi) ^{b}	1 lbf/in^2	= 6.895 $\times$ 10^3	Pa
torr (0°C) (= mmHg)	1 torr	= 1.333 $\times$ 10^2	Pa
Energy, work, quantity of heat			
▶ joule ($\equiv$ W·s)	1 J	[$\equiv$ 1.00 $\times$ 10^0	N·m] ✳
▶ electronvolt	1 eV	[= 1.602 19 $\times$ 10^{-19}	J, approx.]
British thermal unit (International Table)	1 Btu	= 1.055 $\times$ 10^3	J
calorie (thermochemical)	1 cal	= 4.184 $\times$ 10^0	J ✳
calorie (International Table)	1 cal$_{IT}$	= 4.187 $\times$ 10^0	J
erg	1 erg	= 1.00 $\times$ 10^{-7}	J ✳
foot-pound force	1 ft·lbf	= 1.356 $\times$ 10^0	J
kilowatt-hour	1 kW·h	= 3.60 $\times$ 10^6	J ✳
kiloton explosive yield (PNE) ($\equiv$ 10^{12} g-cal)	1 kt yield	$\simeq$ 4.2 $\times$ 10^{12}	J
Power, radiant flux			
▶ watt	1 W	[$\equiv$ 1.00 $\times$ 10^0	J/s] ✳
British thermal unit (International Table) per second	1 Btu/s	= 1.055 $\times$ 10^3	W
calorie (International Table) per second	1 cal$_{IT}$/s	= 4.187 $\times$ 10^0	W
foot-pound force/second	1 ft·lbf/s	= 1.356 $\times$ 10^0	W
horsepower (electric)	1 hp	= 7.46 $\times$ 10^2	W ✳
horsepower (metric) (= ps)	1 ps	= 7.355 $\times$ 10^2	W
horsepower (550 ft·lbf/s)	1 hp	= 7.457 $\times$ 10^2	W
Temperature			
▶ temperature in degrees Celsius, t where T is the thermodynamic temperature in kelvin and T$_0$ is defined as 273.15 K	$t = T - T_0$		
degree Fahrenheit	$t_{°F} - 32$		t *(in degrees Celsius)* ✳
degree Rankine	$T_{°R}$	$\times \left(\dfrac{5}{9} \right)$ gives	T *(in kelvin)* ✳
degrees of temperature difference ^{c}	$\Delta T_{°R}$ (= $\Delta t_{°F}$)		ΔT (= Δt) ✳
Thermal conductivity ^{c}			
1 Btu·in/(ft^2·s·°F)	*(International Table Btu)*	= 5.192 $\times$ 10^2	W·m^{-1}·K^{-1}
1 Btu/(ft·s·°F)	*(International Table Btu)*	= 6.231 $\times$ 10^3	W·m^{-1}·K^{-1}
1 cal$_{IT}$/(cm·s·°C)		= 4.187 $\times$ 10^2	W·m^{-1}·K^{-1}

^{a} atm abs, ata: atmospheres absolute; ^{b} lbf/in^2 (g) (= psig): gauge pressure;
   atm (g), atü: atmospheres gauge.   lbf/in^2 abs (= psia): absolute pressure.
^{c} The abbreviation for temperature difference, deg (= degK = degC), is no longer acceptable as an SI unit.

HOW TO ORDER IAEA PUBLICATIONS

 An exclusive sales agent for IAEA publications, to whom all orders
and inquiries should be addressed, has been appointed
in the following country:

UNITED STATES OF AMERICA   UNIPUB, 345 Park Avenue South, New York, N.Y. 10010

 In the following countries IAEA publications may be purchased from the
sales agents or booksellers listed or through your
major local booksellers. Payment can be made in local
currency or with UNESCO coupons.

ARGENTINA	Comisión Nacional de Energía Atómica, Avenida del Libertador 8250, Buenos Aires
AUSTRALIA	Hunter Publications, 58 A Gipps Street, Collingwood, Victoria 3066
BELGIUM	Service du Courrier de l'UNESCO, 112, Rue du Trône, B-1050 Brussels
C.S.S.R.	S.N.T.L., Spálená 51, CS-113 02 Prague 1
	Alfa, Publishers, Hurbanovo námestie 6, CS-893 31 Bratislava
FRANCE	Office International de Documentation et Librairie, 48, rue Gay-Lussac, F-75240 Paris Cedex 05
HUNGARY	Kultura, Bookimport, P.O. Box 149, H-1389 Budapest
INDIA	Oxford Book and Stationery Co., 17, Park Street, Calcutta, 700016
	Oxford Book and Stationery Co., Scindia House, New Delhi-110001
ISRAEL	Heiliger and Co., 3, Nathan Strauss Str., Jerusalem
ITALY	Libreria Scientifica, Dott. Lucio de Biasio "aeiou". Via Meravigli 16, I-20123 Milan
JAPAN	Maruzen Company, Ltd., P.O. Box 5050, 100-31 Tokyo International
NETHERLANDS	Martinus Nijhoff B.V., Lange Voorhout 9-11, P.O. Box 269, The Hague
PAKISTAN	Mirza Book Agency, 65, Shahrah Quaid-e-Azam, P.O. Box 729, Lahore-3
POLAND	Ars Polona-Ruch, Centrala Handlu Zagranicznego, Krakowskie Przedmiescie 7, Warsaw
ROMANIA	Ilexim, P.O. Box 136-137, Bucarest
SOUTH AFRICA	Van Schaik's Bookstore (Pty) Ltd., P.O. Box 724, Pretoria 0001
	Universitas Books (Pty) Ltd., P.O. Box 1557, Pretoria 0001
SPAIN	Diaz de Santos, Lagasca 95, Madrid-6
	Diaz de Santos, Balmes 417, Barcelona-6
SWEDEN	AB C.E. Fritzes Kungl. Hovbokhandel, Fredsgatan 2, P.O. Box 16358 S-103 27 Stockholm
UNITED KINGDOM	Her Majesty's Stationery Office, P.O. Box 569, London SE1 9NH
U.S.S.R.	Mezhdunarodnaya Kniga, Smolenskaya-Sennaya 32-34, Moscow G-200
YUGOSLAVIA	Jugoslovenska Knjiga, Terazije 27, POB 36, YU-11001 Belgrade

---

 Orders from countries where sales agents have not yet been appointed and
requests for information should be addressed directly to:

 Division of Publications
International Atomic Energy Agency
Kärntner Ring 11, P.O.Box 590, A-1011 Vienna, Austria